CHAPMAN & NAKIELNY'S
GUIDE TO
RADIOLOGICAL
PROCEDURES

"In the memory of Professor Kathirkamanathan Shanmuganathan, a pioneer in radiology, a kind gentle soul and an inspiration to so many" RB

"Dedicated to my colleagues and many wise mentors over the last 30 years" NW

CHAPMAN & NAKIELNY'S

GUIDE TO RADIOLOGICAL PROCEDURES

Edited by

Nick Watson MA, FRCP, FRCR
Consultant Radiologist, University Hospitals of North Midlands,
Stoke-on-Trent, UK
Hon Senior Lecturer, Keele University, Staffordshire, UK

Ravivarma Balasubramaniam MBChB, BSc, FRCR
Consultant Radiologist, University Hospitals of North Midlands,
Stoke-on-Trent, UK

EIGHTH EDITION

ELSEVIER

ELSEVIER

© 2024 Elsevier Ltd. All rights reserved.

Notices

Practitioners and researchers must always rely on their own experience and knowledge in evaluating and using any information, methods, compounds or experiments described herein. Because of rapid advances in the medical sciences, in particular, independent verification of diagnoses and drug dosages should be made. To the fullest extent of the law, no responsibility is assumed by Elsevier, authors, editors or contributors for any injury and/or damage to persons or property as a matter of products liability, negligence or otherwise, or from any use or operation of any methods, products, instructions, or ideas contained in the material herein.

First edition 1981
Second edition 1986
Third edition 1993
Fourth edition 2001
Fifth edition 2009
Sixth edition 2014
Seventh edition 2018
Eighth edition 2024

ISBN 9780323933636

British Library Cataloguing in Publication Data
A catalogue record for this book is available from the British Library

Library of Congress Cataloging in Publication Data
A catalog record for this book is available from the Library of Congress

Content Strategist: Clodagh Holland-Borosh
Content Project Manager: Shivani Pal
Designer: Brian Salisbury

 Working together to grow libraries in developing countries

www.elsevier.com • www.bookaid.org

Printed in Great Britain

Last digit is the print number: 9 8 7 6 5 4 3 2 1

List of contributors

Raneem Albazaz, MBChB (Hons), BSc (Hons), MRCS, FRCR
Consultant Radiologist, Leeds Teaching Hospitals NHS Trust, Leeds, UK
CHAPTER 5

Ravivarma Balasubramaniam, MBChB, BSc, FRCR
Consultant Radiologist, University Hospitals of North Midlands,
Stoke-on-Trent, UK
CHAPTER 4

Matthew Bridge, MBChB, MRCP, FRCA
Consultant Anaesthetist, Liverpool University Hospitals, Liverpool, UK
CHAPTERS 21 AND 22

Megan Bydder, MBChB, MRCP, FRCR
Consultant Radiologist, Nightingale Centre, Manchester University NHS
Foundation Trust, Manchester, UK
CHAPTER 18

Greg Chambers, MBBS, FRCR
Consultant Radiologist and Nuclear Medicine, Leeds Teaching Hospitals NHS
Trust, Leeds, UK
CHAPTER 13

Christopher Day, BSc (Hons), MBBCh, MRCS (Eng), FRCR
Consultant Interventional Radiologist, University Hospitals of North
Midlands, Stoke-on-Trent, UK
CHAPTERS 11 AND 12

Amit Herwadkar, FRCR
Consultant Neuroradiologist, Salford Royal NHS Trust, Salford, UK
CHAPTER 16

Dawn Hopkins, PgCert. (Leadership and Healthcare Management)
Radiology Operations Manager, North Middlesex University Hospital,
London, UK
CHAPTER 19

Samantha B.L. Low, BEng (Hons), MBBS, FRCR
Consultant Radiologist, Norfolk and Norwich University Hospital,
Norwich, UK
CHAPTER 3

Simon Lowes, BSc (Hons), MB BS (Hons), MA, PhD, FRCR
Consultant Radiologist, Gateshead Health NHS Foundation Trust, UK
Honorary Clinical Senior Lecturer, Newcastle University
CHAPTER 18

Pavan Najran, MBChB, FRCR
Consultant Interventional Radiologist, The Christie Hospital NHS Foundation Trust, Manchester, UK
CHAPTER 7

Adam J. Oates, BSc, PhD, MD
Consultant Paediatric Radiologist, Birmingham Children's Hospital, Birmingham, UK
CHAPTER 3

Sofia Otero, BMBCh, FRCR
Consultant Radiologist, University College London Hospital, London, UK
CHAPTER 17

Douglas Pendse, MD, MRCS, FRCR
Consultant Radiologist, University College London;
Associate Professor, Faculty of Medical Sciences, University College London Hospitals, London, UK
CHAPTER 6

Balashanmugam Rajashanker, MBBS, MRCP, FRCR
Consultant Radiologist, Manchester Royal Infirmary and St Mary's Hospital, Manchester, UK
CHAPTER 8

James J. Rankine, MBChB, MRCP, MRaD, FRCR, MD
Consultant Musculoskeletal Radiologist and Honorary Associate Professor, Leeds Teaching Hospitals NHS Trust, Leeds, UK
CHAPTERS 14 AND 15

Samavia Raza, MBBS, FRCR
Consultant Radiologist, Imaging, University Hospitals North Midlands, Stoke-on-Trent, UK
CHAPTER 9

Philip Robinson, MB ChB, MRCP, FRCR
Consultant Musculoskeletal Radiologist, Leeds Teaching Hospitals NHS Trust; Honorary Clinical Associate Professor, Biomedical Research Centre, University of Leeds, Leeds, UK
CHAPTER 14

David M. Rosewarne, PhD, FRCR
Consultant Radiologist, New Cross Hospital, Wolverhampton, UK
CHAPTERS 1 AND 2

Emma Ross, BSc (Hons)
Lead Radiology Nurse, Interventional Radiology, The Christie NHS Foundation Trust, Manchester, UK
CHAPTER 19

Manigandan Thyagarajan, MBBS, MD, FRCR
Consultant Paediatric Radiologist, Birmingham Women's and Children's Hospital NHS Foundation Trust, Birmingham, UK
CHAPTER 3

Sriram Vaidyanathan, MBBS, MRCS, DOHNS, MD, FRCR
Consultant Radiologist and Nuclear Medicine, Honorary Senior Lecturer,
University of Leeds, Leeds, UK; Consultant in Radiology and Nuclear
Medicine, Leeds Teaching Hospitals NHS Trust, Leeds, UK
CHAPTER 13

Nick Watson, MA, FRCP, FRCR
Consultant Radiologist, University Hospitals of North Midlands;
Honorary Senior Lecturer, Keele University, Stoke-on-Trent, UK
CHAPTERS 19 AND 20

Alim Yucel-Finn, MBBS, MSc, FRCR
Consultant Radiologist, University Hospital North Midlands,
Stoke-on-Trent, UK
CHAPTER 10

Preface

The role of diagnostic and therapeutic radiological techniques and procedures has continued to develop and expand. The latest edition has been revised to reflect newer advances in imaging techniques and evolving indications for examinations and procedures, whilst preserving the original concept of the first edition in providing a single compact source to reference imaging techniques and radiological interventional procedures.

The latest edition also introduces an entirely new chapter on Paediatric Radiology to incorporate the complex multi-modality of the subspecialty which utilises a full range of diagnostic and interventional techniques with a bespoke approach tailored to the clinical scenario and age of the paediatric patient group. We envisage this guide being an easily accessible and useful source of information for radiologists, radiographers and nurses, serving as a practical guide to assist in delivering modern radiological practice.

Nick Watson
Ravivarma Balasubramaniam

Acknowledgements

We would like to thank all of the chapter authors for their hard work in preparing this latest edition of the Guide. Several new contributors have been involved to whom we are very grateful, but we would also like to acknowledge the great work of colleagues from the previous edition: I. Britton, F. Coccia, H. Dobson, J. Freedman, P. Guest, H. Jones, Z. Khan, P.S. Richards and T.M. Wah, whose chapters have been revised and updated. We are also extremely thankful for the fantastic support and encouragement we have had from Elsevier – Trinity Hutton (Content Strategist), Cloe Holland-Borosh (Content Strategist), Shivani Pal (Content Project Manager) and Baljinder Kaur (Senior Project Manager).

Contents

1 General notes
David M. Rosewarne
Radiology   1
Radionuclide Imaging   8
  Radiopharmaceuticals   8
Computed Tomography   11
  Renal Protocol   12
Magnetic Resonance Imaging   14
  Safety in Magnetic Resonance Imaging   14
Ultrasonography   19

2 Intravascular contrast media
David M. Rosewarne
Historical Development of Radiographic Agents   21
Adverse Effects of Intravenous Water-Soluble Contrast Media   25
  Toxic Effects on Specific Organs   25
  Idiosyncratic Reactions   27
  Mechanisms of Idiosyncratic Contrast Medium Reactions   29
  Prophylaxis of Adverse Contrast Medium Effects   29
Contrast Agents in Magnetic Resonance Imaging   32
  Historical Development   32
  Mechanism of Action   32
  Gadolinium   34
Contrast Agents in Ultrasonography   38

3 Paediatrics
Samantha B.L. Low, Manigandan Thyagarajan and Adam J. Oates
Paediatric Patients   41
Intravascular Contrast Media Used in Paediatrics: Computed Tomography
  and Magnetic Resonance Imaging   48
Gastrointestinal and Genitourinary Imaging   50
Respiratory and Cardiac   71
Muskuloskeletal   76
Neurological   83

Breast   93

Non-Accidental Injuries   94

4 Gastrointestinal system

Ravivarma Balasubramaniam

Methods of Imaging the Gastrointestinal Tract   97

Introduction to Contrast Media   97

  Water-Soluble Contrast Agents (see also Chapter 2)   97

  Gases   98

  Barium   99

  Pharmacological Agents   100

Contrast Swallow   103

Barium Meal   104

Small Bowel Follow-Through   108

Small Bowel Enema   110

Barium Enema   112

Enema Variants   116

  The 'Instant' Enema   116

  Air Enema   117

Sinogram   117

Retrograde Ileogram   117

Colostomy Enema   117

Loopogram   118

Herniogram   118

Evacuating Proctogram   119

Ultrasound of the Gastrointestinal Tract   121

  Endoluminal Examination of the Oesophagus and Stomach   121

  Transabdominal Examination of the Lower Oesophagus and Stomach   121

  Small Bowel   121

  Appendix   122

  Large Bowel   123

  Endoluminal Examination of the Anus   123

  Endoluminal Examination of the Rectum   123

Computed Tomography of the Gastrointestinal Tract   124

  Rectal Contrast   127

  Computed Tomographic Colonography   127

  Complications   129

  Aftercare   129

  Dual-Energy Computed Tomography   129

Magnetic Resonance Imaging of the Gastrointestinal Tract   132
Radionuclide Gastro-Oesophageal Reflux Study   136
Radionuclide Gastric Emptying Study   137
Radionuclide Meckel's Diverticulum Scan   140
Radionuclide Imaging of Gastrointestinal Bleeding   141
Labelled White Cell Scanning in Inflammatory Bowel Disease   142

5 Liver, biliary tract and pancreas

Raneem Albazaz

Methods of Imaging the Hepatobiliary System   143
Methods of Imaging the Pancreas   143
Plain Films   143
Ultrasound of the Liver   144
Ultrasound of the Gallbladder and Biliary System   146
Ultrasound of the Pancreas   148
Computed Tomography of the Liver and Biliary Tree   149
Computed Tomography of the Pancreas   151
Magnetic Resonance Imaging of the Liver   152
Magnetic Resonance Cholangiopancreatography   155
Magnetic Resonance Imaging of the Pancreas   156
Endoscopic Retrograde Cholangiopancreatography   156
   Intraoperative Cholangiography   158
   Postoperative (T-Tube) Cholangiography   159
Percutaneous Transhepatic Cholangiography   161
External Biliary Drainage   164
   Internal Biliary Drainage   164
   Percutaneous Extraction of Retained Biliary Calculi (Burhenne
      Technique)   165
Angiography   167
   Coeliac Axis, Superior Mesenteric and Inferior Mesenteric
      Arteriography   167
Radionuclide Imaging of the Liver, Gallbladder and Spleen   168
   Liver and Gallbladder   168
   Spleen   170
Investigation of Specific Clinical Problems   171
   Investigation of Liver Tumours   171
   Investigation of Jaundice   172
   Investigation of Pancreatitis   173
   Pancreatitis-Associated Collections   173

6 Urinary tract

Douglas Pendse

Methods of Imaging the Urinary Tract   175

Plain Film Radiography   176

Intravenous Excretion Urography   176

Ultrasound of the Urinary Tract   178

Computed Tomography of the Urinary Tract   181

Low-Dose Computed Tomography of the Kidneys, Ureters and Bladder   182

Computed Tomography Urogram   183

Magnetic Resonance Imaging of the Urinary Tract   184

Multiparametric Prostate Magnetic Resonance Imaging   184

Magnetic Resonance Imaging of the Kidneys   185

Magnetic Resonance Urography   185

Magnetic Resonance Imaging of the Adrenals   186

Magnetic Resonance Renal Angiography   187

Urethrogram (Male)   187

Retrograde Pyeloureterography   189

Conduitogram or Loopogram (in Patients with Ileal Conduit)   190

Perculaneous Renal Biopsy   191

Percutaneous Nephrostomy   191

Percutaneous Nephrolithotomy   193

Dynamic Renal Radionuclide Scintigraphy   196

Direct Radionuclide Micturating Cystography   198

7 Ablation techniques

Pavan Najran

Types of Ablative Technology   201

Radiofrequency Ablation   201

Microwave Ablation   202

Cryoablation   203

Irreversible Electroporation   204

General Procedural Technique   206

Key Challenges & Tips   206

8 Reproductive system

Balashanmugam Rajashanker

Techniques in Imaging the Female Reproductive System   209

Hysterosalpingography   209

Pelvic Ultrasound of the Female Reproductive System   212
Ultrasound of the Scrotum   214
Computed Tomography of the Reproductive System   215
Magnetic Resonance Imaging of the Reproductive System   215
Gynaecological Malignancy   217
   Cervical Cancer   217
   Uterine Carcinoma   218
   Ovarian Cancer   218
Omental Biopsy   219

9 Respiratory system

Samavia Raza

   Methods of Imaging the Respiratory System   221
Computed Tomography of the Thorax   221
Computed Tomography–Guided Lung Biopsy   223
Methods of Imaging Pulmonary Embolism   227
   Radionuclide Lung Ventilation/Perfusion Imaging   228
   Computed Tomography in the Diagnosis of Pulmonary
      Emboli   231
   Pulmonary Arteriography   232
   Magnetic Resonance Imaging of Pulmonary Emboli   233
   Ultrasound of the Diaphragm—The 'Sniff Test'   235
Magnetic Resonance Imaging of the Respiratory System   236
Positron Emission Tomography and Positron Emission Tomography–
   Computed Tomography of the Respiratory System   237

10 Cardiac

Alim Yucel-Finn

   Methods of Imaging the Heart   239
Angiocardiography   239
Coronary Arteriography   241
Cardiac Computed Tomography   244
Cardiac Magnetic Resonance Imaging   251
Radionuclide Ventriculography   254
Radionuclide Myocardial Perfusion Imaging   257

11 Arterial system

Christopher Day

Non-Invasive Imaging   263
Vascular Ultrasound   263

Computed Tomography Angiography   264
Peripheral (Lower Limb) Computed Tomography
   Angiography   264
Magnetic Resonance Angiography   265
Vascular Access   266
General Complications of Catheter Techniques   272
Distant   274
Angiography   275
Angioplasty   276
Stents   278
Catheter-Directed Arterial Thrombolysis   280
Vascular Embolization   282
Thoracic and Abdominal Aortic Stent Grafts   284

12 Venous system

Christopher Day

   Methods of Imaging the Venous System   289
Ultrasound   289
   Lower Limb Venous Ultrasound   290
   Upper Limb Venous Ultrasound   291
Computed Tomography   291
Magnetic Resonance Imaging   292
Peripheral Venography   293
   Lower Limb   293
   Upper Limb   295
Central Venography   296
   Superior Vena Cavography   296
   Inferior Vena Cavography   296
Portal Venography   297
Transhepatic Portal Venous Catheterization   299
Venous Interventions   300
   Venous Angioplasty and Stents   300
Gonadal Vein Embolization   301
Inferior Vena Cava Filters   302
   Patient Preparation   303
Thrombolysis   304
Pulmonary Embolism   306
Thoracic Duct Embolization   307

13 Radionuclide imaging in oncology and infection

Greg Chambers and Sriram Vaidyanathan

Positron Emission Tomography Imaging 311

2-[^{18}F]Fluoro-2-Deoxy-D-Glucose Positron Emission Tomography Scanning 312

Other Positron Emission Tomography Radiopharmaceuticals 315

^{18}F-Fluoroethylcholine 315

^{18}F-Fluoride 315

^{68}Gallium-Labelled Pharmaceuticals 315

^{67}Gallium Radionuclide Tumour Imaging 316

Radioiodine (^{123}I or ^{131}I) Metaiodobenzylguanidine Scan 316

Somatostatin Receptor Imaging 319

Lymph Node and Lymphatic Channel Imaging 320

Ultrasound 320

Computed Tomography 321

Magnetic Resonance Imaging 321

Radiographic Lymphangiography 321

Radionuclide Lymphoscintigraphy 321

Radionuclide Imaging of Infection and Inflammation 324

14 Bones and joints

Philip Robinson and James J. Rankine

Musculoskeletal Magnetic Resonance Imaging: General Points 329

Arthrography: General Points 330

Arthrography 331

Arthrography: Site-Specific Issues 334

Knee 334

Hip 335

Shoulder 338

Elbow 341

Wrist 342

Ankle 344

Tendon Imaging 346

General Points 346

Ultrasound of the Paediatric Hip 346

Thermoablation of Musculoskeletal Tumours 347

Radionuclide Bone Scan 350

15 Spine

James J. Rankine

Imaging Approach to Back Pain and Sciatica 356

Conventional Radiography 357

Computed Tomography and Magnetic Resonance Imaging of the Spine 357

Myelography 359

Contrast Media 359

Cervical Myelography 360

Lumbar Myelography 362

Thoracic Myelography 365

Cervical Myelography by Lumbar Injection 365

Computed Tomography Myelography 365

Paediatric Myelography 366

Facet Joint and Medial Branch Blocks 367

Percutaneous Vertebral Biopsy 367

Bone Augmentation Techniques 369

Nerve Root Blocks 370

Lumbar Spine 370

Cervical Spine 370

16 Brain/Neuro

Amit Herwadkar

Computed Tomography of the Brain 374

Magnetic Resonance Imaging of the Brain 375

Imaging of Intracranial Haemorrhage 377

Computed Tomography 377

Magnetic Resonance Imaging 377

Imaging of Gliomas 378

Computed Tomography 378

Magnetic Resonance Imaging 379

Imaging of Acoustic Neuromas 380

Computed Tomography 380

Magnetic Resonance Imaging 380

Radionuclide Imaging of the Brain 380

Regional Cerebral Blood Flow Imaging 380

Positron Emission Tomography 382

^{201}Thallium Brain Scanning 383

Dopamine Transporter Ligands 384

Cerebral Angiography 385

17 ENT

Sofia Otero

Conventional, Digital Subtraction and Computed Tomography Dacryocystography 389

Magnetic Resonance Imaging of the Lacrimal System 391

Dacryoscintigraphy 391

Plain Film 392

Ultrasound 392

Conventional and Digital Subtraction Sialography 393

Image-Guided Basket Retrieval of Stones and Balloon Dilation of Strictures 395

Magnetic Resonance Imaging Sialography 398

Computed Tomography and Cone-Beam Computed Tomography Sialography 398

Contrast-Enhanced Magnetic Resonance Imaging and Computed Tomography 399

Ultrasound of the Thyroid Gland 400

Ultrasound of the Parathyroid Glands 401

Computed Tomography and Magnetic Resonance Imaging of the Thyroid and Parathyroid Glands 402

Radionuclide Thyroid Imaging 403

Radionuclide Parathyroid Imaging 405

Thyroid Radiofrequency Ablation 407

Thyroid Ethanol Ablation 408

18 Breast

Megan Bydder and Simon Lowes

Overview of Breast Imaging 411

Mammography 414

Ultrasound 416

Magnetic Resonance Imaging 418

Radionuclide Techniques 420

Image-Guided Biopsy of the Breast and Axilla 421

Preoperative Tumour Localization 428

19 Role of the radiographer and the nurse in interventional radiology

Dawn Hopkins, Nick Watson and Emma Ross

Role of the Radiographer in Interventional Radiology 433

Role of the Nurse in Interventional Radiology 436

20 Consent
Nick Watson

Assessment of Capacity   446
Supporting Patients in Decision Making   447
Acting for a Person Who Lacks Capacity   448
Documenting Assessment of Capacity   449
Shared Decision Making   449

21 Sedation and monitoring
Matthew Bridge

Sedation   451
Drugs   453
Local Anaesthesia   453
Inhalational Analgesia   453
Intravenous Analgesia   453
Sedative Drugs   455
Monitoring   457
Sedation and Monitoring for Magnetic
Resonance Imaging   458
Recovery and Discharge Criteria   459

22 Medical emergencies
Matthew Bridge

Equipment   461
Respiratory Emergencies   463
Respiratory Depression   463
Laryngospasm   463
Bronchospasm   463
Aspiration   464
Pneumothorax   464
Cardiovascular Emergencies   465
Hypotension   465
Tachycardia   465
Bradycardia   466
Adverse Drug Reactions   466
Contrast Media Reaction   466
Local Anaesthetic Toxicity   468

Appendix I Dose limits: from The Ionising Radiations Regulations 2017   469

Appendix II The Ionising Radiation (Medical Exposure) Regulations 2017 with the Ionising Radiation (Medical Exposure) (Amendment) Regulations 2018 and the Ionising Radiation (Medical Exposure) (Amendment) Regulations 2011   471

Schedule 1   481

Schedule 2   482

Schedule 3   485

Schedule 4   488

Index   491

General notes
David M. Rosewarne

RADIOLOGY

The procedures within the *Guide* are laid out under a number of subheadings, which follow a standard sequence. The general order is outlined as follows, together with certain points that have been omitted from the discussion of each procedure to avoid repetition. Minor deviations from this sequence will be found in the text where this is believed to be more appropriate.

Methods
A description of the technique for each procedure

Indications
Appropriate clinical reasons for using each procedure

Contraindications
All radiological procedures carry a risk. The risk incurred by undertaking the procedure must be balanced against the benefit to the patient that is expected to be gained from the information obtained. Contraindications may be relative (the majority) or absolute. Factors that increase the risk to the patient can be categorized under three headings: due to radiation, due to the contrast medium and due to the technique.

Risk due to radiation
Radiation effects on humans may be:

- Hereditary—i.e. revealed in the offspring of the exposed individual
- Somatic injuries, which fall into two groups—deterministic and stochastic
    1. Deterministic effects result in loss of tissue function—e.g. skin erythema and cataracts. If the radiation dose is distributed over a period of time, cellular mechanisms allow tissue repair. There is then greater tolerance than if the dose had been administered all at once. This implies a threshold dose above which the tissue will exhibit damage because the radiation dose exceeds the capabilities of cellular repair mechanisms.

2. Stochastic effects refer to random modifications to cell components, such as DNA mutations that can occur at any radiation dose; there is no threshold for stochastic effects.[1] Stochastic effects, such as malignancy, are 'all or none'. The cancer produced by a small dose is the same as the cancer produced by a large dose, but the frequency of occurrence is less with the smaller dose.

The current consensus held by international radiological protection organizations is that for comparatively low doses, the risk of both radiation-induced cancer and hereditary disease is assumed to increase linearly with increasing radiation dose, with no threshold (the so-called *linear no-threshold* model).[2] It is impossible to totally avoid staff and patient exposure to radiation. Therefore, the adverse effects of radiation cannot be completely eliminated but must be minimized. There is a small but significant excess of cancers following diagnostic levels of irradiation—e.g. during childhood[3] and to the female breast[4]— and amongst those with occupational radiation exposure.[5] In the United Kingdom, about 0.6% of the overall cumulative risk of cancer by the age of 75 years could be attributable to diagnostic x-rays. The most important factors that influence the risk of developing cancer after exposure to ionizing radiation are (a) genetic considerations (specific gene mutations and family history), (b) age at exposure (children are, in general, more radiosensitive than adults), (c) sex (there is a slightly increased risk in females), and (d) fractionation and protraction of exposure (higher dose and dose rate increase risk because of the influence of DNA damage).[6]

There are legal regulations which guide the use of diagnostic radiation (see Appendices I and II). These are the two basic principles:

1. Justification that a proposed examination is of net benefit to the patient
2. ALARP—doses should be kept 'as low as reasonably practicable', with economic and social factors being taken into account.[7]

Justification is particularly important when considering the irradiation of women of reproductive age because of the potential risks to a developing foetus. Mammalian embryos and foetuses are highly radiosensitive. The potential risks of in utero radiation exposure on a developing foetus include both teratogenic and carcinogenic effects. The risk of each effect depends on the gestational age at the time of the exposure and the absorbed radiation dose. Developing foetuses are most vulnerable to radiation effects on the central nervous system between 8 and 15 weeks of gestational age, and the risk of development of fatal childhood cancer may be greater if exposure occurs earlier in pregnancy.[8] The teratogenic risk of radiation is dose-dependent, and exposure to ionizing radiation doses of less than 50 mGy has not been shown to be associated with different pregnancy outcomes compared with exposure to background radiation alone.[8] The carcinogenic risk of ionizing radiation is harder to calculate accurately. It is thought that the risk for the general population of developing childhood cancer is 1 in 500.[9] For a foetal radiation dose of 30 mGy, the best estimate is of one excess cancer per 500 foetuses exposed,[10] resulting in a doubling of the natural rate. Most diagnostic radiation procedures lead to a foetal absorbed dose of less than 1 mGy for imaging not directly irradiating the maternal abdomen or pelvis and less than 10 mGy for direct abdominal or pelvic or nuclear medicine imaging.

Almost always, if a diagnostic radiology examination is medically indicated, the risk to the mother of not doing the procedure is likely greater than the risk of potential harm to the foetus. However, whenever possible, alternative investigation techniques that do not involve ionizing radiation should be considered before deciding to proceed with using ionizing radiation in a female patient of reproductive age. It is extremely important to have a robust process in place that prevents inappropriate or unnecessary ionizing radiation exposure to foetuses. Joint guidance from the Health Protection Agency, the College of Radiographers and the Royal College of Radiologists recommends the following:[9]

When a female patient of reproductive age presents for an examination in which the primary beam irradiates the pelvic area or for a procedure involving radioactive isotopes, she should be asked whether she is or might be pregnant. If the patient cannot exclude the possibility of pregnancy, she should be asked if her menstrual period is overdue. Her answer should be recorded, and depending on the answer, the patient should be assigned to one of the following four groups:

1. **No possibility of pregnancy:** Proceed with the examination.
2. **Patient definitely or probably pregnant:** Review the justification for the proposed examination and decide whether to defer until after delivery, bearing in mind that delaying an essential procedure until later in pregnancy may present a greater risk to the foetus, and a procedure of clinical benefit to the mother may also be of indirect benefit to her unborn child. If, after review, a procedure is still considered to be justified and is undertaken, the foetal dose should be kept to the minimum consistent with the diagnostic purpose.
3. **Low-dose examination, pregnancy cannot be excluded:** A low-dose examination is defined as one in which the foetal dose is likely to be below 10 mGy. The vast majority of diagnostic examinations fall into this category. If pregnancy cannot be excluded but the patient's menstrual period is not overdue, proceed with the examination. If the patient's period is overdue, the patient should be treated as probably pregnant, and the advice provided in the previous section should be followed.
4. **High-dose examination, pregnancy cannot be excluded:** A high-dose procedure is defined as any examination that results in a foetal dose greater than 10 mGy (e.g. computed tomography of the maternal abdomen and pelvis). The evidence suggests

that such procedures may double the natural risk of childhood cancer if carried out after the first 3–4 weeks of pregnancy and may still involve a small risk of cancer induction if carried out in the very early stages of an unrecognized pregnancy. There are two options that can be adopted to minimize the likelihood of inadvertent exposure of an unrecognized pregnancy: (a) apply the rule that female patients of childbearing potential are always booked for these examinations during the first 10 days of their menstrual cycles when conception is unlikely to have occurred; or (b) female patients of childbearing potential are booked in the normal way but are not imaged and are rebooked if, when they attend, they are in the second half of their menstrual cycles *and* are of childbearing potential *and* in whom pregnancy cannot be excluded.

If the examination is deemed necessary, evaluation of the foetal dose and associated risks by a medical physicist should be arranged, if possible, and discussed with the patient. A technique that minimizes the number of views and the absorbed dose per examination should be used. However, the quality of the examination should not be reduced to the level at which its diagnostic value is significantly impaired. The risk to the patient of an incorrect diagnosis may be greater than the risk of irradiating the foetus. Radiography of areas that are remote from the pelvis and abdomen may be safely performed during pregnancy, with good collimation and lead protection. The Royal College of Radiologists' guidelines indicate that legal responsibility for radiation protection lies with the employer; the extent to which this responsibility is delegated to the individual radiologist varies. Nonetheless, all clinical radiologists carry a responsibility for the protection from unnecessary radiation of:

- Patients
- Themselves
- Other members of staff
- Members of the public, including relatives and carers[11]

Risk due to the contrast medium

The risks associated with administration of iodinated contrast media and magnetic resonance imaging (MRI) contrast are discussed in detail in Chapter 2, and guidelines are given for prophylaxis of adverse reactions to intravascular contrast.

Contraindications to other contrast media (e.g. barium, water-soluble contrast media for the gastrointestinal (GI) tract and biliary contrast media) are given in the relevant sections.

Risks due to the technique

Skin sepsis at the needle puncture site can occur very rarely.

Specific contraindications to individual techniques are discussed with each procedure.

Contrast Medium

Volumes given are for a 70-kg man.

1

Equipment

For many procedures, equipment should also include a trolley with a sterile upper shelf and a non-sterile lower shelf. Emergency drugs and resuscitation equipment should be readily available (see Chapter 22).

See Chapter 11 for introductory notes on angiography catheters.

If only a simple radiography table and overcouch tube are required, then this information has been omitted from the text.

Patient preparation

1. Will admission to the hospital be necessary?
2. If the patient is a woman of childbearing age, the examination should be performed at a time when the risks to a possible foetus are minimal (as described previously). Any female presenting for radiography or a nuclear medicine examination at a time when her period is known to be overdue should be considered as pregnant unless there is information indicating the absence of pregnancy. If her cycle is so irregular that it is difficult to know whether a period has been missed and it is not practicable to defer the examination until menstruation occurs, then a pregnancy test may be considered. Particular care should be taken to perform hysterosalpingography during the first 10 days of the menstrual cycle so that the risks of mechanical trauma in early pregnancy are reduced.
3. Except in emergencies, in circumstances when consent cannot be obtained, patient consent to treatment is a legal requirement for medical care. Consent should be obtained in a suitable environment and only after the appropriate and relevant information has been given to the patient.[12] Patient consent may take the following forms:
   (a) Implied consent. For a very low-risk procedure, the patient's actions at the time of the examination will indicate whether they consent to the procedure to be performed.
   (b) Express consent. For a procedure of intermediate risk, such as barium enema, express consent should be given by the patient, either verbally or in writing.
   (c) Written consent. This must be obtained for any procedure that involves significant risk or side effects. The ability to consent depends more on a person's ability to understand and weigh the options than on age. At 16 years of age, a young person can be treated as an adult and can be presumed to have the capacity to understand the nature, purpose and possible consequences of the proposed investigation, as well as the consequences of non-investigation. Before the age of 16 years, children may have the capacity to consent depending on their maturity and ability to understand what is involved. The radiologist must assess a child's capacity to decide whether to give consent for or refuse an investigation. If the child lacks the capacity to consent, the

parent's consent should be sought. It is usually sufficient to have consent from one parent. If both parents cannot agree, legal advice should be obtained.[13] When a competent child refuses treatment, a person with parental responsibility or the court may authorize investigations or treatment, which is in the child's best interests. In Scotland, the situation is different: parents cannot authorize procedures that a competent child has refused. Legal advice may be helpful in dealing with these cases. (See Chapter 20 for a fuller discussion of consent.)

4. If an interventional procedure carries a risk of bleeding, then the patient's blood clotting should be measured before proceeding. If impaired coagulation bleeding disorder is discovered, or if the patient is being treated with anticoagulant therapy, the appropriate steps should be taken to manage the patient's clotting periprocedurally, often by liaison with the patient's clinical team. Beware of the possibility of patients being treated with new oral anticoagulants, such as the direct factor Xa inhibitors. Their anticoagulant effects are unreliably measured in the conventional assays of clotting time and must be specifically enquired about because limited checklists assessing whether the patient takes warfarin or not fail to correctly identify that the patient is actively anticoagulated.

5. Cleansing bowel preparations may be used before investigation of the GI tract or when considerable faecal loading obscures other intra-abdominal organs. For other radiological investigations of abdominal organs, bowel preparation is not always necessary, and when given may result in excessive bowel gas. Bowel gas may be reduced if the patient is kept ambulant before the examination, and those who routinely take laxatives should continue to do so.

6. Previous films and notes should be reviewed when possible, and an effort should be made to find missing information where it is thought likely to materially affect the conduct of the procedure.

7. Premedication is necessary for painful procedures or when the patient is unlikely to cooperate for any other reason. Suggested premedication for adults and children is described in Chapters 3 and 21.

Preliminary Images

The purpose of these images is:

1. To make any final adjustments in exposure factors, centring, collimation and patient position, for which purpose the film should always be taken using the same equipment as will be used for the remainder of the procedure

2. To exclude prohibitive factors such as residual barium from a previous examination or excessive faecal loading

3. To demonstrate, identify and localize opacities which may be obscured by the contrast medium

Every radiographic view taken should have on it the patient's name, registration number, date and a side marker. The examination can only proceed if satisfactory preliminary films have been obtained.

1

Technique
1. For aseptic technique, the skin is cleaned with chlorhexidine 0.5% in 70% industrial spirit or its equivalent.
2. The local anaesthetic used most commonly is 1% lidocaine.
3. Gonad protection is used whenever possible unless it obscures the region of interest.

Images
When films are taken during the procedure rather than at the end of it, they have, for convenience, been described under 'Technique'.

Additional Techniques or Modifications of Technique

Aftercare
May be considered as:

1. Instructions to the patient
2. Instructions to the ward

Complications
Complications may be considered under the following three headings:

Due to the anaesthetic

1. General anaesthesia
2. Local anaesthesia:
   (a) Allergic (unusual)
   (b) Toxic

Topical local anaesthetic contributes to the total dose. Symptoms of excessive dose are of paraesthesia and muscle twitching, which may progress to convulsions, cardiac arrhythmias, respiratory depression and death due to cardiac arrest. Treatment is symptomatic and includes adequate oxygenation.

Due to the contrast medium

- Intravascular contrast media (see Chapter 2)
- Barium (see Chapter 4)

Due to the technique

Specific details are given with the individual procedures and may be conveniently classified as:

1. Local
2. Distant or generalized

References
1. Tremblay E, Thérasse E, Thomassin-Nagarra E, et al. Quality initiatives: guidelines for use of medical imaging during pregnancy and lactation. *Radiographics*. 2012;32:897–911.
2. Wakeford R. Cancer risk modelling and radiological protection. *J Radiol Prot*. 2012;32(1):N89–N93.

3. Pearce MS, Salotti JA, Little MP, et al. Radiation exposure from CT scans in childhood and subsequent risk of leukaemia and brain tumours: a retrospective cohort study. *Lancet*. 2012;380(9840):499–505.

4. Einstein AJ, Henzlova MJ, Rajagopalan S. Estimating risk of cancer associated with radiation exposure from 64-slice computed tomography coronary angiography. *J Am Med Assoc*. 2007;298(3):317–323.

5. Muirhead CR, O'Hagan JA, Haylock RGE, et al. Mortality and cancer incidence following occupational radiation exposure: third analysis of the National Registry for Radiation Workers. *Br J Cancer*. 2009;100(1):206–212.

6. Hricak HH, Brenner DJ, Adelstein SJ, et al. Managing radiation use in medical imaging: a multifaceted challenge. *Radiology*. 2011;258:889–905.

7. International Commission on Radiological Protection. The optimization of radiological protection: broadening the process. ICRP publication 101. *Ann ICRP*. 2006;36(3):69–104.

8. Wang PI, Chong ST, Kielar AZ, et al. Imaging of pregnant and lactating patients: evidence-based review and recommendations, parts 1 and 2. *AJR Am J Roentgenol*. 2012;198:778–792.

9. Advice from the Health Protection Agency, The Royal College of Radiologists and the College of Radiographers. *Protection of Pregnant Patients during Diagnostic Medical Exposures to Ionising Radiation*. <https://www.rcr.ac.uk/protection-pregnant-patients-during-diagnostic-medical-exposures-ionising-radiation>; 2009.

10. International Commission on Radiological Protection. Pregnancy and medical radiation. *Ann ICRP*. 2000;30(1):1–43.

11. Royal College of Radiologists. *Good Practice Guide for Clinical Radiologists*. 2nd ed. London: Royal College of Radiologists; 2012.

12. General Medical Council. *Decision Making and Consent*. <https://www.gmc-uk.org/ethical-guidance/ethical-guidance-for-doctors/decision-making-and-consent.> London: General Medical Council; 2020.

13. General Medical Council. *0–18 years: Guidance for all Doctors*. London: General Medical Council; 2007.

RADIONUCLIDE IMAGING

RADIOPHARMACEUTICALS

Radionuclides are shown in symbolic notation, the most frequently used in nuclear medicine being 99m-technetium (^{99m}Tc), a 140-keV gamma-emitting radioisotope of the element technetium with a half-life of 6.0 h.

Radioactive Injections

In the United Kingdome, the Administration of Radioactive Substances Advisory Committee (ARSAC) advises the health ministers on the Medicines (Administration of Radioactive Substances) Regulations 2006 (MARS). These require that radioactive materials may only be administered to humans by a doctor or dentist holding a current ARSAC certificate or by a person acting under their direction. Administration of radioactive substances can only be carried out by an individual who has received appropriate theoretical and practical training, as specified in the Ionising Radiation (Medical Exposure) Regulations 2017 (see Appendix II).[1] These regulations place responsibilities on the referrer to provide medical data to justify the exposure, the practitioner (ARSAC licence holder) to justify individual exposure and operators (persons who carry out practical aspects relating to the exposure).

Activity Administered

The maximum activity values quoted in the text are those currently recommended as diagnostic reference levels in the ARSAC Guidance Notes.[2] The unit used is the SI unit, the megabecquerel (MBq). Millicuries (mCi) are still used in some countries, notably the United States (1 mCi = 37 MBq).

Radiation doses are quoted as the adult effective dose (ED) in millisieverts (mSv) from the ARSAC Guidance Notes.

The regulations require that doses to patients are kept as low as reasonably practicable (the ALARP principle) and that exposure follows accepted practice. Centres are frequently able to administer activities below the maximum, depending upon the capabilities of their equipment and local protocols. Typical figures are given in the text when they differ from the diagnostic reference levels. In certain circumstances, the person clinically directing (ARSAC licence holder) may use activity higher than the recommended maximum for a named patient (e.g. for an obese patient in whom attenuation would otherwise degrade image quality).

The ARSAC recommends that activities administered for paediatric investigations should be reduced according to body weight but no longer in a linear relationship. The guidance notes include a table of suggested scaling factors based on producing comparable quality images to those expected for adults, with a minimum activity of 10% of the adult value for most purposes. However, organs develop at different rates (e.g. the brain achieves 95% of its adult size by age 5 years), and some radiopharmaceuticals behave differently in children, so the administered activity may need to be adjusted accordingly. It should be noted that when scaling activity according to the suggested factors, the radiation dose for a child may be higher than that for an adult.

Equipment

Gamma cameras usually have one or two imaging heads. Double-headed systems have the advantage of being able to capture two sites simultaneously, which in many cases can roughly halve the imaging time. This can be a great advantage for single-photon emission computed tomography (SPECT) scans, in which minimizing patient movement can be critical.

Hybrid systems are commonplace where multislice CT forms part of an integrated system as a single machine with either a double-headed gamma camera (SPECT-CT) or a positron emission tomography (PET) scanner (PET-CT). Advantages include the better anatomical localization of abnormal areas of activity on the co-registered images.

Technique

Patient positioning

The resolution of gamma camera images is critically dependent upon the distance of the collimator surface from the patient, falling off approximately linearly with distance. Every effort should therefore be made to position the camera as close to the patient as possible. For example, in posterior imaging with the patient supine, the thickness of the bed separates the patient from the camera, as well as interposing an attenuating medium. In this case, imaging with the patient sitting or standing directly against the camera is preferable.

Patient immobilization for the duration of image acquisition is very important. If patients are uncomfortable or awkwardly positioned, they will have a tendency to move, which will have a blurring effect on the image. Point marker sources attached to the patient away from areas being examined can help monitor and possibly permit correction of movement artifact.

Images

The image acquisition times quoted in the text should only be considered an approximate guide because the appropriate time depends upon such factors as the sensitivity of the available equipment, the amount of activity injected and the size of the patient. An acceptable acquisition time is usually a compromise between the time available, the counts required for a diagnostic image and the ability of the patient to remain motionless.

Aftercare

Radiation safety

Special instructions should be given to patients who are breast-feeding regarding expression of milk and interruption of feeding.[2] Precautions may have to be taken with patients leaving hospital or returning to wards, depending upon the radionuclide and activity administered.

Complications

With few exceptions (noted in the text), the amount of biologically active substance injected with radionuclide investigations is at trace levels and very rarely causes any systemic reactions. Those that may occasionally cause problems are labelled blood products, antibodies and substances of a particulate nature.

References

1. The Royal College of Radiologists. *IR(ME)R: Implications for Clinical Practice in Diagnostic Imaging, Interventional Radiology and Diagnostic Nuclear Medicine.* 2020.
2. Administration of Radioactive Substances Advisory Committee. *Notes for Guidance on the Clinical Administration of Radiopharmaceuticals and Use of Sealed Radioactive Sources.* UKHSA; 2022.

COMPUTED TOMOGRAPHY

Patient Preparation

Many CT examinations require little physical preparation. An explanation of the procedure, the time it is likely to take, the necessity for immobility and the necessity for breath-holding while scanning the chest and abdomen should be given. Waiting times should be kept to a minimum because a long wait may increase anxiety. The patient should be as pain free as is practical, but sedation or analgesia that is too heavy may be counterproductive; patient cooperation is often required. Children younger than the age of 4 years usually need sedation (see Chapters 3 and 21). Children should also have an intravenous (IV) cannula inserted at the time sedation is administered or local anaesthetic cream applied to two sites if IV contrast medium is needed. If these simple steps are taken, the number of aborted scans will be reduced and the image quality improved.

Intravenous Contrast Medium

Many CT examinations will require IV contrast medium. Essential information should be obtained from the patient and appropriate guidelines followed (see Chapter 2). An explanation of the need for contrast enhancement should be given to the patient.

The dose of contrast (using 300 mg I mL^{-1}) depends on the area examined (e.g. 50 mL for the head; 100 mL for the chest or abdomen). The chest is usually scanned at 20 s after the start of the contrast injection. For arterial phase images of the abdomen or pelvis, the acquisition of the scan is usually commenced 25–30 s after the start of the contrast injection and for portal venous phase images 60–70 s after the start of the contrast injection.

Recent advances in CT scanner technology have led to generally much faster scan acquisition times, and this has resulted in the need for more stringent regimens for IV contrast administration. The use of saline 'chasers' when administering IV contrast allows smaller volumes of contrast to be used; increases peak contrast enhancement; leads to better reproducibility; and, for example in thoracic scanning, can reduce streak artifact from the brachiocephalic veins and right side of the heart. The timing of scanning is now often 'triggered' by enhancement of a specific vascular region of interest to a predetermined threshold or by a timing delay determined by a small test bolus of contrast given immediately before the main scan acquisition. These techniques are particularly important when CT angiography is being performed, but in general, all contrast-enhanced CT will benefit because patient-to-patient variations in body size, cardiac output and so on can be largely overcome. In children, a maximum total iodinated contrast dose of 2 mL kg^{-1} body weight (300 mg I mL^{-1}) should be observed.

Split-bolus multidetector CT is a technique that can merge the enhancement profiles of multiphasic CT into a single acquisition and thereby reduce radiation dose. The method involves 100 to 150 mL of

IV contrast divided over two to three boluses and can be used in the investigation of haematuria:

RENAL PROTOCOL

Indications

1. Haematuria
2. Renal cell carcinoma and transisitonal cell carcinoma
3. Nephrolithiasis

Technique

Unenhanced CT is initially performed followed by 50 mL of IV contrast and subsequently a further 50 mL 8 min later. Images are acquired 55 s after the second doe of contrast, providing a combined nephrographic and renal excretory phases.

The technique can also be used in the assessment of polytrauma and is an emerging method for investigating mesenteric ischemia and the detection of pancreatic and liver malignancies using similar principles. A total of 100 mL of contrast material is injected in the portal venous phase followed by the injection of 40–50 mL of contrast material approximately 35 s later to boost the other phase. Bolus tracking after the second bolus initiates scanning with timing dependant on the rationale for investigation (e.g. immediately for mesenteric ischemia or polytrauma, 15 s after bolus tracking for pancreatic phase, 35 s for hepatic arterial phase).

The advent of new volume-based reconstruction techniques and greater detector fidelity now allows for comparable image noise in acquisitions performed at lower kilovolts, thus using the attenuation characteristics of the 'K-edge' of the iodine, particularly when paired with higher milliampere tube currents. Consequently, this allows similar apparent image contrast with lower iodinated contrast concentrations, useful in patients with impaired renal function. This concept of utilizing the 'K-edge' of the iodine with lower KeV CT image acquisition is also integral to dual-energy CT, an emerging technique that offers potential to reduce the IV contrast volume and radiation dose of the study.

Oral Contrast Medium

For examinations of the abdomen, opacifying the bowel satisfactorily can be problematic. Plain water is recommended as a negative oral contrast medium for CT of the stomach and duodenum. Satisfactory opacification of the small and large bowel can be problematic. Water-soluble contrast medium (e.g. 20 mL Urografin 150 diluted in 1 L of orange squash to disguise the taste, preflavoured contrast such as 20 mL Gastromiro diluted in 1 L of water) or low-density barium suspensions (2% w/v) can be used. Timing of administration is given in Table 1.1. Doses of contrast media in children depend upon age (see also Chapter 3).

Table 1.1   Timing and Volume for Oral Contrast Medium in Computed Tomography[a]

	Volume (mL)	Time Before Scan (min)
Adults		
Full abdomen and pelvis	1000	Gradually over 1 h before scanning
Upper abdomen (e.g. pancreas)	500	Gradually over 0.5 h before scanning
Children		
Newborns	60–90	Full dose 1 h before scanning and a further half dose immediately before the scan
1 mo–1 y	120–240	
1–5 y	240–360	
5–10 y	360–480	
Older than 10 y	As for adults	

[a]If the large bowel needs to be opacified, then give the contrast medium the night before or 3–4 h before scanning.

Pelvic Scanning

Rarely, it may be necessary to opacify the distal bowel using per rectal instillation of contrast medium by catheter. The concentration of contrast medium should be the same as for oral administration.

Computed Tomography Colonography

See Chapter 4.

Further Reading

Beenen LF, Sierink JC, Kolkman S, et al. Split bolus technique in polytrauma: a prospective study on scan protocols for trauma analysis. *Acta Radiol.* 2015;56(7):873–880.

Brook OR, Gourtsoyianni S, Brook A, et al. Split-bolus spectral multidetector CT of the pancreas: assessment of radiation dose and tumor conspicuity. *Radiology.* 2013;269(1):139–148.

Maheshwari E, O'Malley ME, Ghai S, et al. Split-bolus MDCT urography: upper tract opacification and performance for upper tract tumors in patients with hematuria. *AJR Am J Roentgenol.* 2010;194(2):453–458.

Scialpi M, Palumbo B, Pierotti L, et al. Detection and characterization of focal liver lesions by split-bolus multidetector-row CT: diagnostic accuracy and radiation dose in oncologic patients. *Anticancer Res.* 2014;34(8):4335–4344.

Tabari A, Gee S, Singh R, et al. Reducing radiation dose and contrast medium volume with application of dual-energy CT in children and young adults. *AJR Am J Roentgenol.* 2020;214(6):1199–1205.

MAGNETIC RESONANCE IMAGING

Patient Preparation

As for CT scanning, a full description of the purpose and nature of the examination should be given to the patient and waiting times kept to a minimum. Some patients find the interior of the scanner a very disconcerting environment, and combined with the longer imaging duration compared with other modalities such as CT, symptoms of claustrophobia or panic attacks can ensue and are reported in as many as 10% of patients. Most of these patients are able to complete their examinations, but approximately 1% of investigations may have to be curtailed as a result. To decrease the number of scans aborted, the counselling of, explanation to and reassurance of patients by well-trained staff should be routine. A small number of adult patients may require sedation before an MRI scan is undertaken. Sedation or general anaesthesia is often required for MRI scans in young children; details of suggested protocols are given in Chapters 3 and 21.

If IV contrast is required, it is advisable to insert the IV cannula before the examination begins. It is critically important that detailed preparation regarding patient safety is made for each MRI examination.

SAFETY IN MAGNETIC RESONANCE IMAGING

MRI has generally been a very safe process because of the care taken by equipment manufacturers and MRI staff. However, there are significant potential hazards to patients and staff caused by:

1. Electromagnetic fields:
   (a) Static magnetic field
   (b) Gradient magnetic field
   (c) Radiofrequency field
2. Noise
3. Inert gas quench
4. Claustrophobia
5. IV contrast agents (see Chapter 2)

Effects Due to Magnetic Fields

Static field

The strength of the static magnetic field used in MRI is measured in units of gauss or tesla (10,000 gauss = 1 tesla (T)). The earth's magnetic field is approximately 0.6 gauss.

Biological effects

Despite extensive research, no significant deleterious physiological effects have yet been proven.[1] There have been reports of temporary minor changes, such as alteration in electrocardiograms (ECGs; T-wave elevation), presumed to be caused by electrodynamic forces on moving ions in blood vessels. Temporary and dose-correlated vertigo and nausea in patients exposed to static fields higher than 2 T have been found.[2] However, studies of volunteers exposed to 8-T static magnetic fields have shown no clinically significant effect on heart rate, respiratory rate, systolic and diastolic blood pressure, finger pulse oxygenation levels and core body temperature.[3] Teratogenesis in humans is thought unlikely at the field strengths used in clinical MRI.

Non-biological effects

There are two main areas of concern:

1. Ferromagnetic materials (whether iatrogenic or as a result of penetrating injury) may undergo rotational or translational movement as a result of the magnetic field. *Rotational movement* occurs as a result of an elongated object trying to align with the field. This may result in displacement of the object and applies to certain types of surgical clips. Increasingly, iatrogenically implanted materials are non-ferromagnetic and are MR compatible, but it is essential that all implanted devices should be evaluated individually for any such risk. In many cases, postoperative fibrosis (>6 weeks) is strong enough to anchor the material so that no danger of significant displacement exists. *Translational movement* occurs when loose ferromagnetic objects are accelerated by the field. Objects such as paperclips or hairgrips may reach considerable speeds and could potentially cause severe damage to the patient or equipment; this is the so-called *missile effect*. In general, no object or equipment should be brought into the MRI environment unless it is proven to be:
   - MRI safe (no known hazard in all MRI environments); or
   - MRI conditional (no known hazard in a specified MRI environment within specified conditions of use).[4]

     The safety of MRI-conditional items must be verified with the specific scanner and MRI environment in which they are to be used. Most MR departments have access to medical physics staff, whose advice should be sought whenever there is any query regarding the MR compatibility of any patient.

2. Electrical devices such as cardiac pacemakers may be affected by static field strengths. Most modern pacemakers have a sensing mechanism that can be bypassed by a magnetically operated relay triggered by fields as low as 5 gauss. Relay closure can be expected in virtually all conventional cardiac pacemakers placed in the bore of the magnet, and these patients must not enter the controlled MRI area. Recent engineering advances have produced MRI-conditional cardiac pacemaker devices, but great care must still be taken.[5]

Gradient field

Biological effects

The rapidly switched magnetic gradients used in MRI can induce electric fields in a patient, which may result in nerve or muscle stimulation, including cardiac muscle stimulation. The strength of these is dependent on the rate of change of the field and the size of the subject.[6] Studies have shown that the threshold for peripheral nerve stimulation is lower than that for cardiac or brain stimulation.[7] Although possible cardiac fibrillation or brain stimulation are major safety issues, peripheral nerve stimulation is a practical concern because, if sufficiently intense, it can be intolerable and result in termination of the examination. Recommendations for safety limits on gradient fields state that the system must not have a gradient output that exceeds the limit for peripheral nerve stimulation.[6] This also protects against cardiac fibrillation.

Non-biological effects

Rapidly varying fields can induce currents in conductors. Metal objects may heat up rapidly and cause tissue damage. Instances of partial- and full-thickness burns, arising when conducting loops (e.g. ECG electrodes or surface imaging coils) have come into contact with skin, have been recorded.

Radiofrequency field

Radiofrequency energy deposited in the body during an MRI examination is converted to heat, which is distributed by convective heat transfer through blood flow. Energy deposited in this way is calculated as the average power dissipated in the body per unit mass, the specific absorption rate (SAR). SAR values are dependent on the magnetic field strength and may be fourfold higher in a 3-T scanner than a 1.5-T scanner.[8] Guidelines on radiofrequency exposure are designed to limit the rise in temperature of the skin, body core and local tissue to levels below those where systemic heat overload or thermal-induced local tissue damage may occur. The extent to which local temperature rises depends on the SAR and on tissue blood flow. Areas of particular concern include those most sensitive to heat, such as the hypothalamus, and poorly perfused regions, such as the lens of the eye.

For whole-body exposures, no adverse health effects are expected if the increase in body core temperature does not exceed 1°C. In the case of infants and those with circulatory impairment, the temperature increase should not exceed 0.5°C. With regard to localized heating, measured temperature in focal regions of the head should be less than 38° C, in the trunk should be less than 39°C and in the limbs should be less than 40° C.[6]

Noise

During imaging, noise arises from vibration in the gradient coils and other parts of the scanner because of the varying magnetic fields. The amplitude of this noise depends on the strength of the magnetic fields, pulse sequence and scanner design.

Noise levels may reach as much as 95 dB. This level exceeds statutory noise limits in industry, and in most cases, the use of earplugs or headphones by the patient is advised. (Music delivered by closed headphones may both reduce noise level and help the patient relax during the procedure).

Inert Gas Quench

When superconducting magnets are used the coolant gases, liquid helium ± liquid nitrogen could vaporize should the temperature inadvertently rise. This could potentially lead to asphyxiation or exposure to extreme cold. To prevent this, a well-ventilated room with some form of oxygen monitor to raise an alarm should be installed.

Intravenous Contrast Medium

See Chapter 2.

Recommendations for Safety

Detailed MRI safety recommendations have been published by the American College of Radiology.[9] It is essential that all MRI units have clear MRI safety policies and protocols, including a detailed screening questionnaire for all patients and staff (Table 1.2).

Controlled and restricted access

Access to the scanning suite should be limited. Areas should be designated as restricted (5 gauss line) and, closer to the scanner, controlled (10 gauss line). No patient with a pacemaker should be allowed to enter the restricted area. All people who enter this area should be made aware of the hazards—in particular, the 'missile effect'. All persons entering the controlled area should remove all loose ferromagnetic materials, such as paperclips and pens, and it is advisable that wristwatches and magnetic tape and credit cards do not come near the magnet. Other considerations include the use of specially adapted cleaning equipment, wheelchairs and trolleys. Fire extinguishers and all anaesthetic or monitoring equipment must be constructed from non-ferromagnetic materials.

Implants

As mentioned previously, persons with pacemakers must not enter the restricted area. All other persons must be screened to ensure there is no danger from implanted ferromagnetic objects, such as aneurysm clips, prosthetic heart valves, intravascular devices or orthopaedic implants. When an object is not known to be 'MRI safe' or 'MRI conditional', then the person should not be scanned. Lists of safe and unsafe implants are available[10] and should be consulted for each individual object.

Specific questioning is also advisable to assess the risk of shrapnel and intra-ocular foreign bodies being present.

Pregnancy

Developing foetuses and embryos are susceptible to a variety of teratogens, including heat, being most sensitive during organogenesis. Increased static magnetic field strength, flip angle or

Table 1.2   Questions to be Included in a Screening Questionnaire for Magnetic Resonance Imaging Patients and Staff

Question to Patient or Staff Member	Action
Do you have a pacemaker, or have you had a heart operation?	Pacemaker. If present, patient must not enter controlled area.
	Heart operation. Establish if there is any metal valve prosthesis, intravascular device or recent metallic surgical clip insertion and check MR compatibility.
Could you possibly be pregnant?	See text.
Have you ever had any penetrating injury, especially to the eyes, even if it was years ago?	Establish details. If necessary, arrange radiography of the orbits or relevant area to determine if there is any metallic foreign body.
Have you ever had any operations to your head, chest or neck?	Find out details. If there is any metallic aneurysm or haemostatic clips or metallic prosthesis/implant, then check MR compatibility.
Do you have any joint replacements or any other body implants?	Check the details of surgery and MR compatibility of joint replacement or implant.
Have you removed all metal objects and credit cards from your clothing and possessions?	This must be done before entering the controlled area.

MR, Magnetic resonance.

number of radiofrequency pulses and decreased spacing between pulses increase the SAR and therefore the radiofrequency energy deposited as heat on the foetus.[11] Although no conclusive evidence of teratogenesis exists in humans, scanning should be avoided, particularly during the first trimester, unless alternative diagnostic procedures would involve the exposure of the foetus to ionizing radiation. Before a pregnant patient is accepted for an MRI examination, a risk–benefit analysis of the request should be made. When MRI examinations are performed in pregnant patients, the scan time should be limited as much as possible to reduce the SAR and can be shortened sometimes by direct supervision and on table image review. Staff members who are pregnant are advised to remain outside the controlled area (10 gauss line) and to avoid exposure to gradient or RF fields.

MRI contrast agents should generally be avoided during pregnancy and only used with extreme caution (see Chapter 2).[11]

References

1. Hartwig V, Giovannetti G, Vanello N, et al. Biological effects and safety in magnetic resonance imaging: a review. *Int J Res Public Health*. 2009;6(6):1778–1798.
2. De Vocht F, Stevens T, van Wendel De Joode B, et al. Acute neurobehavioral effects of exposure to static magnetic fields: analysis of exposure–response relations. *J Magn Reson Imaging*. 2006;23:291–297.
3. Chakeres DW, Kangarlu A, Boudoulas H, et al. Effect of static magnetic field exposure of up to 8T on sequential human vital sign measurements. *J Magn Reson Imaging*. 2003;18(3):346–352.
4. Shellock FG, Spinazzi A. MRI safety update 2008: part 2, screening patients for MRI. *AJR Am J Roentgenol*. 2008;191(4):1140–1149.
5. Shinbane JS, Colletti PM, Shellock FG. Magnetic resonance imaging in patients with cardiac pacemakers: era of "MR Conditional" designs. *J Cardiovasc Magn Reson*. 2011;13(1):63.
6. The International Commission on Non-Ionizing Radiation Protection. Medical magnetic resonance (MR) procedures: protection of patients. *Health Phys*. 2004;87(2):197–216.
7. Nyenhuis JA, Bourland JD, Kildishev AV, et al. Health effects and safety of intense gradient fields. In: Shellock FG, ed. *Magnetic Resonance Procedures: Health Effects and Safety*. CRC Press. 2001:31–53.
8. Chavhan GB, Babyn PS, Singh M, et al. MR imaging at 3.0T in children: technical differences, safety issues, and initial experience. *Radiographics*. 2009;29(5):1451–1466.
9. Kanal E, Barkovich AJ, Bell C, et al. ACR guidance document for safe MR practices. *J Magn Reson Imaging*. 2013;37(3):501–530.
10. Shellock FG. *Reference Manual for Magnetic Resonance Safety, Implants, and devices*. Biomedical Research Publishing Group; 2020. <http://www.mrisafety.com>.
11. Wang PI, Chong ST, Kielar AZ, et al. Imaging of pregnant and lactating patients: part 1, evidence-based review and recommendation. *AJR Am J Roentgenol*. 2012;198(4):778–784.

ULTRASONOGRAPHY

Patient Preparation

For many ultrasound examinations, no preparation is required. This includes examination of tissues such as thyroid, breast, testes, musculoskeletal, vascular and cardiac. In certain situations, simple preparatory measures are required.

Abdomen

For optimal examination of the gallbladder, it should be dilated, which usually requires fasting for 6–8 h before scanning. If detailed assessment of the pancreas is required, it can be helpful to have clear fluid filling the stomach, acting as an 'acoustic window'.

Pelvis

To visualize the pelvic contents optimally, bowel gas must be displaced. This can be facilitated by filling the urinary bladder to capacity, which then acts as an acoustic window. The patient should be instructed to drink 1–1.5 L of water during the hour before scanning and to not empty the bladder. In practice, both abdominal and pelvic scanning are often performed at the same attendance. Oral intake of clear fluids does not provoke gallbladder emptying, so the two examinations can usually be combined. However, it should be noted that in normal patients who drink a large volume of oral fluid before the scan to fill their bladders, the renal collecting systems may appear slightly dilated. If this is the case, the patient should be asked to empty the bladder, and the kidneys should be rescanned. If the renal collecting system dilatation is significant, it will persist after the bladder is emptied.

Endoscopic

Endoscopic ultrasound examination of the rectum or vagina requires no physical preparation, but clearly, an explanation of the procedure in a sympathetic manner is needed.

Examination of the oesophagus or transoesophageal echocardiography requires preparation similar to upper GI endoscopy. The patient should be appropriately starved before the procedure. Anaesthesia and sedation are partly a matter of personal preference of the operator. Local anaesthesia of the pharynx can be obtained using 10% lidocaine spray. Care to avoid overdose is essential because lidocaine is rapidly absorbed via this route. The maximum dose of lidocaine should not exceed 200 mg. Sedation using IV benzodiazepines may also be necessary. If local anaesthetic has been used, then the patient must be instructed to avoid hot food and drink until the effect has worn off (1–2 h) to avoid both heat injury and potential aspiration.

Children

Ultrasound examination in children can, in most cases, be performed with no preparation apart from explanation and reassurance to both child and parent. In some cases, when a child is particularly anxious or when immobility is required, sedation may be necessary. With echocardiography in infants, sedation is essential to obtain optimal recordings. The sedation regimens described in Chapters 3 and 21 may be used.

Intravascular contrast media

David M. Rosewarne

HISTORICAL DEVELOPMENT OF RADIOGRAPHIC AGENTS

The first report of opacification of the urinary tract after intravenous (IV) injection of a contrast agent appeared in 1923 using an IV injection of 10% sodium iodide solution, which was at that time prescribed for treatment of syphilis and was excreted in the urine. In 1928, German researchers synthesized a compound with a number of pyridine rings containing iodine in an effort to detoxify the iodine. This mono-iodinated compound was developed further into di-iodinated compounds, and subsequently, in 1952, the first tri-iodinated compound, sodium acetrizoate (Urokon), was introduced into clinical radiology. Sodium acetrizoate was based on a six-carbon ring structure, tri-iodo benzoic acid, and was the precursor of all modern water-soluble contrast media.

Until the early 1970s, all contrast media were ionic compounds and were hypertonic with osmolalities of 1200–2000 mosmol kg^{-1} water, four to seven times the osmolarity of blood. These are referred to as *high-osmolar contrast media* (HOCM) and are distinguished by differences at position 5 of the anion and by the cations sodium, meglumine, or both. In 1969, Almén[1] first postulated that many of the adverse effects of contrast media were the result of high osmolality and that by eliminating the cation, which does not contribute to diagnostic information but is responsible for up to 50% of the osmotic effect, it would be possible to reduce the toxicity of contrast media.

Conventional ionic contrast media had a ratio of three iodine atoms per molecule to two particles in solution, that is, a ratio of 3:2 or 1.5 (Table 2.1) to decrease the osmolality without changing the iodine concentration, the ratio between the number of iodine atoms and the number of dissolved particles must be increased.

The development to produce *low-osmolar contrast medium* (LOCM) agents proceeded along two separate paths (see Table 2.1). The first was to combine two tri-iodinated benzene rings to produce an ionic dimer with six iodine atoms per anion, ioxaglate (Hexabrix). The alternative, more successful, approach was to produce compounds that do not ionize in solution and therefore do not provide radiologically useless cations. LOCM of this type are referred to as *non-ionic*. These include the non-ionic monomers iopamidol (Niopam, Iopamiron, Isovue,

Table 2.1   Schematic Illustration of the Development of Contrast Media

Description	Name	Chemical Structure	Ratio of No. of Iodine Atoms/Ions: No. of Particles in Solution	Osmolarity of a 280 mg I mL⁻¹ Solution	Osmolarity Group
	Sodium iodide	Na⁺ I−	0.5		
	Diodone	[structure: Na⁺, RCOO–N pyridine ring with I, I, O]	1		
Ionic monomer	Diatrizoate (Urograffin, Hypaque) Metrizoate (Isopaque) Iothalamate (Conray)	[structure: Na⁺/Meg⁺, COO−, benzene ring with I, I, I, R, R] monomeric-monoacidic	1.5	1500	High

2

Ionic dimer	Ioxaglate (Hexabrix)	dimeric-monoacidic	3	490	Low
Non-ionic monomer	Iopamidol (Niopam, Isovue) Iohexol (Omnipaque) Iomeprol (Iomeron) Ioversol (Optiray) Iopromide (Ultravist)	monomeric-non-ionic	3	470	Low
Non-ionic dimer	Iotrolan (Isovist) Iodixanol (Visipaque)	dimeric-non-ionic	6	300	Iso

Meg, Meglumine; *R*, an unspecified side chain.

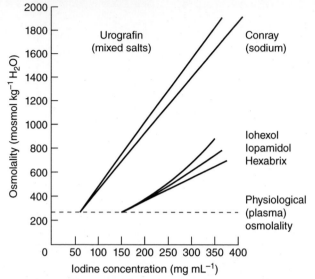

Fig. 2.1 A plot of osmolality against iodine concentration for new and conventional contrast media. (From Dawson P, Grainger RG, Pitfield J. The new low-osmolar contrast media: a simple guide. *Clin Radiol.* 1983;34:221–226; reproduced by courtesy of the editor of *Clinical Radiology.*)

and Solutrast), iohexol (Omnipaque), iopromide (Ultravist), iomeprol (Iomeron) and ioversol (Optiray), which are widely used today.

For both types of LOCM, the ratio of iodine atoms in the molecule to the number of particles in solution is 3:1, and osmolality is theoretically halved in comparison with HOCM. However because of aggregation of molecules in solution, the measured reduction is only approximately one-third (Fig. 2.1).

Further research led to the introduction of non-ionic dimers, iotrolan (Isovist) and iodixanol (Visipaque). These have a ratio of six iodine atoms for each molecule in solution with satisfactory iodine concentrations at iso-osmolality; they are thus called *iso-osmolar contrast media*. The safety profile of the iso-osmolar contrast agents is at least equivalent to LOCM, but any significant advantage of iso-osmolar contrast remains controversial.[2,3]

The low- and iso-osmolar contrast media are 5–10 times safer than the HOCM and are used routinely in clinical practice. With development having reached the stage of iso-osmolality, further research is now targeted on decreasing the chemotoxicity and viscosity of iodinated contrast media.

References

1. Almén T. Development of nonionic contrast media. *Invest Radiol.* 1985;20:S2–9.
2. Dawson P, Grainger RG, Pitfield J. The new low-osmolar contrast media: a simple guide. *Clin Radiol.* 1983;34:221–226.
3. Morcos SK. Contrast-induced nephropathy: are there differences between low osmolar and iso-osmolar iodinated contrast media? *Clin Radiol.* 2009;64:468–472.

ADVERSE EFFECTS OF INTRAVENOUS WATER-SOLUBLE CONTRAST MEDIA

The toxicity of contrast media is a function of osmolarity, ionic charge (ionic contrast agents only), chemical structure (chemotoxicity) and lipophilicity.

Adverse reactions after administration of non-ionic iodinated contrast media are rare, occurring in fewer than 1% of all patients.[1] Of these reactions, the vast majority are mild and self-limiting. The incidence of moderate or severe non-ionic contrast reactions is less than 0.001%.[2]

TOXIC EFFECTS ON SPECIFIC ORGANS

Vascular Toxicity

Venous

1. Pain at the injection site, usually the result of extravenous leak.
2. Transient pain extending up the arm caused by stasis of contrast medium in the vein. It may be relieved by abducting the arm.
3. Delayed limb pain caused by thrombophlebitis as a result of the toxic effect on endothelium.

Arterial

Arterial endothelial damage and vasodilatation are mostly related to hyperosmolality. Contrast medium injected during peripheral arteriography often causes a sensation of heat or, occasionally, pain.

Soft Tissue Toxicity

Pain, swelling, erythema and even sloughing of skin may occur from extravasated contrast medium. The risk is increased when pumps are used to inject large volumes of contrast medium during computed tomography (CT) examinations. Treatment should consist of the application of cold packs and elevation of the limb. If symptoms do not resolve quickly, admit and monitor the patient; a surgical referral may be needed in the case of skin blistering, paraesthesia, altered tissue perfusion or pain lasting more than 4 hours.

Cardiovascular Toxicity

1. Intracoronary injection of contrast media may cause significant disturbance of cardiac rhythm.
2. Increased vagal activity may result in depression of the sinoatrial and atrioventricular nodes, causing bradycardia or asystole.
3. Injection of hypertonic contrast medium causes significant fluid and ion shifts. Immediately after injection, there is a significant increase in serum osmolality. This causes an influx of water from the interstitial space into the vascular compartment, an increase in blood volume, an increase in cardiac output and a brief increase of systemic blood pressure. Peripheral dilation may cause a more prolonged decrease in blood pressure. Injection into the right heart or pulmonary artery causes transitory pulmonary hypertension and systemic hypotension; injection into the left ventricle or aorta causes brief systemic hypertension followed by a more prolonged fall.

Nephrotoxicity

Contrast-induced nephropathy (CIN) is one of the most serious adverse effects associated with the use of intravascular contrast media and is defined as an impairment of renal function (urine output <0.5 mL kg^{-1}h^{-1} for 6 h, an increase in serum creatinine by >25 µmoles L^{-1} within 48 h, or an increase in serum creatinine >50% baseline value within 1 week of administration)[3,4] in the absence of an alternative aetiology. In affected patients, the serum creatinine concentration starts to rise within the first 24 h, reaches a peak by 2–3 days and usually returns to baseline by 3–7 days. In rare cases, patients may need temporary or permanent dialysis.

It was hoped that the iso-osmolar contrast agents might be less nephrotoxic than LOCM; however, clinical trials have so far yielded conflicting results,[5] and there are insufficient reasons to select iso-osmolar agents on the basis of CIN risk.

There are a number of predisposing factors in CIN:

1. The single most important risk factor is preexisting impairment of renal function; patients with normal renal function are at very low risk.
2. Diabetes
3. Heart failure
4. Hypovolaemia
5. Sepsis
6. Increasing age is cited in some studies but is not regarded as an independent risk factor in current Royal Australian and New Zealand College of Radiologists recommendations.
7. High dose of contrast medium
8. Renal transplant
9. Intraarterial administration of contrast.

A further hazard for patients who have impairment of renal function as a result of intravascular iodinated contrast is reduced renal clearance of other drugs (e.g. metformin). The resultant accumulation of metformin can theoretically result in the development of the potentially fatal complication lactic acidosis, though this is not a significant consideration when estimated glomerular filtration rate is greater than 45 mL min^{-1}1.76 m^2.

See Table 2.2 for guidelines on prophylaxis of renal adverse reaction to iodinated contrast.

Thyroid Function

Iodinated contrast media may rarely cause thyroid dysfunction, and intravascular contrast should be avoided when possible in hyperthyroidism[6] with careful evaluation of the risk–benefit ratio. The administration of contrast precludes the use of radioiodine in the treatment of thyroid cancer for 2 months, and similarly, radioiodine imaging should be avoided for 2 months after iodinated contrast administration.

Table 2.2   Guidelines for Prophylaxis of Renal Adverse Reactions to Iodinated Contrast Medium

Renal Adverse Reactions

Identification of Patients at Increased Risk

1. The referring clinician should identify patients with preexisting renal impairment and inform the radiology department.
2. eGFR (or serum creatinine) should be measured before the administration of contrast in patients:
   (a) With previously known renal impairment
   (b) Who have diabetes and are taking metformin
   (c) Who will undergo intra-arterial contrast injection
   (d) With clinical history suggesting increased risk of renal impairment (e.g. diabetes, renal surgery or administration of nephrotoxic drugs)

Precautions for Patients with Significant Renal Impairment (Any Patient with eGFR< 60 mL min^{-1})

1. Consider an alternative imaging method not using iodinated contrast media.
2. The risk of IV CI-AKI is likely to be non-existent for patients with eGFR >45 mL min^{-1}1.73 m^{-2}. No special precautions are recommended in this group before or following IV administration of iodinated contrast media.
3. The risk is of IV CI-AKI is also very likely to be low or non-existent for patients with eGFR of 30–45 mL min^{-1}1.73 m^{-2}. Universal use of periprocedural hydration in this group to prevent the theoretical risk of CI-AKI cannot be recommended, but patients with impaired function in this range that is acutely deteriorating rather than stable may benefit from this intervention.
4. In patients with severe renal function impairment (eGFR <30 mL^{-1} min^{-1} 1.73 m^{-2} or actively deteriorating renal function (acute kidney injury)), careful weighing of the risk versus the benefit of iodinated contrast media administration needs to be undertaken. Consideration should be given to periprocedural renal protection using IV hydration with 0.9% saline. There is insufficient evidence to support the use of prophylactic administration of N-acetyl cysteine for patients at high risk of contrast nephropathy.
5. Severe renal function impairment should not be regarded as an absolute contraindication to medically indicated iodinated contrast media administration.
6. Use low- or iso-osmolar contrast medium in the lowest dose of contrast consistent with a diagnostic result.
7. Patients with normal renal function (eGFR >45 mL min^{-1}) receiving contrast can continue metformin treatment normally. Others should have metformin paused for 48 h after the study and renal function tested before restarting.

CI-AKI, Contrast media-related acute kidney injury; *eGFR*, estimated glomerular filtration rate; *IV*, intravenous.

IDIOSYNCRATIC REACTIONS

Adverse reactions can be classified in terms of severity as:

1. Mild: nausea, vomiting, urticaria
2. Moderate: mild bronchospasm, vasovagal reaction, tachycardia, diffuse erythema

Table 2.3   Categories of Adverse Effects of Low-Osmolar Contrast Medium Contrast Doses[12]

Category of Adverse Effect[12]	Proportion of Adverse Effect Events (n = 458) (%)	Proportion of Total Patient Group (n = 298,000) (%)
Mild	81.6	0.125
Moderate	15.1	0.02
Severe	3.3	0.005

3. Severe: cardiovascular collapse, moderate or severe bronchospasm, laryngeal oedema, loss of consciousness or seizure

Mild and moderate reactions are uncommon; major adverse reactions are very rare for both LOCM[7] and iso-osmolar iodinated contrast.[8] Adverse effects of low-osmolar iodinated contrast are found in approximately 0.15% of all patients. In a large study of LOCM contrast doses,[9] the adverse effects were categorized (Table 2.3).

The vast majority of adverse effects were managed with patient reassurance or antihistamine treatment, and only one death was presumed caused by LOCM (0.0003% of the total patient group).

Fatal Reactions

Deaths caused by iodinated contrast agents are very rare, occurring at a rate of 1.1–1.2 per million contrast media packages distributed. Most are attributed to renal failure, anaphylaxis or allergic reaction.[2,10]

Other than renal failure, almost every fatal reaction will occur within minutes after injection; therefore, all patients must be under close observation during this time. The fatal event may be preceded by trivial events, such as nausea and vomiting, or may occur without warning. The majority of deaths occur in those older than 50 years of age. Causes of death include cardiac arrest, pulmonary oedema, respiratory arrest, consumption coagulopathy, bronchospasm, laryngeal oedema and angioneurotic oedema.

Non-fatal Reactions

1. Flushing, metallic taste in the mouth, nausea, sneezing, cough and tingling are common and related to dose and speed of injection.
2. Perineal burning, a desire to empty the bladder or rectum and an erroneous feeling of having been incontinent of urine are more common in women.
3. Urticaria
4. Angioneurotic oedema. This most commonly affects the face. Its onset may be delayed for several hours after administration and may persist for up to 3 days.
5. Rigors

6. Necrotizing skin lesions are rare and mostly in patients with preexisting renal failure (particularly those with systemic lupus erythematosus).
7. Bronchospasm: Predisposed to by a history of asthma and by therapy with beta-blockers. In most patients, the bronchospasm is subclinical. Mechanisms include the following:
   (a) Direct histamine release from mast cells and platelets
   (b) Cholinesterase inhibition
   (c) Vagal overtone
   (d) Complement activation
   (e) Direct effect of contrast media on bronchi.
8. Non-cardiogenic pulmonary oedema during acute anaphylaxis or hypotensive collapse and possibly caused by increased capillary permeability
9. Arrhythmias
10. Hypotension: Usually accompanied by tachycardia, but in some patients, there is vagal overreaction with bradycardia. The latter is rapidly reversed by atropine 0.6 mg IV. Hypotension is usually mild and is treatable by a change of posture. Rarely, it is severe and may be accompanied by pulmonary oedema.
11. Abdominal pain: May be a symptom in anaphylactic reactions or vagal overactivity. It should be differentiated from the loin pain that may be precipitated in patients with upper urinary tract obstruction.
12. Delayed-onset reactions (occurring between 1 h and 1 week after injection) include nausea, vomiting, rashes, headaches, itching and parotid gland swelling. Late adverse reactions are commoner by a factor of three to four after iso-osmolar contrast medium injection. Risk factors for delayed reaction are previous contrast medium reaction, history of allergy and interleukin-2 treatment.[11]

MECHANISMS OF IDIOSYNCRATIC CONTRAST MEDIUM REACTIONS

Idiosyncratic contrast medium reactions are usually labelled *anaphylactoid* because they have all the features of anaphylaxis but are negative for immunoglobulin E in more than 90% of cases. However, patients who experience a severe anaphylactoid reaction to iodinated contrast should be referred for an immunology opinion.

PROPHYLAXIS OF ADVERSE CONTRAST MEDIUM EFFECTS

Guidelines for prophylaxis of renal and non-renal adverse contrast media reaction are given in Table 2.4 (see also Table 2.2). Sources used in these tables include documents of the Royal Australian and New Zealand College of Radiologists,[3] Canadian Association of Radiologists[4] and European Society of Urogenital Radiology[12] on contrast medium administration. General safety issues include the following:

Table 2.4   Guidelines for Prophylaxis of Non-renal Adverse Reactions to Iodinated Contrast Medium

Non-renal Adverse Reactions

Identification of Patients at Increased Risk of Anaphylactoid Contrast Reaction

It is essential that before administration of iodinated contrast, every patient must be specifically asked whether they have a history of:

1. *Previous contrast reaction*: Associated with a sixfold increase in reactions to contrast medium.[14] Determine the exact nature and specific agent used.
2. *Asthma*: A history of asthma associated with a 6- to 10-fold increase in the risk of severe reaction. Determine whether the patient has true asthma or COPD and whether asthma is currently well controlled. If asthma is not currently well controlled and examination is non-emergency, the patient should be referred back for appropriate medical therapy.
3. *Previous allergic reaction requiring medical treatment*: Determine the nature of the allergies and their sensitivity. (There is no specific cross-reactivity with shellfish or topical iodine in acute reactions.)

Precautions for Patients at Increased Risk of Anaphylactoid Contrast Reaction

1. Consider an alternative test not requiring iodinated contrast.
2. If the injection is considered necessary:
   (a) For previous reactors to iodinated contrast, use a different non-ionic low- or iso-osmolar contrast to that used previously.
   (b) Maintain close supervision.
   (c) Leave the cannula in place and observe for 30 min.
   (d) Be ready to promptly treat any adverse reaction and ensure that emergency drugs and equipment are ready (see Chapter 22).

There are no conclusive data supporting the use of premedication with corticosteroids or antihistamines in the prevention of severe reactions to contrast media in patients at increased risk.[3] Pretreatment with antihistamines is associated with an increased incidence of flushing.

Other Situations

Pregnancy: Iodinated contrast may be given if the clinical situation dictates; see text.
Lactation: No special precaution is required.
Thyrotoxicosis: Intravascular contrast should not be given if the patient is hyperthyroid. Avoid thyroid radio-isotope tests and treatment for 2 mo after iodinated contrast medium administration.

COPD, Chronic obstructive pulmonary disease.

- A doctor should be immediately available in the department to deal with severe reactions.
- Facilities for treatment of patients with acute adverse reaction should be readily available and regularly checked.
- Patients must not be left alone or unsupervised for the first 5 minutes after injection of the contrast agent.
- The patient should remain in the department for at least 15 minutes after the contrast injection. In patients at increased risk of reaction, this should be increased to 30 minutes.

Iodinated Contrast in Pregnancy and Lactation

There is no evidence of mutagenic or teratogenic effects after IV administration of iodinated contrast to the mother during pregnancy, but there is a potential impact on the neonatal thyroid gland. The foetal thyroid develops early in pregnancy and plays an important role in the development of the nervous system. It is recommended that iodinated contrast be only used in pregnant women when (a) no alternative test is available, (b) information obtained from the study is useful to both the mother and foetus during the pregnancy and (c) the referring physician considers it imprudent to delay the imaging study until after delivery.[13] A single in utero exposure to low-osmolar iodinated contrast is unlikely to have any effect on thyroid function at birth;[14] in any case, neonatal thyroid function is routinely tested to detect congenital hypothyroidism in all newborn babies.

Only small amounts of IV contrast medium reach the breast milk during lactation: approximately 0.5% of the dose received by the mother. It is considered safe for both the mother and infant to continue breastfeeding after iodinated contrast administration.[13]

References

1. Mortelé KJ, Oliva MR, Ondategui S, et al. Universal use of nonionic iodinated contrast medium for CT: evaluation of safety in a large urban teaching hospital. *AJR Am J Roentgenol.* 2005;184(1):31–34.
2. Hunt CH, Hartman RP, Hesley GK. Frequency and severity or adverse effects of iodinated and gadolinium contrast materials: retrospective review of 456,930 doses. *AJR Am J Roentgenol.* 2009;193:1124–1127.
3. The Royal Australian and New Zealand College of Radiologists. *Iodinated Contrast Media Guideline.* Author; 2018.
4. Canadian Association of Radiologists. *Consensus Guidelines for the Prevention of Contrast Induced Nephropathy.* 2nd ed. Canadian Association of Radiologists; 2011.
5. Seeliger E, Sendeski M, Rihal CS, et al. Contrast induced kidney injury: mechanisms, risk factors and prevention. *Eur Heart J.* 2012;33(16):2007–2015.
6. Heinrich MC, Häberle L, Müller V, et al. Nephrotoxicity of iso-osmolariodixanol compared with non-ionic low-osmolar contrast media: meta-analysis of randomized controlled trials. *Radiology.* 2009;250(1):68–86.
7. Rhee CM, Bhan I, Alexander EK, et al. Association between iodinated contrast media exposure and incident hyperthyroidism and hypothyroidism. *Arch Intern Med.* 2012;172(2):153–159.
8. Kopp AF, Mortele KJ, Cho YD, et al. Prevalence of acute reactions to iopromide: postmarketing surveillance study of 74,717 patients. *Acta Radiol.* 2008;49(8):902–911.
9. Haussler MD. Safety and patient comfort with iodixanol: a postmarketing surveillance study in 9515 patients undergoing diagnostic CT examinations. *Acta Radiol.* 2010;51(8):924–933.
10. Wysowski DK, Nourjah P. Deaths attributed to X-ray contrast media on US death certificates. *AJR Am J Roentgenol.* 2006;186:613–615.
11. Bellin MF, Webb JA, Thomsen HS, et al. Late adverse reactions to intravascular iodine based contrast media: an update. *Eur Radiol.* 2011;21(11):2305–2310.

12. European Society of Urogenital Radiology Contrast Media Safety Committee. *ESUR Guidelines on Contrast Media*, Version 10.0. 2018.
13. American College of Radiology. *ACR Manual on Contrast Media*. Author; 2022.
14. Bourjeily G, Chalhoub M, Phornphutkl C, et al. Neonatal thyroid function: effect of single exposure to iodinated contrast medium in utero. *Radiology*. 2010;256(3):744–750.

CONTRAST AGENTS IN MAGNETIC RESONANCE IMAGING

HISTORICAL DEVELOPMENT

Shortly after the introduction of clinical magnetic resonance imaging (MRI), the first contrast-enhanced human MRI studies were reported in 1981 using ferric chloride as a contrast agent in the gastrointestinal (GI) tract. In 1984, Carr et al.[1] were the first to demonstrate the use of a gadolinium compound as a diagnostic intravascular MRI contrast agent. Currently, around one-quarter of all MRI examinations are performed with contrast agents.

MECHANISM OF ACTION

MRI contrast agents act indirectly by altering the magnetic properties of hydrogen ions (protons) in water and lipid, which form the basis of the image in MRI. The paramagnetic effect of the contrast agent rather than the agent itself is imaged. To increase the inherent contrast between tissues, MRI contrast agents must alter the rate of relaxation of protons within the tissues. The changes in relaxation vary, and therefore different tissues produce differential enhancement of the signal (Figs. 2.2 and 2.3). These figures show that, for a given time t, if the T1 relaxation is more rapid, then a larger signal is obtained (brighter images), but the opposite is true for T2 relaxation, in which more rapid relaxation produces reduced signal intensity (darker images). There are different means by which these effects on protons can be produced using a range of MRI contrast agents.

MRI contrast agents interact with the magnetic moments of the protons in the tissues by exerting a large magnetic field density (a property imparted by their unpaired electrons) and thereby altering their T1 relaxation time (longitudinal relaxation rate), producing a change in signal intensity (see Fig. 2.2). The electron magnetic moments also cause local changes in the magnetic field, which promote more rapid proton dephasing and therefore shorten the T2 relaxation time (transverse relaxation rate). All contrast agents shorten both T1 and T2 relaxation times, but some predominantly affect T1 and others predominantly T2.

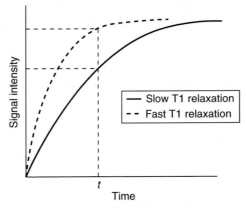

Fig. 2.2 Signal intensity and T1 relaxation time.

Agents with unpaired electron spins are potential contrast material for use in MRI. These may be classified under three headings:

1. **Ferromagnetic:** These retain magnetism even when the applied field is removed. This may cause particle aggregation and interfere with cell function and are therefore unsafe for clinical use as MRI contrast agents.
2. **Paramagnetic** (e.g. gadolinium contrast agents): These are by far the most widely used MRI contrast agents. Their maximum effect is on protons in the water molecule, shortening the T1 relaxation time and hence producing increased signal intensity (white) on T1 images (see Fig. 2.2).
3. **Superparamagnetic** (e.g. particles of iron oxide—Fe_3O_4): These cause abrupt changes in the local magnetic field, which results in rapid proton dephasing and reduction in the T2 relaxation time and hence producing decreased signal intensity (black) on T2 images (see Fig. 2.3). Superparamagnetic compounds are available in preparations for providing GI contrast.

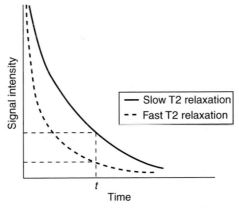

Fig. 2.3 Signal intensity and T2 relaxation time.

GADOLINIUM

Gadolinium (Gd) is a toxic heavy metal with seven unpaired electrons. It is rendered non-toxic and soluble by chelation with large organic molecules, forming a stable complex around the gadolinium. Gadolinium chelates represent the largest group of MRI contrast media and can either be injected intravenously or used as an oral preparation.

Gadolinium contrast agents are available in three forms:

1. **Extracellular fluid (ECF) agents:** These are far the most commonly used form of gadolinium. They include:
   (a) Gd-diethylenetriamine penta-acetic acid (DTPA), gadopentetate dimeglumine (Magnevist)
   (b) Gd-DTPA-bis methylamide, gadodiamide (Omniscan)
   (c) Gd-DO3A, Gadoteridol (ProHance)
   These all contain a central, strongly paramagnetic gadolinium ion within an eight-coordinate ligand and a single water molecule forming a stable nine-coordinate complex. After IV injection, they circulate within the vascular system and are excreted unchanged by the kidneys. There is a wide range of indications for ECF agents, including improved detection rates and more accurate delineation and characterization of tumours. The ECF agents do not cross the normal, intact blood–brain barrier but extravasate across where it is abnormal, and thus they are very effective in demonstrating many forms of central nervous system pathology. ECF agents are used for angiography but rapidly leak out of the vascular space into the interstitial space and thus are used only for dynamic arterial studies.

2. **Liver agents:** The excretion pathway of the gadolinium chelates can be modified to produce compounds such as Gd-BOPTA, gadobenate (MultiHance) and Gd-DTPA and gadoxetate disodium (Primovist), which are taken up by hepatocytes and excreted intact via the hepatobiliary system. These agents are used to (a) improve the detection of liver lesions that do not contain hepatocytes (and therefore do not take up the contrast), such as liver metastases, and (b) to characterize lesions that do take up the contrast, such as some hepatocellular carcinoma and focal nodular hyperplasia (FNH). They can also be used to provide positive contrast (T1 weighted) imaging of the biliary system via a delayed hepatobiliary phase.

3. **Blood pool agents:** These bind reversibly to human albumin, forming large molecules with higher relaxivity and longer persistence in the vascular space than ECF agents, allowing a wider range of vascular imaging (e.g. gadofosveset trisodium, Vasovist).

Dose

For ECF gadolinium agents, usually 0.1 mmol kg^{-1} body weight is given. Up to 0.2 mmol kg^{-1} is given when used in low-field magnets.

Table 2.5 Acute Adverse Reaction Rates for Gadolinium Contrast Agents

Study	Number of Examinations	Mild (%)	Moderate (%)	Severe (%)	Fatal
Morgan et al.[2]	28,078	0.63	0.02	0.014	None
Abujudeh et al.[3]	32,659	0.13	0.018	0.006	None
Dillman et al.[4]	78,353	0.05	0.012	0.005	None
Hunt et al.[5]	158,439	0.03	0.007	0.0025	None

Adverse Reactions

Gadolinium contrast agents are very safe and well tolerated; they have a lower incidence of adverse reactions than iodinated contrast agents.[2,3] Adverse reactions to gadolinium are mostly mild and self-limiting.[4,5] These can be divided into acute and delayed reactions.

Acute adverse reactions

These are rare (Table 2.5) and are classified as:

1. **Mild:** nausea, vomiting, headache, dizziness, shaking, altered taste, itching, rash, facial swelling
2. **Moderate:** tachycardia or bradycardia, hypertension, generalized erythema, dyspnoea, bronchospasm, wheezing, mild hypotension
3. **Severe:** laryngeal oedema (severe or rapidly progressive), unresponsiveness, cardiopulmonary arrest, convulsions, clinically manifest cardiac arrhythmias

Patients with a history of previous adverse reaction to gadolinium contrast agents have an increased likelihood of experiencing adverse reactions, with a 30% recurrence rate of hypersensitivity reactions in those with previous reactions.[6] Those with asthma, documented allergies or previous adverse reaction to iodinated contrast are also at increased risk of adverse reaction.[7]

Delayed adverse reactions

1. **Renal impairment:** When used at the standard doses listed previously, gadolinium contrast agents do not cause significant impairment of renal function.
2. **Nephrogenic systemic fibrosis (NSF):** This rare but significant systemic disorder, first described in 2000, is characterized by increased deposition of collagen with thickening and hardening of the skin; contractures; and in some patients, clinical involvement of other tissues.[8] Most cases are mild, but an estimated 5% have a

progressive debilitating course.[9] NSF occurs in patients with renal disease, and almost all patients with NSF have been exposed to gadolinium-based contrast agents within 2–3 months before the onset of the disease. The mechanism by which renal failure and gadolinium-based contrast agents trigger NSF is not known.

In 2009, the European Medicines Agency Committee for Medicinal Products for Human Use Scientific Advisory Group categorized gadolinium products according to risk of causing nephrogenic systemic fibrosis:

1. **Low risk:** macrocyclic chelates, including gadoterate meglumine (Dotarem), gadoteridol (ProHance) and gadobutrol (Gadovist)
2. **Medium risk:** linear ionic chelates, including gadoxetic acid (Primovist) and gadobenate dimeglumine (Multilane)
3. **High risk:** linear non-ionic chelates, including gadodiamide (Omniscan), and linear ionic chelates, including gadopentetate dimeglumine (Magnevist)

Preventative guidelines have been shown to be extremely effective in protection of patients from NSF.[10]

Precautions for prevention of adverse reactions

Detailed guidelines are available from the American College of Radiology,[7] Royal College of Radiologists[11] and European Society of Urogenital Radiology.[12] These form the basis for the following advice.

Acute adverse reactions

1. Identify patients at increased risk of reaction because of previous gadolinium reaction, asthma, allergies and previous adverse reaction to iodinated contrast.
2. For those at increased risk, consider an alternative test not requiring a gadolinium agent.
3. If proceeding with IV gadolinium contrast:
   (a) Patients who have previously reacted to one gadolinium-based contrast agent should be injected with a different agent if they are restudied.
   (b) Those with an increased risk of adverse reaction should be monitored more closely after injection.

Delayed adverse reactions

1. Identify patients at risk of NSF, particularly patients with renal impairment, patients in the perioperative period after liver transplant, infants, neonates, older adults and women who are pregnant or breastfeeding according to current Royal College of Radiologist (RCR) guidelines.
2. For patients at increased risk, consider an alternative test not requiring a gadolinium agent.
3. If proceeding with gadolinium contrast, the use of high-risk gadolinium contrast medium is to be avoided unless absolutely

necessary (see previous notes). The lowest possible dose of low- or medium-risk gadolinium-based contrast agent should be used. The dose should not be repeated within 7 days.

Magnetic Resonance Imaging Contrast Agents in Pregnancy and Lactation

2

MRI contrast agents should not be routinely given to pregnant patients.[7] Although there are no reports of teratogenic or mutagenic effects in humans, there are no case-controlled prospective studies in large numbers of patients, and the precise risk to foetuses is not known. Gadolinium chelates may accumulate in the amniotic fluid and remain there for an indefinite period of time, with potential dissociation of the toxic free gadolinium ion. The decision to administer an MRI contrast agent to a pregnant patient should be made on a case-by-case basis dependant on a risk–benefit analysis.

The use of gadolinium contrast agents is considered safe during lactation.[13] Only tiny amounts of gadolinium-based contrast medium given intravenously to a lactating mother reach the milk, and a minute proportion entering the baby's gut is absorbed.

References

1. Carr DH, Brown J, Bydder GM, et al. Intravenous chelated gadolinium as a contrast agent in NMR imaging of cerebral tumours. *Lancet*. 1984;1(8375):484–486.
2. Morgan DE, Spann JS, Lockhart ME, et al. Assessment of adverse reaction rates during gadoteridol-enhanced MRI imaging in 28,078 patients. *Radiology*. 2011;259(1):109–116.
3. Abujudeh HH, Kosaraju VK, Kaewlai R. Acute adverse reactions to gadopentetatedimeglumine and gadobenatedimeglumine: experience with 32,659 injections. *AJR Am J Roentgenol*. 2010;194(2):430–434.
4. Dillman JR, Ellis JH, Cohan RH, et al. Frequency and severity of acute allergic-like reactions to gadolinium-containing IV contrast media in children and adults. *AJR Am J Roentgenol*. 2007;189(6):1533–1538.
5. Hunt CH, Hartman RP, Hesley GK. Frequency and severity or adverse effects of iodinated and gadolinium contrast materials: retrospective review of 456,930 doses. *AJR Am J Roentgenol*. 2009;193:1124–1127.
6. Jung JW, Kang HR, Kim MH, et al. Immediate hypersensitivity reaction to gadolinium based MR contrast media. *Radiology*. 2012;264(2):414–422.
7. American College of Radiology. *ACR Manual on Contrast Media*, Version 2022. Author; 2022.
8. Cowper SE, Robin HS, Steinberg SM, et al. Scleromyxoedema-like cutaneous diseases in renal dialysis patients. *Lancet*. 2000;356(9234):1000–1001.
9. Reiter T, Ritter O, Prince MR, et al. Minimising risk of nephrogenic systemic fibrosis in cardiovascular magnetic resonance. *J Cardiovasc Magn Reson*. 2012;14(1):31.
10. Wang Y, Alkasab TK, Narin O, et al. Incidence of nephrogenic systemic fibrosis after adoption of restrictive gadolinium based contrast guidelines. *Radiology*. 2011;260(1):105–111.
11. The Royal College of Radiologists. *Standards for Intravascular Contrast Administration to Adult Patients BFCR(15)1*. The Royal College of Radiologists; 2015.

12. European Society of Urogenital Radiology Contrast Media Safety Committee. *ESUR Guidelines on Contrast Media*, Version 10.0. 2018.
13. Tremblay E, Thérasse E, Thomassin-Naggara I, Trop I. Quality initiatives: guidelines for use of medical imaging during pregnancy and lactation. *Radiographics*. 2012;32(3):897–911.

CONTRAST AGENTS IN ULTRASONOGRAPHY

Since the first reported use of ultrasound (US) contrast was published in the late 1960s, describing the intracardiac injection of agents during echocardiography, considerable progress has been made in the development and clinical application of US contrast agents, and they are now used increasingly to assess vascularity and tissue perfusion. US contrast agents contain microbubbles of air, nitrogen or fluorocarbon gas coated with a thin shell of material such as albumin, galactose or lipid. The contrast is usually injected intravenously, but to cross the pulmonary capillary bed and reach the systemic arterial circulation, the microbubbles must be 3–5 μm in diameter, approximately the size of a red blood cell. Bubbles of this size only remain intact for a very short time in blood. The bubbles do not pass through the vascular endothelium and therefore provide pure intravascular contrast. The effect of a bolus injection is to increase the echo signal from blood by a factor of 500–1000. After about 5 minutes, the gas from the bubbles diffuses into the blood, and the very small mass of shell material is then metabolized.[1]

Clinical applications of US contrast agents include the following:[2,3]

1. Identification and characterization of solid lesions, particularly in the liver,[4] but also in the spleen, pancreas, kidney, prostate, ovary and breast
2. To assist US-guided interventions such as biopsy
3. Voiding urosonography can be used to detect vesicoureteric reflux in children; here, US contrast is administered directly into the bladder
4. Assessment of fallopian tubal patency at hysterosonosalpinography
5. Determination of disease activity in patients with inflammatory bowel disease

A number of different microbubble contrast agents are available. Levovist consists of microbubbles of air enclosed by a thin layer of palmitic acid in a galactose solution and is stable in blood for 1–4 minutes. SonoVue, another microbubble contrast agent, is an aqueous suspension of stabilized sulphur hexafluoride microbubbles.

The US agents in clinical use are well tolerated, and serious adverse reactions are rarely observed. These agents are not nephrotoxic and may be used in patients with any level of renal function.[5] Allergic-type reactions occur rarely, and adverse events are usually mild and self-resolving.[6]

References

1. Wilson S, Burns PN. Microbubble-enhanced US in body imaging: what role? *Radiology.* 2010;257:24–39.
2. Quaia E. Microbubble ultrasound contrast agents: an update. *Eur Radiol.* 2007;17(8):1995–2008.
3. Furlow B. Contrast-enhanced ultrasound. *Radiol Technol.* 2009;80(6):547–561.
4. Piscaglia F, Lencioni R, Sagrini E, et al. Characterization of focal liver lesions with contrast enhanced ultrasound. *Ultrasound Med Biol.* 2010;36(4):531–550.
5. Wilson S, Greenbaum L, Goldberg BB. Contrast enhanced ultrasound: what is the evidence and what are the obstacles? *AJR Am J Roentgenol.* 2009;193(1):55–60.
6. Jakobsen JA, Oyen R, Thomsen HS, et al. Safety of ultrasound contrast agents. *Eur Radiol.* 2005;15(5):941–945.

Further Reading

Burns PN, Wilson SR. Microbubble contrast for radiological imaging 1. *Principles. Ultrasound Q.* 2006;22(1):5–13.

Wilson SR, Burns PN. Microbubble contrast for radiological imaging 2. *Applications. Ultrasound Q.* 2006;22(1):15–18.

2

Paediatrics

Samantha B.L. Low, Manigandan Thyagarajan and
Adam J. Oates

PAEDIATRIC PATIENTS

Children are not small adults. The emotions triggered in a child's visit to the radiology department are variable and are influenced by factors such as their age, developmental stage, previous experience, being in pain, feeling a loss of control (physical and emotional), a new environment, fear of the unknown and parental anxiety.

It is essential to create a positive experience for the child because this will not only facilitate the radiological examination but also prevent negative associations for future events. To achieve this, the patient-facing healthcare professional must obtain the cooperation of the child and family whilst creating a child-friendly environment.

Preparing the Environment

1. Ensure sufficient time for each examination to facilitate a stress-free environment for the child and family.
2. Allow the child to bring significant attachment items, such as a favourite toy or blanket, to the radiology department to promote security.
3. Provide positive ambience in the waiting and examination rooms with visual and audio distractions such as environmental features that provide an appropriate level of sensory stimulation such as murals with nature scenes (Figs. 3.1 and 3.2), mood lighting (Fig. 3.3) and calming background music.
4. Have a selection of toys, screen media and mobile devices available to allay anxiety and serve as distractions to help pass the time.
5. As with adult patients, late cancellations of appointments by the radiology department can cause significant additional anxiety and clearly should be avoided when possible.

Preparing the Child and Family

Preprocedure

1. Recognize and understand the age of the child, sequential stages of child development and behaviour of the child, which all influence the level of cooperation during the procedure.

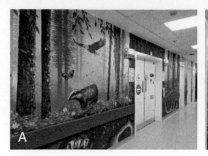
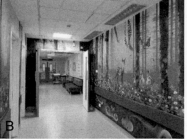

Fig. 3.1 **A** and **B,** Colourful wall (reproduced here in black and white) murals along the corridor of the radiology department. (Images courtesy of the Birmingham Children's Hospital Radiology Department.)

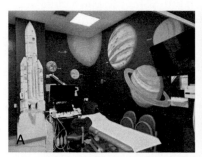
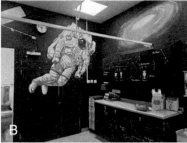

Fig. 3.2 **A** and **B,** Wall murals in the ultrasound room. (Images courtesy of the Birmingham Children's Hospital Radiology Department.)

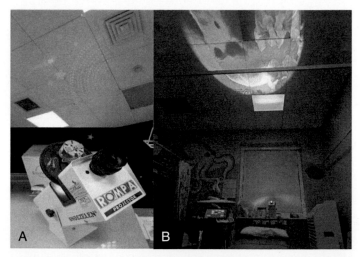

Fig. 3.3 **A** and **B,** Sensory projector projecting different scenes on the ceiling, providing sensory simulation and distraction. (Images courtesy of the Birmingham Children's Hospital Radiology Department.)

2. Balance the demands of the procedure with the risks of patient management techniques. Would the child be suitable for behavioural techniques (e.g. reassurance, education, play therapy, natural sleep, sedation or anaesthesia)? Involve the caregiver in this decision-making process because family-centred care is best practice.

3. Before scanning, children and parents should be given information, such as information or picture booklets, videos, link to websites with answers to common questions, to prepare themselves for the procedure. Advance or pre-arranged visits to the radiology department could also be helpful to dismiss fear of the unknown.

4. Play therapy can be especially useful in anxious children who do not respond to routine reassurance. Rehearsing scans through play can help children to gain confidence, although success may require ample planning and hours of preparation. Unfortunately, given the time constraints, play specialists are less likely to be appropriate for urgent situations.

During the procedure

1. Establish a good rapport early with the child and family through open communication and interaction.

2. Involve the caregiver in the procedure or allow them to stay with child as long as permissible. Caregivers can elicit the child's cooperation while the attention of the healthcare professional is directed toward the equipment or screen. Caregivers can assist with restraint or immobilization after appropriate discussion with the healthcare professional. Caregivers also serve as witness to the treatment of the child, minimizing future dispute about the professional conduct of the healthcare professional.

3. Talk softly and in a reassuring manner to the child.

4. Prepare the child and family for the procedure, tailored to the developmental level of the child. Explain what is happening and what the child can expect to see, hear, feel or taste during the exam.

5. Give encouragement and ample praise for cooperation with the procedure and for maintaining immobilization during the procedure.

6. Emphasize the benefits of the procedure and ongoing encouragements such as referring to reward stickers and certificates of achievement (dependent on the child's age) to be received at the end of the study.

Post-procedure

Encourage the child to express their feelings about the procedure; praise and reward them for completing the procedure.

Sedation in children

Procedural sedation aims to reduce fear and anxiety, augment pain control and minimize movement during medical procedures. Each child should be individually assessed for her or his suitability for sedation by staff trained in delivering, monitoring and dealing with the complications of sedation. In most circumstances, parents should stay with the child, and with patience and encouragement, the need for sedation may sometimes be avoided.

Table 3.1   Commonly Used Agents for Pharmacological Sedation in Paediatric Patients

Agent	Dose
Chloral hydrate	Refer to the local Trust policy or the British National Formulary for Children
Dexmedetomidine	
Alimemazine	
Midazolam	

Short procedures such as computed tomography (CT) can often be achieved in neonates by keeping them awake and then feeding the child and swaddling just before the procedure. Often, children older than the age of 4–5 years do not need sedation and will cooperate. If venous access is required, local anaesthetic cream (e.g. Ametop) can be applied to a suitable vein before insertion of a cannula. Oral sedation does not work well in children older than the age of 4 years, and older children who are unable to cooperate usually require general anaesthetic.

It is important to ensure that all monitoring and resuscitation equipment is suitable for paediatric use. A nurse who is experienced in the care of sedated children should be present throughout. Staff should have knowledge, understanding and competency in sedative drug action, child assessment, monitoring, recovery care, immediate management of complications and paediatric life support. Further training in intermediate or advanced life support may be needed if deeper level of sedation is required. When drugs are given that are likely to result in loss of consciousness, the primary care of the patient should be under the direct supervision of an anaesthetist and adhering to local guidelines (Table 3.1).

For many years, chloral hydrate (per oral or per rectal) has been the mainstay for sedation of young children for a variety of procedures. It is a hypnotic drug with no analgesic properties. An alternative agent is alimemazine, a sedating antihistamine with anticholinergic effects that can also be administered per orally or per rectally.

Other sedating agents include midazolam, which can be given via the oral, intranasal or intravenous (IV) routes. It has a rapid onset of effect, within 1–5 min and a variable duration of effect of 1–4 h. The effects of midazolam can be reversed by the competitive antagonist flumazenil; onset of flumazenil is within 1–3 min, with a half-life of 4–15 min. The clinical effect depends on the dose of flumazenil and sedative given. Note that the half-life of flumazenil is shorter than that of midazolam; therefore, resedation effects can occur.

Dexmedetomidine is an agonist of α_2-adrenergic receptors; it can provide sedation, analgesia and anxiolysis without respiratory depression and can be used via intranasal and IV routes. Last, the use of IV anaesthetic agents, such as ketamine and propofol, can result in the patient's moving quickly from a state of sedation to anaesthesia with concomitant risks and should only be used by those who have undergone appropriate specialist training.

Vomiting is common after oral sedation is given. If the child vomits within 10 min of administration, the dose can be repeated. The dose should not be repeated after 20 min because significant absorption may have already occurred.

On the night before the procedure or scan, parents should be asked to try to keep the child awake for as long as possible. The child should be woken early on the relevant day, and no 'naps' should be allowed on the journey to the hospital. This will ensure that the child is already tired before administration of the sedation. The sedative medication usually takes about 45 min to take effect.

Starvation is not required for procedures involving minimal sedation or moderate sedation in which verbal contact will be maintained (National Institute for Health and Care Excellence (NICE) CG112). Outside of this, the starvation guidance is as per elective procedures:

1. 1 h for clear fluids
2. 4 h for breast milk
3. 6 h for formula feed and food

Complications of sedation

Early recognition and treatment of complications is essential to reduce morbidity and mortality from sedation in all patients.

Minor complications include:

1. Syncope
2. Phlebitis
3. Emesis
4. Agitation
5. Rash

Major complications are rare but include:

1. Bradycardia
2. Hypotension
3. Hypoxia
4. Death

Sedation causes a reduction in muscle tone of the oropharynx, and at deeper levels of sedation, the glottic reflexes may fail. Major complications of sedation are most often caused by airway obstruction and respiratory depression.

The following patient groups are at high risk:

1. Obese patients with risk of obstructive sleep apnoea: These patients have a blunted ventilator drive. Supine position impairs chest wall function and oxygenation. Patients may need supplemental oxygen and bronchodilators. Local anaesthesia should be used for pain whenever possible, and sedative drugs should be used sparingly.

2. Hepatic dysfunction or renal failure: altered drug metabolism in renal and liver disease increases the risk of overdose when using opioids and benzodiazepines. These drugs should be used in reduced doses. In renal impairment, dose reduction should be considered.

Monitoring

Monitoring should be used:

1. In all patients receiving any form of sedation
2. For patients at risk of haemorrhage
3. In all prolonged or complicated procedures

The purposes are to observe and assess the response of the patient to any psychological or physiological stress imposed by the procedure or sedative agents administered and allow appropriate therapeutic action to be taken.

Consent (see also Chapter 20)

The consent process is a continuum beginning with the referring healthcare professional who requests the radiological examination and ending with the practitioner who carries it out.

The legal position concerning consent and refusal of treatment by those younger than the age of 18 years is different from the position for adults. Like adults, young people (aged 16 or 17 years) are presumed to have sufficient capacity to be able to consent to their own medical treatment. However, unlike adults, the refusal of a competent person aged 16–17 years may in certain circumstances be overridden by either a person with parental responsibility or a court.

Children younger than the age of 16 years can also consent to their own treatment if they are believed to have enough intelligence and understanding to fully appreciate what is involved in their treatment. This is known as being Gillick competent.

When a child younger than the age of 16 years lacks capacity to consent (i.e. is not Gillick competent), consent can be given on their behalf by any one person with parental responsibility or by the court. This could be:

1. The child's mother or father
2. The child's legally appointed guardian
3. A person with a residence order concerning the child
4. A local authority designated to care for the child
5. A local authority or person with an emergency protection order for the child

It is the responsibility of the referring professional to provide sufficient information to the patient to enable the latter to consent to the examination being requested. It is the responsibility of the imaging practitioner to ensure that the patient understands the scope of the examination before giving his or her consent. Verbal consent must be obtained for all examinations.

For detailed advice on best practice around consent, privacy and confidentiality, refer to relevant professional guidance and the online reference guide published by the Department of Health and Social Care.

Respecting the Child's Dignity

When building a healthcare relationship with children and young people:

1. Introduce yourself and explain your role, why the examination is necessary and what the examination will involve.
2. Listen to and be seen to believe their experiences (e.g. symptoms such as discomfort, how they are feeling).
3. Reassure them that you will take their concerns seriously.
4. Provide calm and positive emotional support and encouraging words.
5. Discuss with them how you will act on what they have said.
6. Regularly confirming with their child or young person that they can change their mind at any time about how involved they want them to be.
7. Give all children and young people opportunities to express their opinions about their health needs independently, including:
   (a) Giving them opportunities to ask questions
   (b) Offering to see them separately from their parents or carers for part of the consultation
8. Maintain privacy and dignity during the examinations such as attaching a 'Do Not Enter' sign to the outside of the scan room door or locking the door to stop patients and staff entering. If the patient has to be undressed for the examination, ensure a sheet has been given to the patient to cover up. Ensure a chaperone is present before carrying out an intimate examination. It is preferable to have a healthcare professional act as a chaperone.

Duty of Candour

As in adult radiology practice, duty of candour is fundamental, and we refer readers to General Medical Council guidance for more information.

Further Reading

American College of Radiology. *ACR-SIR Practice Guideline for Sedation/Analgesia.* <http://www.acr.org/media/F194CBB800AB43048B997A75938AB482.pdf>.

Beth Linder JM, Schiska AD. Imaging children: tips and tricks. *J Radiol Nurs.* 2007;26(1):23–25.

Department of Health and Social Care. *Reference Guide to Consent for Examination or Treatment.* 2nd ed. <https://www.gov.uk/government/publications/reference-guide-to-consent-for-examination-or-treatment-second-edition>.

General Medical Council. *Intimate examinations and chaperones.* <https://www.gmc-uk.org/ethical-guidance/ethical-guidance-for-doctors/intimate-examinations-and-chaperones>.

General Medical Council. *Openness and honesty when things go wrong: the professional duty of candour.* <https://www.gmc-uk.org/ethical-guidance/ethical-guidance-for-doctors/candour—openness-and-honesty-when-things-go-wrong>.

Hardwick J, Gyll C. *Radiography of Children: A Guide to Good Practice*: Churchill Livingstone; 2004.

Martin ML, Lennox PH. Sedation and analgesia in the interventional radiology department. *J Vasc Interv Radiol.* 2003;14(9 Pt 1):1119–1128.

National Institute for Health and Care Excellence. *NICE Clinical Guideline 112. Sedation for Diagnostic and Therapeutic Procedures in Children and Young People.* <http://www.nice.org.uk/guidance/CG112>.

National Institute for Health and Care Excellence. *NICE guideline [NG204] Babies, Children and Young People's Experience of Healthcare.* <https://www.nice.org.uk/guidance/ng204>.

Patatas K, Koukkoulli A. The use of sedation in the radiology department. *Clin Radiol.* 2009;64:655–663.

Quan X, Joseph A, Nanda U, et al. Improving pediatric radiography patient stress, mood, and parental satisfaction through positive environmental distractions: a randomized control trial. *J Pediatr Nurs.* 2016;31(1):e11–e22.

Royal College of Anaesthetists. *Chapter 7: Guidelines for the Provision of Anaesthesia Services in the Non-theatre Environment 2023.* <https://rcoa.ac.uk/gpas/chapter-7>.

Royal College of Anaesthetists. *Guidance on the Provision of Sedation Services.* <https://rcoa.ac.uk/chapter-7>.

Royal College of Radiologists. *Safe Sedation, Analgesia and Anaesthesia Within the Radiology Department.* London: The Royal College of Radiologists; 2003. <https://www.rcr.ac.uk/publication/safe-sedation-analgesia-and-anaesthesia-within-radiology-department>.

Royal Radiologists/Royal College of College of Anaesthetists Joint Publication. *Sedation and Anaesthesia in Radiology.* London: The Royal College of Radiologists; 1992.

Sury MRJ, Harker H, Begent J, et al. The management of infants and children for painless imaging. *Clin Radiol.* 2005;60(7):731–741.

INTRAVASCULAR CONTRAST MEDIA USED IN PAEDIATRICS: COMPUTED TOMOGRAPHY AND MAGNETIC RESONANCE IMAGING

The information regarding the use of computed tomography (CT) and magnetic resonance (MR) contrast media in adults applies equally to children. See Chapter 2.

Further Reading

Bhargava R, Hahn G, Hirsch W, et al. Contrast-enhanced magnetic resonance imaging in pediatric patients: review and recommendations for current practice. *Magn Reson Insights.* 2013;6:95–111.

Rozenfeld MN, Podberesky DJ. Gadolinium-based contrast agents in children. *Pediatr Radiol.* 2018;48(9):1188–1196.

Shah R, D'Arco F, Soares B, et al. Use of gadolinium contrast agents in paediatric population: Donald Rumsfeld meets Hippocrates! *Br J Radiol.* 2019;92(1094):20180746.

Ultrasound

Sulfur hexafluoride lipid-type A microspheres for injectable suspension has been distributed outside the United States since 2001 under the name SonoVue. Since 2019, SonoVue has been approved by the US Food and Drug Administration under the name of Lumason to be used in echocardiography and hepatic investigations for both adults and children, as well as intravesically, for the evaluation of pediatric vesicoureteral reflux.

In Europe and the United Kingdom, ultrasound (US) contrast in children remains an off-label drug, although there have been promising results when used in abdominal trauma initial diagnosis and follow-up; characterization and differential diagnosis of focal liver lesions; characterization of lung, pleura, renal and splenic pathology; and detection of complications after paediatric transplantation. There remains scope to develop its role in evaluating inflammatory activity, assessing tumour response to antiangiogenic therapy, diagnosis of vascular anomalies and characterization of scrotal lesions.

According to the manufacturer recommendation, the dose of SonoVue should be based on the body weight and is 0.03 mL/kg, with a maximum of 2.4 mL per injection.

In an article by Rafailidis et al.,[1] the authors have adapted doses to the patient body size, broadly correlating with the child age. They report administering 0.6 mL in children younger than 6 years old, 1.2 mL in children between 6 and 12 years of age and 2.4 mL in children older than 12 years of age. Other previously published dosage schemes include (a) 0.1 mL of SonoVue for every year of age and (b) standard single doses of 0.1, 0.5, 1.0, 1.2, 2.4 and 4.8 mL of SonoVue.

The microbubbles are administered through an IV 20-gauge cannula placed in the antecubital fossa and flushed with 5–10 mL of normal saline. The microbubbles can be administered through 16- to 24-gauge catheters or 18- to 25-gauge needles, although the manufacturer recommendation is for a catheter larger than 20 gauge. There has been no significant difference on enhancement or microbubble concentration with catheter or needle sizes ranging from 18 to 21 gauge.

Contrast-specific US imaging modes are deployed, which specifically discriminate the non-linear response from microbubbles and suppress the linear signal originating from the static tissues, thus creating an image containing only signals from the microbubbles.

Reference

1. Rafailidis V, Deganello A, Watson T, et al. Enhancing the role of paediatric ultrasound with microbubbles: a review of intravenous applications. *Br J Radiol*. 2017;90(1069):20160556.

Further Reading

Antrim A. FDA approves ultrasound enhancing agent for use in pediatric patients. Pharmacy Times. <https://www.pharmacytimes.com/view/fda-approves-ultrasound-enhancing-agent-for-use-in-pediatric-patients>.

Bracco. LUMASON (sulfur hexafluoride lipid-type A microspheres) for injectable suspension, for intravenous use or intravesical use. *Bracco Imaging*. 2021. <https://imaging.bracco.com/us-en/products/contrast-enhanced-ultrasound/Lumason>.

Laugesen NG, Nolsoe CP, Rosenberg J. Clinical applications of contrast-enhanced ultrasound in the pediatric work-up of focal liver lesions and blunt abdominal trauma: a systematic review. *Ultrasound Int Open*. 2017;3(1):E2–E7.

GASTROINTESTINAL AND GENITOURINARY IMAGING

Fluoroscopy

Contrast swallow

Indications

1. To identify any pathology intrinsic to the oesophagus and includes gastroesophageal reflux, trachea-oesophageal fistula, achalasia and oesophageal web.
2. Alternatively, any abnormality causing extrinsic compression to the oesophagus such as a vascular ring or enteric duplication cyst.

Contrast medium

Barium or water-soluble contrast agent, as appropriate

Patient preparation

Aim for a 4-h fast before administration of contrast; however, in an acutely unwell child, stomach contents can be aspirated by a nasogastric (NG) tube.

Technique

1. Depending upon the age of child, commence in upright or supine position. Typically, in an older child (in whom the clinical presentation does not support a malrotation), a standing upright position is adopted. In an infant, the patient will be supine.
2. Before beginning the exam, ensure any in situ NG tube is adequately positioned.
3. Give the patient contrast orally and take a capture or a fluoroscopic run of the anteroposterior (AP) oesophagus. Barium can be given to the infant through a bottle with an enlarged teat opening or in an older child through a straw with his or her head turned to the side.
4. Turn the patient to the right lateral position, give the patient contrast and take a fluoroscopic run of the lateral oesophagus.
5. Follow the contrast as it starts to empty from the stomach; in our practice, we also track it into the duodenum.
6. When contrast is seen to enter the third or fourth part of the duodenum, turn the patient supine and document the position of the duodenal–jejunal junction with a fluoroscopic run or exposure.
7. Move the patient from right to left lateral and back again to attempt to induce gastroesophageal reflux.

Additional techniques and modification of techniques

1. To demonstrate a tracheo-oesophageal fistula in infants, a tube oesophagogram may be performed if the standard oesophagogram result is negative.
2. A tube oesophagram can be challenging in an unsettled patient and caution is always required to avoid aspiration, and water-soluble contrast should be used.
3. The patient is positioned prone with the arms up and the table may be tilted slightly head down. An NG tube is introduced into the distal oesophagus.
4. Inject contrast through the tube to distend the oesophagus, which will force the contrast medium through any small fistula that may be present.
5. If no fistula is seen, retract the tube for a few centimetres and repeat until the upper oesophagus has been examined. It is important to actively monitor for aspiration into the airway from overspill, which can lead to diagnostic confusion.
6. Obtain high-frame rate fluoroscopic runs or AP and lateral images of the oesophagus at each level of injection.
7. Failure to radiologically demonstrate an H-type tracheoesophageal fistula does not mean that a very subtle abnormal communication does not exist.

Further Reading

American College of Radiology-Society for Pediatric Radiology. *Practice Parameter for the Performance of Contrast Esophagrams and Upper Gastrointestinal Examinations in Infants and Children.* <https://www.acr.org/-/media/ACR/Files/Practice-Parameters/UpperGI-Infants.pdf>.
Hiorns MP. Gastrointestinal tract imaging in children: current techniques. *Pediatr Radiol.* 2011;41(1):42–54.

Videofluoroscopy

Indications

1. Clinical evidence from the speech and language team (SALT) bedside assessment of oropharyngeal dysphagia requiring further investigation
2. Differential diagnosis of dysphagia (e.g. neurogenic vs structural, repeated chest infection or pneumonia suspected to be caused by aspiration)
3. As a baseline in a progressive neurological condition
4. To provide feedback or education to the patient and carer
5. To monitor the effectiveness of therapeutic interventions

Contrast medium

Foods of different consistency and texture mixed or coated with barium, often prepared by the SALT team

Patient preparation

Fast for 4 h for younger patients who will only drink when hungry; otherwise not required

Technique

1. Set video to a high frame-rate mode (e.g. 8 frames s^{-1}).
2. Obtain a lateral image, centred at the uvula, and magnify the image to fill the screen.
3. Capture screening loops as the patient swallows the different consistencies of barium-coated food.
4. Assess images for airway penetration and aspiration and whether a spontaneous cough reflex is elicited with aspiration.
5. Typically, a formal, detailed report will be provided by the attending SALT specialist.

Aftercare

Advise the patient to drink plenty of liquids to wash barium out of system and that barium will lighten the colour of stools.

Further Reading

Batchelor G, McNaughten B, Bourke T, et al. How to use the videofluoroscopy swallow study in paediatric practice. *Arch Dis Child Educ Pract.* 2019;104(6): 313–320.

Hiorns MP, Ryan MM. Current practice in paediatric videofluoroscopy. *Pediatr Radiol.* 2006;36(9):911–919.

Neonatal contrast meal

Indications

1. Contrast meal: duodenal atresia, duodenal stenosis, malrotation, midgut volvulus, jejunal atresia, jejunal stenosis
2. Contrast follow-through: to assess motility or strictures post necrotizing enterocolitis (NEC), gastroschisis
3. Short bowel syndrome after bowel infarction
4. To delineate bowel anatomy in patients with or without bowel distension who show no stool passage even after contrast enema

Contrast medium

Barium or water-soluble contrast agent as appropriate

Equipment

Ensure the grid is taken out of fluoroscopy machine if the patient weighs less than 20 kg.

Patient preparation

Ensure the NG tube is in situ if the study is being performed to exclude neonatal malrotation.

Technique

1. With the patient in the supine position, administer a small volume of contrast down the NG tube (3–5 mL) so that it just fills the fundus (paradoxically, overfilling can delay gastric emptying).
2. Turn the patient right lateral such that gravity assists in the transit of the contrast through the pylorus. If transit is particularly slow, the

child can be turned slightly more prone, which may promote gastric emptying. Gastric emptying is prolonged if the child is upset, and a dummy coated with sugar water may assist in settling the infant.

3. When contrast enters the first part of the duodenum, it is key to ensure a retroperitoneal course (i.e. the duodenum extends posteroinferiorly towards the spine).

4. When contrast begins to ascend (in a retroperitoneal course), the infant is returned promptly to the supine position, and with the child perfectly straight, the position of the duodenojejunal flexure can be ascertained and should be to the left of the midline at the level of the duodenal bulb. Captured images or runs should include costophrenic angles with the spine running perfectly vertical in the middle of the image to verify that the child is straight (Table 3.2).

5. Although contrast studies are considered the gold standard to diagnose malrotation, in cases in which there is an associated volvulus, to provide additional reassurance before committing a child to an emergency laparotomy, US can be performed to assess for the 'whirlpool' sign and the spiralling of the superior mesenteric vein (SMV) and superior mesenteric vein artery (SMA) vessels.

6. When malrotation has been excluded, a further volume of barium is administered until the stomach is reasonably full such that other forms of upper intestinal partial or complete obstruction (e.g. duodenal atresia, duodenal stenosis or web or annular pancreas) may be assessed for.

7. At the end of the procedure, the stomach should be aspirated of residual contrast under fluoroscopic guidance (because it can be associated gastro-oesophageal reflux) and the tube flushed with water to ensure it does not become blocked.

Table 3.2 Pictorial Representation of the Neonatal Contrast Meal Technique with Corresponding Fluoroscopic Findings and *Arrowheads* Demonstrating the Normal Flow of Contrast

Position of Baby	Supine	Right Lateral	Supine
Pictorial representation			
Fluoroscopic finding			

Additional techniques and modification of techniques

1. For a follow-through, serial plain radiographs of the abdomen are obtained at regular intervals (30-minute to 1-h intervals) to follow progress of contrast up to terminal ileum. This can be performed as routine outpatient radiographs without needing the fluoroscopy suite (although assessing bowel peristalsis under fluoroscopic screening is highly desirable). Ensure that the patient and family are aware that they would need to be present in the hospital for up to 3 h after the contrast meal study.
2. If an abnormality is seen or if the ileocaecal valve is poorly visualized on the radiographs, it needs further fluoroscopic evaluation with the patient lying prone or with manual compression devices.

Further Reading

Daneman A. Malrotation: the balance of evidence. *Pediatr Radiol.* 2009;39(2):164–166.

Daneman A. Malrotation: techniques, spectrum of appearances, pitfalls, and management. In: Hodler J, ChL Zollikofer, Von Schulthess GK, eds. *Diseases of the Abdomen and Pelvis 2010–2013: Diagnostic Imaging and Interventional Techniques 42nd International Diagnostic Course in Davos (IDKD).* Davos, March 21–26, 2010. Springer; 2010:247–251.

Long FR, Kramer SS, Markowitz RI, et al. Radiographic patterns of intestinal malrotation in children. *Radiogr Rev Publ Radiol Soc N Am Inc.* 1996;16(3): 547–556, discussion 556–560.

Oates AJ, Suleman NJ, Low SBL, et al. The radiological diagnosis of midgut volvulus—wow, it's difficult! *Pediatr Radiol.* 2021;51(10):1936–1937.

Intussusception reduction

Contraindications

Peritonitis, bowel perforation, shock (inadequate resuscitation)

Equipment

16- or 18-gauge needle to reduce a tension pneumoperitoneum in case of perforation

Patient preparation

1. The patient has been reviewed by the paediatric surgeons and adequately resuscitated.
2. The patient has had sonographic confirmation of ileocolic intussusception.
3. Analgesia for pain relief is given before air enema reduction.

Technique

1. The child can be placed in either the prone or supine position. Some may find with the former that it is easier to maintain the catheter in the rectum, although some children may become distressed when they are facing the table rather than individuals in the room.
2. A 14- to 22-Fr (dependent on size of child) Foley catheter is inserted per rectum after the application of a small amount of lubricating

gel. If there is subsequent leakage of air during the procedure, the buttocks can be taped together, but in our practice, this is not usually an issue because we inflate the balloon (under fluoroscopic guidance), and gentle traction on the catheter can be applied to obtain a good seal.

3. Obtain a pre-insufflation scout view to exclude perforation and to identify the lead point.

4. Air is instilled by a hand or mechanical pump, and the intussusception is pushed back by a sustained pressure of up to 120 mmHg (or as per manufacturer's guidance if a mechanical pump is used). Pressure should be monitored at all times, and there should be a fail-safe pressure-release valve in the system to ensure that excessive pressures are not delivered.

5. Reduction is successful when there is free flow of air into the distal ileum.

6. If the intussusception does not move after 3 min of sustained pressure, the pressure is reduced. Two further attempts are made, again with pressures up to 120 mmHg (or as per manufacturer's guidance if a mechanical pump is used) for 3 min. If the intussusception is still immovable, it is considered irreducible, and arrangements are made for surgery.

7. The intussusception is only considered completely reduced when the terminal ileum is filled with air. However, it is common for there to be a persisting filling defect in the caecum at the end of the procedure, with or without reflux of air into the terminal ileum. This is often caused by an oedematous ileocaecal valve. In the presence of a soft tissue caecal mass, a clinically well and stable child should be returned to the ward to await a further attempt at reduction after a period of 2–8 h rather than proceed to surgery.

8. Repeat US to reassess for intussusception if patient redevelops symptoms.

9. A second enema is often successful at complete reduction or showing resolution of the oedematous ileocaecal valve.

Supporting information

1. When air (or contrast) dissects between the two layers of the intussusception (the dissection sign) or when trapped fluid is seen between the intussusceptum and the intussuscipiens on US, reduction is less likely.

2. Most failed enema reductions are idiopathic, and pathologic lead points are noted in 25% of cases, the most common of which are lymphoid hyperplasia, Burkitt lymphoma, Meckel diverticulum, enteric duplication cyst, juvenile polyp and adenovirus appendicitis.

Complications

Perforation may result in a tension pneumoperitoneum, resulting in respiratory compromise. The peritoneal cavity must be punctured with a large bore needle to facilitate decompression.

Further Reading

Daneman A, Navarro O. Intussusception. Part 1: a review of diagnostic approaches. *Pediatr Radiol.* 2003;33(2):79–85.

Daneman A, Navarro O. Intussusception. Part 2: an update on the evolution of management. *Pediatr Radiol.* 2004;34(2):97–108.

Fishman M, Borden S, Cooper A. The dissection sign of nonreducible ileocolic intussusception. *AJR Am J Roentgenol.* 1984;143(1):5–8.

Lioubashevsky N, Hiller N, Rozovsky K, et al. Ileocolic versus small-bowel intussusception in children: can US enable reliable differentiation? *Radiology.* 2013;269(1):266–271.

Navarro O, Daneman A. Intussusception. Part 3: diagnosis and management of those with an identifiable or predisposing cause and those that reduce spontaneously. *Pediatr Radiol.* 2004;34(4):305–312.

Navarro OM, Daneman A, Chae A. Intussusception: the use of delayed, repeated reduction attempts and the management of intussusceptions due to pathologic lead points in pediatric patients. *AJR Am J Roentgenol.* 2004;182(5):1169–1176.

Ntoulia A, Tharakan SJ, Reid JR, et al. Failed intussusception reduction in children: correlation between radiologic, surgical, and pathologic findings. *AJR Am J Roentgenol.* 2016;207(2):424–433.

Neonatal contrast enema

Indications

1. Low intestinal obstruction in a newborn: Hirschsprung's disease, functional immaturity of the colon (small left colon syndrome, meconium plug syndrome), colonic atresia, meconium ileus and ileal atresia
2. Preoperative evaluations: for ostomy takedown, evaluation of fistulae or for colon abnormalities before small bowel surgery

Contraindications

Perforation, ischemic colon, toxic megacolon, hypovolemic shock, peritonitis, or other potentially unstable clinical condition

Contrast medium

Dilute ionic contrast medium as is used for cystography (e.g. Urografin 150). This has the advantage of not provoking large fluid shifts and being dense enough to provide satisfactory images. Non-ionic contrast media and barium offer no advantages (and the latter is contraindicated with perforation as a possibility). Infants with meconium ileus or functional immaturity benefit from a water-soluble contrast enema, so their therapeutic enema commences with the diagnostic study.

Technique

1. A 14- to 22-Fr (dependent on size of child) Foley catheter is inserted per rectum after the application of a small amount of lubricating gel. Secure the catheter without inflating the balloon.
2. Use gravity or gentle hand injection to instil contrast.
3. Start contrast injection with the patient in the left lateral position to evaluate the rectosigmoid ratio.
4. Turn the patient supine and advance the catheter into the sigmoid colon.

5. If it is not possible to maintain a firm anal seal externally, consider inflating the catheter balloon under fluoroscopic guidance to create an internal seal.
6. Continue contrast injection to opacify the colon and monitor for contrast refluxing into the terminal ileum.
7. If the enema demonstrates that the entire colon is small (a microcolon; <1 cm in diameter), then the diagnosis is likely to be meconium ileus or ileal atresia. The microcolon of prematurity and total colonic Hirschsprung's disease are alternative rare diagnoses.

Additional techniques and modification of techniques

For the treatment of meconium ileus, the aim is to run the water-soluble contrast medium into the small bowel to surround the meconium. An attempt should be made to get the contrast medium back into the dilated small bowel. If successful, meconium should be passed in the next hour. If no result is seen and the infant's condition deteriorates, then surgical intervention is required. If the passage of meconium is incomplete and the clinical condition remains stable, multiple enemas over the succeeding few days will be necessary to ensure complete resolution of the obstruction.

Further Reading

Baad M, Delgado J, Dayneka JS, et al. Diagnostic performance and role of the contrast enema for low intestinal obstruction in neonates. *Pediatr Surg Int.* 2020;36(9):1093 1101.
Copeland DR, St Peter SD, Sharp SW, et al. Diminishing role of contrast enema in simple meconium ileus. *J Pediatr Surg.* 2009;44(11):2130–2132.
Tsitsiou Y, Calle-Toro JS, Zouvani A, et al. Diagnostic decision-making tool for imaging term neonatal bowel obstruction. *Clin Radiol.* 2021;76(3):163–171.

Colostogram (fistulogram)

Indications

Anorectal malformation: to delineate anatomy (i.e. location of the distal rectal pouch, distance of the rectum to the anus), to identify the presence and level of a recto-urogenital fistulae, to assess the anatomy of the posterior urethra and other anomalies in adjacent structures (e.g. distal colonic strictures)

Contrast medium

Refer to the Neonatal contrast enema section.

Technique

1. Obtain a precontrast, scout view as a baseline and to exclude intraabdominal pathology.
2. An appropriate-sized (6–10 Fr, dependent on the size of the sinus) Foley catheter is inserted into the orifice of the sinus after the application of a small amount of lubricating gel. The balloon may be inflated inside the sinus to prevent retrograde flow. Alternatively, the balloon may be inflated outside the orifice and pushed to the

skin using a forceps or similar device to secure a seal (and keep the operator's fingers outside the field of view).

3. The contrast medium is injected carefully under fluoroscopic guidance (either with gravity or gentle hand injection) with care taken to avoid leakage at the skin surface where possible. The operator may find it beneficial to use multiple absorbent sheets ('Inco pads') under the patient that can be serially removed if leakage does occur to avoid obscuring the image.

4. Ensure that a tight seal is established and maintained. Inject contrast to fully distend calibre of colon from mucous fistula to rectum. It is important to ensure that high enough pressures are generated in the length of colon (between the mucous fistula to rectum) to demonstrate the fistula.

5. Fluoroscopic 'runs' are obtained supplemented by proper exposures as required, including tangential views.

Additional techniques and modification of techniques

1. Consider the 'double urethral catheter technique' if the bladder cannot be sufficiently distended to assess the posterior urethra or exclude vesicoureteric reflux.

2. Pass a 6-Fr urinary catheter via the urethra; if the recto-urogenital fistula is wide, the catheter will preferentially go into the rectum via the fistula. Leave the urethral–rectal catheter in situ and pass a second 6-Fr urinary catheter up the urethra. This will pass into the bladder because the first catheter is occluding the fistula.

Further Reading

Abdalla WMA, De La Torre L. The high pressure distal colostogram in anorectal malformations: technique and pitfalls. *J Pediatr Surg.* 2017;52(7):1207–1209.

Kraus SJ, Levitt MA, Peña A. Augmented-pressure distal colostogram: the most important diagnostic tool for planning definitive surgical repair of anorectal malformations in boys. *Pediatr Radiol.* 2018;48(2):258–269.

Soccorso G, Thyagarajan MS, Murthi GV, et al. Micturating cystography and 'double urethral catheter technique' to define the anatomy of anorectal malformations. *Pediatr Surg Int.* 2008;24(2):241–243.

Micturating cystogram

Indications

1. Hydronephrosis or hydroureter
2. Abnormal US (any degree of hydronephrosis, uroepithelial thickening, scarring) after first urinary tract infection (UTI), especially if febrile or non–*Escherichia coli* (E. coli)
3. Recurrent UTI
4. Congenital anomalies of the urinary tract
5. Dysfunctional voiding, such as neurogenic dysfunction of the bladder
6. Urinary incontinence
7. Bladder outlet obstruction
8. Post-operative evaluation of the urinary tract
9. Dysuria or difficulty voiding
10. Haematuria

11. Trauma
12. Suspected patent urachus or posterior urethral valves

Contraindication

Acute UTI

Contrast medium

Dilute ionic contrast medium as is used for cystography (e.g. Urografin 150)

3

Equipment

1. Fluoroscopy unit with spot film device and tilting table
2. Bladder catheter

Patient preparation

1. Explain the procedure to the patient and parents. Explain that the urethra will be anaesthetized with lidocaine gel as the catheter is being passed into the urethra; however, when the catheter is in, it does not hurt. Emphasize that the child will have to be immobilized throughout the examination and will be more upset about being immobilized than the discomfort from the catheter.
2. The patient will need to have the full treatment course of antibiotics for 3 days. If the patient is not on prophylactic antibiotics, they will need to take treatment dose antibiotics for 3 days, from the day before the scan until and including the day after the scan. If the patient is already on prophylaxis, the prophylactic antibiotic dose will need to be doubled for 3 days, from the day before the scan until and including the day after the scan. This can either be as one single larger dose per day or an extra dose in the morning or evening. Refer to your local trust guidance.

Technique

1. Using aseptic technique, the bladder is catheterized with a 4- to 6-Fr (dependent on size of child) feeding tube or catheter. Secure the catheter without inflating the balloon. In girls, the catheter may be secured in place with tape to the perineum or in older girls to the thigh. In boys, after the catheter is inserted, a strip of tape may be placed on the catheter extending longitudinally along the dorsum of the penis to the symphysis. Avoid circumferential placement of tape around the penis because this may be locally traumatic when removing the tape.
2. Residual urine is drained. This can be sent to the lab for microscopy, culture and sensitivities (if needed).
3. Use gravity or gentle hand injection to instil contrast.
4. Contrast medium slowly dripped in with the patient supine, and bladder filling is observed by intermittent fluoroscopy. It is important that early filling is monitored by fluoroscopy in case the catheter is malpositioned (e.g. in the distal ureter or vagina and to assess for the presence of ureterocoeles).

5. Filling continues slowly until the patient has the urge to void or, in the case of infants, spontaneous micturition occurs. Attention should be paid to filling to age-adjusted bladder capacity and allowing the child adequate time to void during performance of the cystogram.
6. In infants, cycles of filling and micturition may be needed. Initially, with voiding around the catheter and then after subsequent filling, the catheter can be removed at the start of micturition, and voiding images of the urethra are obtained.
7. In older children with bladder control, the catheter is removed, and patients are later asked to void on command. Older children are given a urine receiver, but smaller children should be allowed to pass urine onto absorbent pads on which they can lie.
8. Obtain right and left oblique fluoroscopic views during filling and voiding to identify ureteral diverticulum.
9. Intermittent monitoring is also necessary to identify transient reflux. Any reflux should be recorded.
10. Obtain oblique lateral views to assess the full length of the urethra as the patient micturates with the feeding tube or catheter in situ. In infants and children with neuropathic bladders, micturition may be accomplished by suprapubic pressure.
11. Finally, a full-length view of the abdomen is taken to demonstrate any undetected reflux of contrast medium that might have occurred into the kidneys and to record the post-micturition residue.

Supporting information

1. The patient should be filled to their estimated bladder capacity to prevent bladder overdistension, which may cause rupture, overgrading and overdiagnosing of vesicoureteric reflux, as well as overestimation of post-void residual. Formulas used to estimate age-adjusted bladder capacity: infants younger than 1 years: Capacity (mL) = (2.5 × age (months)) + 38; children older than 1 year: Capacity (mL) = (2 + age (years)) × 30
2. If the patient is younger than 2 years old, a cyclic study may be considered to increase the sensitivity to detecting reflux. This is done by performing several cycles of filling and voiding before removal of the catheter during voiding and the final image of the urethra is obtained.

Aftercare

No special aftercare is necessary, but patients and parents of children should be warned that dysuria, possibly leading to retention of urine, may rarely be experienced. In such cases, a simple analgesic is helpful, and children may be helped by allowing them to micturate in a warm bath. Very rarely ascending infections may occur and parents should be advised to seek prompt medical attention if their child becomes unwell e.g. febrile etc.

Complications

1. UTI
2. Catheter trauma may lead to dysuria, frequency, haematuria and urinary retention

3. Complications of bladder filling (e.g. perforation from overdistension)
4. Catheterization of the vagina or an ectopic ureteral orifice

Further Reading
Agrawalla S, Pearce R, Goodman TR. How to perform the perfect voiding cystourethrogram. *Pediatr Radiol.* 2004;34(2):114–119.
American College of Radiology-Society for Pediatric Radiology. *Practice Parameter for the Performance of Fluoroscopic and Sonographic Voiding Cystourethrography in Children.* <https://www.acr.org/-/media/ACR/Files/Practice-Parameters/VoidingCysto.pdf>.
Higgins JJ, Urbine JA, Malik A. Beyond reflux: the spectrum of voiding cystourethrogram findings in the pediatric population. *Pediatr Radiol.* 2022;52(1):134–143.

3

Ultrasound

US is the main stay of imaging in the paediatric population. Because of the lower proportion of fat and body habitus of children, US is able to acquire high-resolution diagnostic images, allowing the identification and monitoring of disease in different parts of the body without the need for ionizing radiation.

Stomach

Indications

Clinical features that would be suggestive of hypertrophic pyloric stenosis such as projectile, non-bilious vomiting, an olive-shaped mass in the epigastrium, failure to thrive, weight loss and so on.

Equipment

1. Linear, high-frequency probe
2. Bottle of water for the patient to feed

Technique

1. The pylorus is viewed in two planes at 90 degrees to each other: Longitudinal view through the pylorus, cross-sectional transverse view (target sign).
2. The baby lies in the right posterior oblique position (left side raised). This encourages the stomach contents to lie against the gastropyloric junction, aiding identification and encouraging gastric emptying.
3. Scan the epigastrium in the transverse plane and identify the gallbladder. The pylorus is visualized medial to this.
4. Rotate the transducer as necessary into the sagittal oblique plane until the long axis of the pylorus is achieved.
5. Often, a pyloric stenosis is immediately apparent on subjective assessment but measure the pyloric muscle thickness, length and diameter in centimetres on the same image.
6. A dynamic assessment of the pylorus should be undertaken using a small volume (15 mL) of the Dioralyte or sterile water to observe if the pylorus opens up and fluid passes through into the duodenum.
7. Observe in real time with US to confirm gastric emptying. It can take 15–20 min for the pyloric muscle to open, so continue scanning at intervals if there is no gastric emptying for up to 20 min.

8. If a pyloric stenosis is confirmed, then check both kidneys for any associated hydronephrosis or renal abnormalities.
9. If the scan is negative for pyloric stenosis, other causes of vomiting should be assessed (e.g. position of the SMV or SMA to look for malrotation or gross hydronephrosis or lesion causing mass effect).

Small and large bowel

Indications

Acute appendicitis, inflammatory bowel disease, intussusception

Equipment

Linear, high-frequency probe

Technique

1. Start at an area of bowel with a known fixed location to find reliable anatomy and follow the lumen. For example, for suspected acute appendicitis and intussusception, start in the right iliac fossa to identify the caecum and terminal ileum. For inflammatory bowel disease, start at the rectum.
2. Use the US transducer to apply graded compression to bowel to be able to visualize the posterior bowel wall and the more posteriorly located bowel loops.
3. The bowel should be examined for its location, wall thickness and symmetry, transmural changes, motility and vascularity. The surrounding mesentery and lymph nodes should also be assessed.
4. A single wall layer thickness of 2 mm is considered normal in a distended healthy segment of bowel. Bowel wall is made of five distinct sonographic layers (inner to outer being lumen, mucosa, submucosa, muscularis propria and serosa). The layers should be symmetrical and clearly delineated in healthy bowel. Normal small bowel should exhibit peristalsis.
5. The normal appendix should be compressible and have a maximum diameter of 6 mm. It should also exhibit peristalsis.
6. Note that the sigmoid, transverse colon and caecum can move, or be longer than expected.

Sonographic features for an intussusception include:

1. Concentric parallel rings of bowel wall (bowel-within-bowel appearance, target, or doughnut sign) on transverse views
2. Multiple long, parallel, hypoechoic, and echogenic stripes (sandwich sign) or eccentric mesenteric fat that is dragged into the intussusception, mimicking the renal hilum, with the renal parenchyma formed by the oedematous bowel (pseudokidney sign) on longitudinal views. Ensure the kidneys have been identified separately to the intussusception.
3. Assess for the presence of trapped hypoechoic fluid between compressed bowel segments (suspicious for ischemia), central lead

point lesion and perforation (presence of large-volume ascites, debris and free gas).

Further Reading
Gongidi P, Bellah RD. Ultrasound of the pediatric appendix. *Pediatr Radiol.* 2017;47(9):1091–1100.
Quigley AJ, Stafrace S. Ultrasound assessment of acute appendicitis in paediatric patients: methodology and pictorial overview of findings seen. *Insights Imaging.* 2013;4(6):741–751.

3

Liver and gallbladder

Indications

Suspected or known liver disease (e.g. ascites, jaundice, itching, pruritus, altered liver function test (LFT) results, portal cavernoma, surgical portosystemic shunts, choledochal cyst, Budd-Chiari, Wilson's disease, cirrhosis, focal nodular hyperplasia), liver lesions, before and after liver transplant, cystic fibrosis surveillance

Patient preparation

1. All patients are required to fast including milk (unless clinically contraindicated) depending on age before the US. Only sips of clear fluid are allowed. Exceptions include after liver transplant, after Kasai procedure and after cholecystectomy.
2. The number of hours to fast vary according to the patient's age:
   (a) Younger than 1 years: 3-h fast
   (b) Age 1–4 years: 4-h fast
   (c) Older than 5 years: 6-h fast

Technique

1. Liver: Assess its shape, contour, size and echo texture. Doppler assessment of the portal, hepatic and splenic veins; inferior vena cava (IVC); and hepatic artery is required for hepatobiliary referrals including biliary atresia, portal hypertension, pre and post liver transplant, abnormal LFT results or if indicated on US examination.
2. Gallbladder: size, shape, contour and surrounding area; US characteristics of the wall and the nature of any contents
3. Common duct: maximum diameter and contents; optimally, it should be visualized throughout its length to the head of pancreas

Supporting information

1. Common bile duct dilation is defined as a diameter greater than 2 mm in infancy, 4 mm in childhood (up to 12 years) and 7 mm in patients older than 16 years of age.
2. Check for intrahepatic biliary dilation; if the intrahepatic bile ducts are visible, measure the AP diameter of the intrahepatic bile duct (IHBD) and the AP diameter of the adjacent intrahepatic branch of the portal vein (IHPV). Intrahepatic biliary dilatation confirmed if the IHBD is greater than 50% the diameter of the adjacent IHPV.

Further Reading

Lee HC, Yeung CY, Chang PY, et al. Dilatation of the biliary tree in children: sonographic diagnosis and its clinical significance. *J Ultrasound Med.* 2000;19(3):177–182.

Son YJ, Lee MJ, Koh H, et al. Asymptomatic bile duct dilatation in children: is it a disease? *Pediatr Gastroenterol Hepatol Nutri.* 2015;18(3):180–186.

Pancreas

Indications

Cystic fibrosis (fibrosis and fatty replacement of pancreas), pancreatitis, pancreatic lesions

Technique

1. Pancreas: size, shape, contour and US characteristics of head, body and tail
2. Check SMV–SMA axis

Spleen

Indications

Assessment of spleen size in any disease that affects the spleen (e.g. haematological conditions and malignancies; infections, e.g. infective mononucleosis, tropical diseases)

Technique

Spleen: size, shape, contour and US characteristics of the parenchyma. Measure the longest length. Patency of the splenic vein should be assessed in instances of splenomegaly, portal hypertension, chronic liver disease, before and after liver transplant or otherwise clinically indicated.

Kidneys

Indications

1. Foetal renal pelvis dilation, atypical or recurrent UTI
2. UTI in infant younger than 6–12 months that responds to treatment
3. Continuous wetting
4. Neuropathic bladder
5. Urinary tract obstruction (pelviureteric junction obstruction, vesico-ureteric junction obstruction)
6. Cystic disease
7. Haematuria
8. Chronic renal disease
9. Hypertension
10. Loin pain (calculi, renal mass lesions)
11. VACTERL (vertebral defects, anal atresia, cardiac defects, tracheo-oesophageal fistula, renal anomalies, and limb abnormalities) or deafness screening
12. Varicocele
13. Renal transplant assessment and follow-up

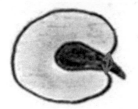
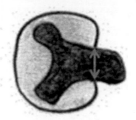

Fig. 3.4 Image of the kidney in the transverse view, with the patient in the prone position, demonstrating correct caliper placement. An isolated renal pelvic dilatation (RPD) of 10 mm or less (i.e. in a normal kidney with no pelvicalyceal or ureteric dilation and good cortical thickness) is deemed normal. (Image courtesy of the Birmingham Children's Hospital Referral and justification criteria for urinary tract ultrasound document.)

Technique

1. Kidneys: size, shape, position and orientation; outline and US characteristics of cortex, medulla, collecting system. Measure the longest renal length and mention if this has been measured with the patient in supine or prone position for ease of future follow-up. Correlate renal length with corresponding renal centile calculated for child's age (except in presence of hydronephrosis or kidney transplant). If the renal pelvis appears full, if there is pelvicalyceal dilation or hydronephrosis, a baseline transverse AP diameter of the renal pelvis should be made with the patient in the prone position (Fig. 3.4). If hydronephrosis is present it can be graded according to the morphology of the calices and renal cortex (Table 3.3).
2. If a single kidney is seen, assess renal size for age. If hypertrophic, this suggests that the other kidney is involuted or absent. If of normal size, check carefully for an ectopic kidney.
3. Check for a horseshoe kidney (bridge of tissue connecting two lower poles across the midline)
4. Bladder: size and wall thickness. Note any collection or free fluid posterior to the bladder or in either iliac fossa. Consider pre- and post-micturition views as necessary.

Further Reading

National Institute for Health and Care Excellence. *Urinary Tract Infection In Under 16s: Diagnosis and Management (NG 224)*. <https://www.nice.org.uk/guidance/ng224>.

Obrycki Ł, Sarnecki J, Lichosik M, et al. Kidney length normative values in children aged 0–19 years—a multicenter study. *Pediatr Nephrol*. 2022;37(5):1075–1085.

Female pelvis

Indications

Pelvic inflammatory disease, Turner's syndrome, pelvic pain, abnormal bleeding, ovarian torsion, pelvic mass, ambiguous genitalia and anomalies of pelvic organs, early or delayed puberty in girls, follow-up of simple cyst greater than 4 cm in diameter, primary or secondary amenorrhoea, polycystic ovary syndrome

Table 3.3   Guidance for Reporting of Renal Hydronephrosis on Ultrasound

Normal	Mild	Moderate	Severe
No evidence of pelvicalyceal dilation	Isolated dilatation of the renal pelvis >10 mm in APD diameter scanned in prone position	Dilation of the renal pelvis *and* major and minor calices	Gross dilation of the renal pelvis and major and minor calices
Isolated dilation of the renal pelvis <10 mm in APD diameter scanned in **prone** position	Dilation of the renal pelvis *and* major calices	Evidence of blunting of calyces	Borders between renal pelvis and calyces are missing
	Attenuated sinus reflex		Significant signs of renal atrophy (thin parenchyma)
	No signs of parenchymal atrophy		

APD, Anteroposterior diameter.
Images courtesy of the Birmingham Children's Hospital Referral and justification criteria for ultrasound of the female pelvis document.

Polycystic ovary syndrome is a clinical and biochemical diagnosis. At least two of these criteria are required:

1. Oligomenorrhoea or anovulation
2. Clinical or biochemical hyperandrogenism with measurement of the free androgen index
3. Polycystic ovaries, with the exclusion of other causes. The diagnosis of a polycystic ovary on US requires the demonstration of at least 12 follicles measuring 2–9 mm in diameter or an ovarian volume in excess of 10 mL.

Patient preparation
1. Full bladder
2. The patient should drink at least 750 mL (three glasses) of clear fluid at least 1 h before the examination time and not empty her bladder until after the examination. If it is not possible for the patient to consume the recommended volume of fluid, then she should be encouraged to drink as much as possible.

3

Technique
1. Uterus: Assess the myometrium for presence of pathology. Measurements (Fig. 3.5):
   (a) Longitudinal section (LS): Because of the difficulty in identifying the internal os in paediatric patients, the LS measurement should extend from the fundus to the external os rather than internal os.
   (b) AP at the cervix and the fundus
   (c) Transverse section
2. Endometrium: If visualized, endometrial thickness should be measured and assessed for pathology (Fig. 3.6).
3. Ovaries: If visualized, the ovaries should be measured in three planes and ovarian volume calculated (Fig. 3.7). Assess for position, follicular activity if appropriate and presence of pathology. If an ovarian cyst or mass is identified, follow local or British Society for Paediatric & Adolescent Gynaecology guidance for subsequent management.
4. Adnexae: Assess for the presence or absence of cysts or masses. Hydrosalpinx can mimic loculated cysts; scan in two planes to identify a tubular cystic structure. Iliac vessels can mimic ovaries or cysts. Use colour Doppler to differentiate.
5. Pouch of Douglas: Assess for the presence or absence of free fluid or masses.
6. Renal tract: The urinary tract must be assessed when a pelvic mass is identified (to look for hydronephrosis) and when a Müllerian duct uterine anomaly is suspected. The renal tract should always be examined because of the association with renal tract abnormalities.

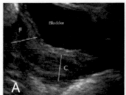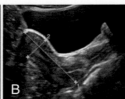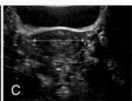

Fig. 3.5 Caliper placements for paediatric uterine measurements. The anteroposterior diameter of the fundus (APF) and anteroposterior diameter of the cervix (APC) measurements on a longitudinal view of the uterus (**A**), craniocaudal length of the uterus (**B**) and transverse length of the uterus (**C**). (Image courtesy of the Birmingham Children's Hospital Referral and justification criteria for ultrasound of the female pelvis document.)

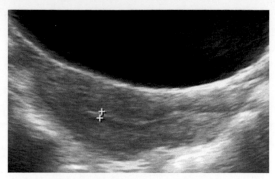

Fig. 3.6 Caliper placement for post-pubertal endometrial thickness. (Image courtesy of the Birmingham Children's Hospital Referral and justification criteria for ultrasound of the female pelvis document.)

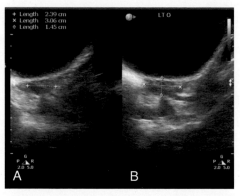

Fig. 3.7 **A** and **B,** Caliper placement for post-pubertal ovarian volume.

Guidance for assessing the post-pubertal endometrium:

1. In longitudinal view, carefully sweep to the right and left of the midline examining the uterus in its entirety.
2. Magnify image and heel/toe the probe to ensure endometrium perpendicular to beam.
3. Magnify and measure endometrial thickness.
4. Correlate endometrial thickness with stage in menstrual cycle and use of oral contraceptives.

Further Reading

Ritchie J, O'Mahony F, Garden A. *British Society for Paediatric & Adolescent Gynaecology (BritSPAG) Guideline for the Management of Ovarian Cysts in Children and Adolescents.* <https://britspag.org/wp-content/uploads/2019/02/Ovarian-cyst-management-in-PAG-guideline-Dec-2018-1.pdf>.

Groin and scrotum

Indications

Pain, unilateral or bilateral swelling, trauma, palpable lump (urgent if malignancy is suspected), undescended testes, ambiguous genitalia, varicoceles (performed in conjunction with a renal US)

Technique

1. Both testicles: size, volume, shape, position, outline and US characteristics, vascularity.
2. Both epididymides.
3. Scrotal wall: If a varicocele is found, image the urinary tract.

Computed Tomography

Abdomen and pelvis

Indications

Evaluation of parenchymal injury after trauma; tumour diagnosis, staging and follow-up; diagnosis and monitoring of infectious or inflammatory disorders as an adjunct to US; characterization of bony pathology as an adjunct to MRI.

Contraindications

In the event of contrast administration: history of reactions to contrast agents, radioactive iodine treatment for thyroid disease, chronic or acutely worsening renal disease.

Contrast medium

Consider using the Camp Bastion protocol to achieve simultaneous arterial and venous enhancement while ensuring adequate parenchymal enhancement in the same scan, negating the need to reirradiate the same volume of tissue to obtain different contrast phases. The Camp Bastion protocol is a biphasic injection in which two-thirds of the contrast medium volume is injected at a slow rate followed by the remaining third volume injected at approximately double the rate, with the scan triggering at 70s whilst the contrast medium is still flowing in. Contrast volume and rates can be approximated from the Camp Bastion Contrast Calculator Wheel based on the patient's weight (Fig. 3.8).

Technique

1. Acquired: 0.625-mm soft tissue
2. Reconstruction: 0.625-mm bone
3. Multiplanar reconstructions (MPRs): three planes, 3-mm thickness

Additional techniques and modification of techniques

The extent of CT coverage should be tailored to the clinical question. This is in contrast to adult trauma practice in which whole-body CT is the default imaging of choice in severely injured patients and in oncological staging.

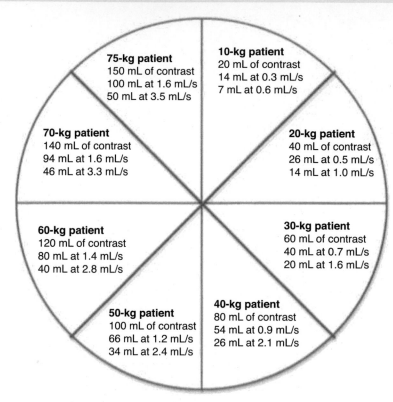

Fig. 3.8 Camp Bastion contrast calculator. (Image courtesy of the Royal College of Radiologists Paediatric trauma protocols, 2014.)

Further Reading

Low SBL, Tan Y, Patel H, et al. Four-year experience of paediatric penetrating injuries: findings from a paediatric major trauma centre in the UK. *Clin Radiol.* 2022. S0009926022000459.

Royal College of Radiologists. *BFCR(14)8 Paediatric Trauma Protocols.* <https://www.rcr.ac.uk/publication/paediatric-trauma-protocols>.

Magnetic Resonance Imaging

Magnetic resonance urography

MR urography is used for assessing disorders of the urinary tract and permits a comprehensive evaluation of the kidneys and urinary tract, providing anatomical and functional information without the need for ionizing radiation.

Indications

Common indications for paediatric MR urography include evaluation of complex renal and urinary tract anatomy, suspected urinary tract obstruction, operative planning and post-operative assessment. T2-weighted imaging of urine allows the assessment of dilated or obstructed urinary systems, and post-contrast imaging (gadolinium-enhanced T1-weighted imaging of the kidneys and urinary system) depicts non-dilated or non-obstructed urinary systems. In addition, post-contrast MR urography provides a functional evaluation of the kidneys and urinary tract that includes estimation of differential renal function.

Patient preparation

The patient is asked to change into a gown, remove all metal belongings and empty their bladder immediately before the scan.

Technique

1. Furosemide is administered at 1 mg kg^{-1} (maximum, 20 mg) and Buscopan (dose, 1 mL age for age 11 years and older and 0.5 mL for age 7–11 years).
2. The patient is imaged in the supine position, and the following sequences are used:
    (a) Precontrast: axial T2-weighted fat-suppressed (FS) breath-hold (BH), T2-weighted three-dimensional (3D) volume coronal respiration triggered, T2-weighted FS coronal BH, axial T2-weighted half Fourier acquisition single-shot turbo spin echo (HASTE), T2-weighted sagittal pelvis high-resolution, T1-weighted Vibe Dixon coronal
    (b) Post-contrast (if no renal impairment): T1-weighted Vibe Dixon coronal, STAT and at 5 min; T1-weighted Vibe Dixon coronal and axial at 8 and 12 min; additional Vibe Dixon sequences if required

RESPIRATORY AND CARDIAC

Fluoroscopy

Bronchography

Indications

1. To assess for structural or functional abnormalities of the larynx, trachea or bronchi (e.g. tracheobronchomalacia)
2. To determine the minimal positive end-expiratory pressure (PEEP) needed to manage the patient as an outpatient

The diagnosis of tracheobronchomalacia has been replaced by bronchoscopy and newer imaging techniques such as dynamic four-dimensional multidetector CT and cine MRI.

Bronchography is mainly performed to facilitate patient management on discharge rather than diagnosis and should only be performed by experienced paediatric radiologists with the onsite support of a dedicated paediatric airway management team, at the time of the procedure.

Ultrasound

Lung

Indications

1. To evaluate the neonatal lung (neonatal point of care US)
2. To follow up and evaluate antenatally detected lung abnormalities

3. To evaluate and follow up consolidation
4. To assess an opaque hemithorax
5. To clarify inconclusive plain film findings

Equipment

1. High-frequency linear probe to examine the pleura in detail
2. Lower-frequency curvilinear probe for assessment of the lungs and deeper thorax.

Technique

1. The thorax should be examined in a systematic fashion, with the patient in a supine or semirecumbent position and with the arm raised if tolerated. If the patient is breathless, image in semirecumbent position, sitting up position or any position possible.
2. When possible, the whole thorax should be scanned bilaterally, and specific attention should be given to any area of concern identified on previous imaging.
3. The whole of the affected hemithorax should be imaged from the parasternal region, extending laterally and posteriorly to the paravertebral region.
4. There are varying techniques advocated for examination of the paediatric thorax. The probe can be positioned in the xiphisternum and angled superiorly. The thorax can be further divided into six zones and scanned in an overlapping manner 'mowing the lawn'.
    (a) Zones 1 and 2: anteriorly in the mid clavicular line with the probe placed in the longitudinal position between the costal spaces
    (b) Zones 3 and 4: laterally in the mid axillary line with the probe angled between the costal spaces
    (c) Zones 5 and 6: posteriorly, scanning around the scapula
5. The thorax should be examined to assess the pleural line for sharpness or areas of irregularity or nodularity, presence and thickness of pleural rind, presence or absence of lung collapse or consolidation and presence or absence and type of pleural fluid.
6. There may be focal areas of abnormality within the lung such as air bronchograms, abscess, necrosis or mass lesions.
7. Use colour or power Doppler to identify the presence or absence of vascularity within the lung or lung lesion. Absence of vascularity may indicate lung necrosis in the consolidated lung.
8. M-mode imaging may be used to identify pleural sliding.

Further Reading

Calder A, Owens CM. Imaging of parapneumonic pleural effusions and empyema in children. *Pediatr Radiol*. 2009;39(6):527–537.

Dietrich CF, Mathis G, Cui XW, et al. Ultrasound of the pleurae and lungs. *Ultrasound Med Biol*. 2015;41(2):351–365.

Heffner JE, Klein JS, Hampson C. Diagnostic utility and clinical application of imaging for pleural space infections. *Chest*. 2010;137(2):467–479.

Joshi P, Vasishta A, Gupta M. Ultrasound of the pediatric chest. *Br J Radiol*. 2019;92(1100):20190058.

King S, Thomson A. Radiological perspectives in empyema. *Br Med Bull.* 2002;61:203–214.

Mayo PH, Copetti R, Feller-Kopman D, et al. Thoracic ultrasonography: a narrative review. *Intensive Care Med.* 2019;45(9):1200–1211.

Mong A, Epelman M, Darge K. Ultrasound of the pediatric chest. *Pediatr Radiol.* 2012;42(11):1287–1297.

Diaphragm

Indications

Assessment of diaphragmatic function. Paralysis of the diaphragm is associated with damage to the phrenic nerve and may occur after thoracic surgery. US helps differentiate other causes of an apparently high hemidiaphragm, such as subpulmonary fluid, diaphragmatic defects or eventration.

Technique

1. The patient should be breathing without mechanical assistance as ventilator support fills the lungs with air, which will cause the diaphragms to move down with inspiration even when paralyzed.
2. Perform the examination with the child in quiet respiration. Scan both diaphragms in longitudinal and transverse planes. High transverse scans must be undertaken with both diaphragms in view for comparison of movement.
3. Consider using the M-mode to measure the direction of diaphragmatic motion and the amplitude of excursion.
4. The diaphragm normally moves down on inspiration and up on expiration. With paralysis of the diaphragm, it will either remain high and fixed or may exhibit paradoxical movement so that on inspiration, it moves upwards.
5. With M-mode, diaphragmatic movement is considered normal if the diaphragm moves towards the transducer during inspiration, with excursion of greater than 4 mm and difference in excursion between the domes of less than 50%.

Further Reading

Chavhan GB, Babyn PS, Cohen RA, et al. Multimodality imaging of the pediatric diaphragm: anatomy and pathologic conditions. *Radiographics.* 2010;30(7):1797–1817.

De Bruyn R. *Paediatric Ultrasound: How, Why and When.* Elsevier, Churchill Livingstone; 2005.

Nason LK, Walker CM, McNeeley, et al. Imaging of the diaphragm: anatomy and function. *Radiographics.* 2012;32(2):E51–E70.

Thymus

Indications

To confirm the presence of the thymus, to identify the nature of a suspected thymic mass, to help in image-guided aspiration or biopsies of thymic lesions

Equipment

1. High-frequency linear probe
2. Small footprint, high-frequency curvilinear probe, which can be positioned in the sternal notch

Technique

US evaluation can be done via the suprasternal or parasternal approach because of the incompletely ossified costal cartilage and sternum.

Normal sonographic appearances of the thymus

1. The thymus is a gland that lies anterior to the aortic arch and is commonly visualized in children up to 2 years of age in the superior mediastinum. In later childhood, it atrophies.
2. There is quite a wide variation in size of the thymus. In all patients, the thymus has a smooth margin that is sharply defined. It is hypovascular (on Doppler) and hypoechoic with multiple brightly echogenic internal structures and punctate foci presenting connective tissue septae and vessels.
3. With lower-frequency probes, the thymus can appear homogeneous, with echogenicity comparable with the liver or spleen; however, higher-frequency probes reveal its hyperechoic internal structures to be distinct from those within the liver, spleen or thyroid.
4. The thymus is either centrally located with symmetric appearances or has a left-sided predominance. It is often rectangular on transverse scanning and triangular on longitudinal scanning.
5. The thymus is deformable and normally moulds to underlying structures such as the great vessels and should never cause obstruction to the structures in the superior mediastinum.

Further Reading

De Bruyn R. *Paediatric Ultrasound: How, Why and When.* Elsevier, Churchill Livingstone; 2005.
Gravel CA, Bachur RG. Point-of-care ultrasound differentiation of lung consolidation and normal thymus in pediatric patients: an educational case series. *J Emerg Med.* 2018;55(2):235–239.
Manchanda S, Bhalla AS, Jana M, et al. Imaging of the pediatric thymus: clinicoradiologic approach. *World J Clin Pediatr.* 2017;6(1):10–23.

Computed Tomography

Thorax

Indications

1. To evaluate complications from pneumonia and surgical planning
2. To detect or characterize primary or secondary lung tumours
3. To assess for the extent and pattern of congenital or acquired airway disease and malformation
4. To assess trauma to blood vessels or the lung

Contraindications

In the event of contrast administration: history of reactions to contrast agents, radioactive iodine treatment for thyroid disease, chronic or acutely worsening renal disease

Technique

1. Acquired: 0.625-mm soft tissue
2. Recons: 2.5 mm lung (whole chest); 1.25-mm lung (high-resolution CT style)
3. MPRs: three planes, 3-mm thickness soft tissue

Additional techniques and modification of techniques

1. The need for contrast, phase of contrast and extent of CT coverage should be tailored to the clinical question. The use of inspiratory and expiratory phase imaging is dependent on the ability of the child to understand and perform breathing instructions.
2. For fungal infection or infiltration, consider non-contrast CT of the chest.
3. For vascular rings, consider arterial phase CT of the chest.
4. For congenital lung lesions, consider arterial phase CT of the chest, including the coeliac axis to assess for the extrathoracic origin of the systemic arterial supply.
5. For tumour staging, consider a Bastion protocol CT of the chest for the first chest staging scan as a baseline and to facilitate nodal assessment. Subsequent CT of the chest can be performed without contrast for nodule assessment and follow-up.
6. For patients with bronchiolitis obliterans or graft-versus-host disease or after bone marrow transplant, consider inspiratory and expiratory phase imaging.

Cardiac

Indications

1. To diagnose and delineate the cardiac and extracardiac anatomy in children with complex congenital or acquired cardiac pathology
2. To guide treatment and surgical planning

Technique

Readers are referred to dedicated texts; however, an electrocardiography-gated technique is suggested:

1. Babies (age younger than 12 months): 80 kVp, 100 mA; children: 80 kVp, 160 mA; teenagers: 100 kVp, 200 mA
2. Centre R-peak delay, 40%; padding, 70 ms, with adaptive gating
3. Contrast 2 mL kg^{-1}, contrast column of 20 s with a saline flush; bolus tracked from the aorta (depending on indication)
4. Acquired: 0.625 mm voxels, cardiac cine scan
5. Recons: reconstructed at 5% phases and with 1 mm, three-plane MPRs from a chosen phase

Further Reading

DiGeorge NW, El-Ali AM, White AM, et al. Pediatric cardiac CT and MRI: considerations for the general radiologist. *AJR Am J Roentgenol.* 2020;215:1464–1473.

Mortensen KH, Tann O. Computed tomography in paediatric heart disease. *Br J Radiol.* 2018;91(1092):20180201.

Magnetic Resonance Imaging

Cardiac

Cardiac MRI is increasingly used to provide anatomical and radiation-free functional assessment, flow measurements and a degree of tissue characterization that cannot be performed with CT or echocardiography. Further details and protocols are beyond the scope of this chapter, so readers are referred to the recommended reading in the Cardiac section.

MUSKULOSKELETAL

Ultrasound

Neonatal hips for developmental dysplasia of the hip

There is no universally accepted standard technique for US examination of the infant hip. However, this section describes the Graf technique because this is the technique with which the authors are most familiar.

The Graf technique requires the sonographer to be able to identify important landmarks in the coronal plane and from these landmarks to measure the alpha and beta angles. This technique requires some training and practice, and sonographers should ensure that they are adequately trained by an experienced practitioner in this method before it is used.

Indications

Suspicion of developmental dysplasia of the hip based on family history, birth history and clinical examination in an infant younger than 6 months of age or for follow-up

Technique

1. It is recommended that a positioning device is used to immobilize the patient. The infant is placed on their side with the examined limb exposed. The examined limb is rotated slightly inward and adducted to avoid the knee protruding above the cradle bolster, and the transducer is placed over the greater trochanter.
2. The following main reference points need to be identified: chondro-osseous border, femoral head, synovial fold, joint capsule, labrum, cartilage, bony roof and bony rim (turning point) (Table 3.4). Even if only one structure is missing, the sonogram is not diagnostic and must not be used.
3. For hip sonograms to be comparable, it is necessary to establish a standardized cross section of the hip joint with three landmarks. The

Table 3.4   Checklist for Anatomical Identification

Anatomical Identification

1. Chondro-osseous border
2. Femoral head
3. Synovial fold
4. Joint capsule
5. Labrum
6. Cartilage
7. Bony roof
8. Bony rim
9. Lower limb of ilium

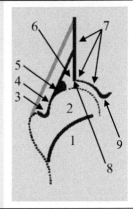

Image courtesy of Graf R, Lercher K, Baumgartner F, et al. *Essentials of Infant Hip Sonography According to Graf.* Stolzalpe: Edition Stolzalpe Sonocenter 2017.

Table 3.5   Checklist for the Standard Plane

Standard Plane

1. Uppermost point of cartilaginous roof
2. Acetabular labrum
3. Bony rim
4. Lower limb of Ilium

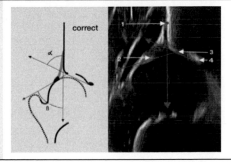

Image courtesy of Graf R, Lercher K, Baumgartner F, et al. *Essentials of Infant Hip Sonography According to Graf.* Stolzalpe: Edition Stolzalpe Sonocenter 2017.

standard plane is defined when the 1ower limb of the ilium, cross section through the midportion of the bony roof and acetabular labrum are identified (Table 3.5). Only sonograms that are in the standard plane can be measured.

4. Draw the baseline (point where the echo of the proximal perichondrium meets with the echo from the Ilium), bony roof line (line tangent from the lower limb of the ilium just touching the bony roof) and cartilaginous roofline (line from the turning point/bony rim through the middle of the labrum). The three lines seldom cross at one point.

5. The base line and bony roof line form the alpha or bony roof angle. The alpha angle evaluates the size of the bony socket. The

base line and cartilaginous roof line form the beta angle that assesses the size of the cartilaginous roof and is not universally used.
6. Repeat these steps for the contralateral hip.

Further Reading

De Bruyn R. *Paediatric Ultrasound: How, Why and When*. Elsevier, Churchill Livingstone; 2005.

Graf R. *Hip Sonography: Diagnosis and Management of Infant Hip Dysplasia*. 2nd ed. Springer; 2006.

Graf R, Lercher K, Scott S, et al. *Essentials of Infant Hip Sonography According to Graf*. Sonocenter Stolzalpe; 2017.

Royal College of Radiologists. *iRefer: Making the Best Use of Clinical Radiology*, 8th ed, Guidelines P37. <https://www.irefer.org.uk/guidelines/list/paediatrics>.

Lumps and bumps

Indication

Any soft tissue lump

Equipment

Linear, high-frequency probe

Technique

1. Any discrete mass should be characterized and measured in three dimensions, including colour or power Doppler imaging.
2. Identify its morphology: well-circumscribed or ill-defined; its internal characteristics: solid, cystic, contains fluid, fat or calcification; its location: subcutaneous, subfascial, inter- or intramuscular; and its relationship to bone (if applicable).

Joints

Indications

1. To assess for joint inflammation by detecting synovial thickening, synovitis or effusion
2. To identify adjacent bone involvement
3. To guide aspiration of a joint for diagnostic or therapeutic purposes
4. To map the distribution of joints affected by systemic arthropathies

Equipment

Linear, high-frequency probe

Technique

1. Always scan both limbs using the asymptomatic side as a control or baseline if appropriate. Take care to position the asymptomatic side similar to the symptomatic side.
2. Position the long axis of the probe along the long axis of the limb over the area where the capsule is most slack.
   (a) In the hip, this is along the anterior femoral neck in an oblique sagittal plane.

Table 3.6   Key Sonographic Differences Between Synovial Fluid or Effusion and Synovial Thickening

Synovial Fluid or Effusion	Synovial Thickening
• Abnormal hypoechoic or anechoic but sometimes may be isoechoic or hyperechoic (relative to subdermal fat) intraarticular material • Displaceable and compressible • No Doppler vascularity	• Abnormal hypoechoic but sometimes may be isoechoic or hyperechoic (relative to subdermal fat) intraarticular tissue • Non-displaceable and poorly compressible • May have Doppler vascularity

(b) In the knee, this is along the suprapatellar space in the midline, bearing in mind the knee joint also extends infrapatellar and into both medial and lateral joint recesses.

(c) In the ankle, this is at the midline of the anterior ankle crease.

3. Most fluid is echo free, but some effusions can contain particulate matter with internal echoes. When there is doubt, one should first compare the potential area of fluid with known areas of fluid at the same depth, such as a vessel or the bladder. The gain setting should then be adjusted to make the known fluid appear just echogenic and then turning the gain back to the point at which it appears just echo free and reexamining the suspect areas. This allows an objective comparison and aids characterization of the fluid in question.

4. Although US can accurately detect effusions, it cannot determine the nature of the fluid (Fig. 3.9). There is no single feature that is specific for blood, pus or transudate. This discrimination can only be made by aspirating the fluid.

5. Use power Doppler in addition to gray scale ultrasound features to assess for active synovitis/synovial hypertrophy. Ensure that there is an adequate gel pad over the skin so that only minimal pressure is applied when the power Doppler is turned on because the low-volume, low-velocity synovial microvascularity can be easily obviated with pressure (Table 3.6 and Fig. 3.10).

6. Assess the adjacent bone for periosteal reaction or erosions. Healthy cortical bone appears as a regular, highly hyperechoic line with posterior acoustic shadowing and some reverberation artefacts. In children, the normal periosteum is visualized as thin and avascular (apart from nutrient vessels that perforate the periosteum and enter the bone cortex). An erosion is an intraarticular discontinuity of the bone surface that is visible in two perpendicular planes.

Further Reading

D'Agostino MA, Terslev L, Aegerter P, et al. Scoring ultrasound synovitis in rheumatoid arthritis: a EULAR-OMERACT ultrasound taskforce—part 1: definition and development of a standardised, consensus-based scoring system. *RMD Open*. 2017;3(1):e000428.

Dumitriu D, Menten R, Clapuyt P. Ultrasonography of the bone surface in children: normal and pathological findings in the bone cortex and periosteum. *Pediatr Radiol*. 2022;52(7):1392–1403.

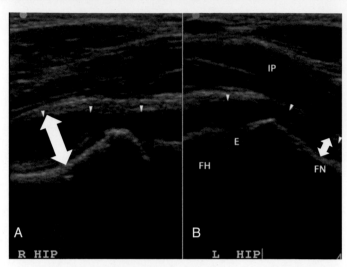

Fig. 3.9 **A,** Right hip joint effusion. **B,** Normal left hip. *Two-headed arrows* showing the depth of the joint effusions in the right and left hips. *Arrowheads* demarcate the joint capsule of the respective hips. *FH,* Femoral head; *FN,* femoral neck; *IP,* iliopsoas muscle. (Image courtesy of the British Society of Paediatric Radiology (BSPR) paediatric ultrasound on-call guide, First edition, June 2020.)

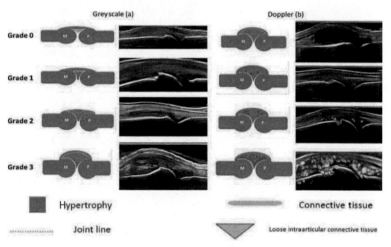

Fig. 3.10 A semiquantitative way of describing synovial hypertrophy and Doppler activity. Schematic drawings of the individual grades of hypoechoic greyscale synovial hypertrophy (**A**) and Doppler activity (**B**) with the corresponding ultrasound image. (Image courtesy of the EULAR-OMERACT Ultrasound Taskforce.)

Koski JM, Saarakkala S, Helle M, et al. Power Doppler ultrasonography and synovitis: correlating ultrasound imaging with histopathological findings and evaluating the performance of ultrasound equipments. *Ann Rheum Dis.* 2006;65(12):1590–1595.

McDonald L, Siddle K, Starzyk B, et al. *Paediatric Ultrasound On-Call Guide—* prepared for the British Society of Paediatric Radiology (BSPR) by the

Newcastle Team, following the BSPR ASM of 2020. 1st ed. British Society of Paediatric Radiology; 2020. <https://www.bspr.co.uk/documents/on-call-guide-for-registrars-and-others>.

Wakefield RJ, Balint PV, Szkudlarek M, et al. Musculoskeletal ultrasound including definitions for ultrasonographic pathology. *J Rheumatol.* 2006;33(2):440.

Wilson D. *Paediatric Musculoskeletal Disease: With an Emphasis on Ultrasound (Medical Radiology).* Springer; 2005.

Windschall D, Malattia C. Ultrasound imaging in paediatric rheumatology. *Best Pract Res Clin Rheumatol.* 2020;34(6):101570.

Neck

Indications

1. Salivary glands (submandibular and parotid): inflammatory sialadenitis, suspected abscess formation, obstructing calculus, discrete solitary mass, anterior floor-of-the-mouth lesion (which may be solid or cystic), a simple or plunging ranula, diffuse enlargement and dry mouth (Sjogren's syndrome), autoimmune condition
2. Thyroid (and parathyroid) glands: evaluation of the location and characteristics of palpable neck masses or abnormalities detected by other imaging examinations or laboratory studies; assessment of the presence, size (thyroid volume; volume of each lobe and total volume) and location of the thyroid gland; screening of high-risk patients for occult thyroid malignancy; follow-up of thyroid nodules, when indicated; indicate presence of thyroid hyperaemia and associated lymphadenopathy when thyroiditis or autoimmune thyroiditis (Hashimoto's thyroiditis/Graves' disease) is suspected
3. Lymph nodes: identification and characterization of lymph nodes, cause of unilateral or bilateral neck swelling, differentiating lymphadenitis from abscess formation (Fig. 3.11)
4. Congenital lesions: localization of lymphangioma, haemangioma; parotid, branchial cleft, thyroglossal duct, parathyroid or thymic cysts and cervical cleft

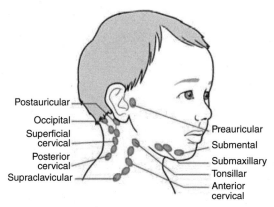

Fig. 3.11 Lymph nodes in the head and neck region. (Image courtesy of the Royal Children's Hospital Melbourne Clinical Practice Guidelines: Cervical Lymphadenopathy.)

Equipment

Linear, high-frequency probe

Technique

1. Salivary glands: The salivary glands should be evaluated in transverse and longitudinal planes, noting parenchymal echogenicity and the presence of focal abnormalities, hyperaemia, duct dilatation and calculi with or without lymphadenopathy. Each salivary gland examined should be compared with the asymptomatic contralateral gland.
2. Lymph nodes: Assess the location, number and distribution of nodes, size and morphology.
3. Thyroid (and parathyroid) glands: Record the size of each thyroid lobe in three dimensions (AP, transverse and longitudinal) and the thickness (anteroposterior measurement) of the isthmus on the transverse view. Document any thyroid (e.g. nodules) or adjacent soft tissue abnormalities (e.g. abnormal lymph nodes, thrombosed veins) with respect to the location, size, number and character of significant abnormalities. Also note the presence of any extra thyroid collection or abscess indicating acute suppurative thyroiditis.
4. Congenital lesions: Assess the location (e.g. intra- or extraparenchymal) and lesion characteristics, including Doppler vascularity, to facilitate identification.

Guidance on sonographic lymph node assessment:

1. Maximum size in short axis (normal <10 mm in short-axis diameter)
2. Shape of node (normal lymph nodes: oval rather than rounded)
3. Presence of normal central echogenic hilum with reduced echogenicity peripherally (normal and reactive nodes are predominantly hypoechoic compared with the adjacent muscles; malignant or metastatic nodes can be hypo- or hyperechoic)
4. Presence of intranodal necrosis or calcification with posterior acoustic shadowing is abnormal. The presence of microcalcification is a strong indicator for malignancy but can also be seen in tuberculosis and atypical infections.
5. Nodal borders: Unsharp and smooth borders are common in reactive nodes caused by the oedema and inflammation of the surrounding soft tissue in comparison with metastatic and lymphomatous nodes, which tend to have sharp borders. Sharp borders are believed to be caused by the tumour infiltration and the reduced fatty deposition within the lymph nodes, which increase the acoustic impedance difference between the lymph node and the surrounding tissues; however, capsular spread may result in loss of border.
6. Presence or absence of normal central vascularity on Doppler insonation. (Peripheral vascularity, regardless of sole peripheral or mixed vascularity, is highly suspicious of malignancy.)

Further Reading
Ahuja AT, Ying M, Ho SY, et al. Ultrasound of malignant cervical lymph nodes. *Cancer Imaging*. 2008;8(1):48–56.
Lakshmi C, Madala S, Ravikiran A, et al. Evaluation of reliability of ultrasonographic parameters in differentiating benign and metastatic cervical group of lymph nodes. *ISRN Otolaryngol*. 2014;2014:238740.
Ludwig BJ, Wang J, Nadgir RN, et al. Imaging of cervical lymphadenopathy in children and young adults. *AJR Am J Roentgenol*. 2012;199(5):1105–1113.
Meier JD, Grimmer JF. Evaluation and management of neck masses in children. *Am Fam Physician*. 2014;89(5):353–358.
Raja Lakshmi C, Sudhakara Rao M, Ravikiran A, et al. Evaluation of reliability of ultrasonographic parameters in differentiating benign and metastatic cervical group of lymph nodes. *ISRN Otolaryngol*. 2014;2014:238740.
Ying M, Bhatia KSS, Lee YP, et al. Review of ultrasonography of malignant neck nodes: greyscale, Doppler, contrast enhancement and elastography. *Cancer Imaging*. 2014;13(4):658–669.

Radiography

Skeletal dysplasia

Indications

Common indications include but are not limited to unexplained short stature, facial dysmorphism and bony abnormality (e.g. small thorax, bowed long bones) identified on the antenatal US.

Technique

1. In 2015, the Skeletal Dysplasia Group for Teaching and Research proposed that standardized radiographic protocols should be used to image children because this would ensure uniformity of practice when patients are referred for expert tertiary radiology opinion.
2. This differs from the skeletal survey performed in cases of suspected or confirmed non-accidental injury or child abuse and includes the following radiographs: skull (AP and lateral), thoracolumbosacral spine (lateral), chest (AP), pelvis (AP), one upper limb (AP, left or right), one lower limb (AP, left or right) and left hand Dorsopalmer (DP).

Further Reading
Offiah AC, Hall CM. Radiological diagnosis of the constitutional disorders of bone. As easy as A, B, C? *Pediatr Radiol*. 2003;33(3):153–161.
Watson S, Calder A, Offiah A, et al. A review of imaging protocols for suspected skeletal dysplasia and a proposal for standardisation. *Pediatr Radiol*. 2015; 45:1733–1737.

NEUROLOGICAL

CT and MRI are used when imaging the foetal, neonatal and paediatric brain for the identification and treatment follow-up of neurological conditions, including congenital malformations; phakomatoses; neoplasms; traumatic and vascular lesions; and metabolic, infectious and inflammatory disorders.

CT is the first-line cross-sectional modality in acute neurological deterioration, principally because of its available at nearly all centres 24/7. It can provide a guide to the need of prompt neurosurgical input (e.g. shunt insertion in hydrocephalus or evacuation for large-volume haemorrhage). Given the speed of acquisition, often even a young child (particularly if neurologically compromised or 'knocked off') is sufficiently motionless to obtain diagnostic images without the need for sedation or general anaesthetic. Although requiring the need for IV contrast, assessing the venous sinuses with CT venogram is considered optimal compared with MR venograms in our experience.

The main drawback of CT, in addition to the involvement of ionizing radiation, is that it is relatively poor at assessing the brain parenchyma. In cases of early ischaemia, demyelination or encephalitis, CT has limited sensitivity. Conventional MRI has the benefit of no radiation exposure and superior assessment of the brain substance given the excellent soft tissue contrast but is highly susceptible to movement artefact. MRI requires the child to stay motionless for several minutes and possibly in excess of 30 min, although the ongoing development of shorter acquisition sequences may change the landscape.

It is beyond the scope of this chapter to cover all CT and MRI protocols; instead, discussions are restricted to those that have particular relevance to paediatric imaging and commonly used applications.

Computed Tomography

Routine head

Indications

Head injury (according to NICE CG176 guidance), acute stroke, intracranial space-occupying lesion, brain abscess. Consider contrast administration in situations in which vascular injury, vasculopathy, infection or a space-occupying lesion is suspected or has been identified on the precontrast imaging.

Contraindications

In the event of contrast administration: history of reactions to contrast agents, radioactive iodine treatment for thyroid disease, chronic or acutely worsening renal disease

Technique

1. Patients should be positioned with the chin down and organ dose modulation used over the eyes to reduce lens dose when appropriate. MPRs to be reconstructed done to the patient's anatomical planes as per MRI (e.g. axials to the corpus callosum) not orthogonally through the volume. Five-mm MPRs should be considered on larger patients.
2. Non-contrast CT of the head
   (a) Acquired: 1.25-mm brain

(b) Recons: 0.625-mm bone
(c) MPRs: three planes, 3-mm thickness; 3D model if assessing for a
fracture or ventriculoperitoneal shunt in position
3. Post-contrast CT of the head: performed after 2 mL/kg of IV contrast
and scanned 90 s after the start of the contrast administration, as per
CT venogram
(a) Post-contrast acquisition: 1.25-mm brain
(b) MPRs: three planes, 3-mm thickness

Hydrocephalus

Indications

Hydrocephalus: suspected shunt malformation

Technique

Low-dose scan primarily to assess ventricular size

1. Acquired: 1.25-mm brain
2. Recons: 1.25-mm bone
3. MPRs: three planes, 5-mm thickness; 3D model to demonstrate valve
and shunt tubing

Venogram

Indication

Suspected cerebral venous thrombosis

Contraindications

History of reactions to contrast agents, radioactive iodine treatment
for thyroid disease, chronic or acutely worsening renal disease

Technique

Performed after 2 mL/kg of IV contrast and scanned 90 s after the start
of contrast administration:

1. Acquired: 0.625-mm venogram
2. MPRs: axial 1.25-mm brain, three planes in 3 mm thickness

Cerebral arterial angiogram

Indications

Haemorrhagic or non-haemorrhagic stroke

Contraindications

History of reactions to contrast agents, radioactive iodine treatment
for thyroid disease, chronic or acutely worsening renal disease

Technique

1. If haemorrhagic stroke, scan from skull base to vertex. If non-
haemorrhagic stroke, scan from aortic arch to vertex.

2. Performed after 2 mL kg^{-1} of IV contrast with bolus tracking (region of interest at aortic arch) for arterial phase imaging. Scan may be triggered automatically or manually by a radiologist or senior radiographer.
   (a) Acquired: 0.625-mm angiography
   (b) MPRs: three planes, 2-mm thickness

Magnetic Resonance Imaging

Brain MRI protocols should be tailored to maximize the specificity of pathology detection according to the brain's developmental stage from foetus to adult. For infants, a focus on myelin maturation is key, with T1-weighted sequences included in all protocols. For children when myelin maturation is complete, adult-type sequences can be used but optimized for the clinical question. For infants younger than 6 months, the maturation of myelin is best assessed using T1-weighted images. Beyond 6 months until the completion of myelination at around 2–3 years of age, T2-weighted images are more useful.

Volumetric imaging is optimal for tumour follow-up, improving accuracy in tumour size measurements between examinations. Volumetric Fluid-attenuated inversion recovery (FLAIR) sequence helps to increase sensitivity in epilepsy imaging such as for the identification of focal cortical dysplasia, which are often subtle. 3D Steady-state free precession (SSFP) (e.g. Fast imaging employing steady-state acquisition (FIESTA), Three-dimensional (3D) constructive interference in steady state (CISS)) images remove cerebrospinal fluid (CSF) flow artefact and provide high spatial resolution for the assessment of a CSF interface (e.g. aqueductal stenosis, post-endoscopic third ventriculostomy). Susceptibility-weighted imaging is highly sensitive for detecting haemorrhagic foci in the brain parenchyma, allowing assessment of the vascular supply to tumours and malformations.

Standard brain

Indications

Developmental delay, headaches, neurocutaneous syndromes, suspected congenital malformations, infection, metabolic and inflammatory disorders, tumours, metastases, CSF and cranial nerve pathologies, vascular pathologies

Contraindications

Absolute

Pulmonary artery monitoring catheters and temporary transvenous pacing leads, intraaortic balloon pumps, left and right ventricular assist devices, epicardial leads, retained transvenous leads, fractured leads, ferromagnetic vascular clips, metallic foreign body (e.g. shrapnel, metal splinters, welding splinters, bullets, grenade fragments), spinal cord neurostimulators, vascular access port, implants (e.g. insulin pump, prostheses)

Relative

Cochlear implants, implanted pacemakers and implantable cardio-verter-defibrillators are considered a strong relative contraindication; intracranial endovascular clips (as per neurosurgeon); endovascular stent grafts depending on the material; renal insufficiency (if contrast needed); cardiac valves; joint replacement; IVC filters (early within 6 weeks of implantation)

3

Technique

1. Non-contrast MRI of the head
   (a) Acquired: three planes, T2, 5-mm slice thickness; axial T2-weighted FLAIR, diffusion and susceptibility weighted, gradient-echo sequences; sagittal T1 volume
   (b) Reconstructed: T1 volume reconstructed in the axial and coronal planes
2. Post-contrast MRI of the head
   (a) Post-contrast acquisition: axial T1-weighted and sagittal T1-weighted volume with reconstructions in the axial and coronal planes

Neonatal head

The neonatal brain has a high relative water content compared with the mature brain, and inversion recovery sequences may complement the standard brain protocols used for older children.

Indications

Neonatal brain up to 1 h old, Hypoxic-ischaemic encephalopathy (HIE), germinal matrix haemorrhage, prognostication

Technique

Acquired: axial T1, T2, T1 FLAIR, diffusion and susceptibility-weighted, gradient-echo sequences, sagittal T1, coronal T2

Epilepsy

Indication

Epilepsy

Technique

1. Acquired: sagittal and axial T2, coronal T2 3-mm slice thickness angled to hippocampi, coronal FLAIR 4-mm slice thickness, axial diffusion, sagittal T1 volume
2. Reconstructed: sagittal T1 volume-reconstructed in the axial and coronal planes (angled to hippocampi)

Spine

Indications

Scoliosis, tumours, metastases, neurocutaneous syndromes, suspected congenital malformations including spinal dysraphism, infection, metabolic and inflammatory disorders, tumours, metastases, CSF, cord and nerve root pathologies, vascular pathologies

Technique

1. Acquired: sagittal T1, T2 and T2 fat-suppressed of the whole spine to below coccyx, axial T1 from conus to below the coccyx.
2. Include axial T2 through sites of signal abnormality (e.g. syrinx or cord signal abnormality)
3. Consider sagittal CISS of lumbosacral spine to below coccyx, with axial MPR.
4. Consider contrast administration with post-contrast sagittal and axial T1 fat-suppressed sequences when there is an abnormality.

Additional techniques and modification of techniques

For scoliosis: include coronal T2, segmented according to curvature with overlap

Further Reading
Kozak BM, Jaimes C, Kirsch J, et al. MRI techniques to decrease imaging times in children. *Radiographics*. 2020;40:485–502.

Ultrasound

Neonatal cranium

Indications

1. Preterm (<30–32 wks) and extremely low-birth-weight (<1500 g) infants: screening and serial cranial US for germinal matrix and intraventricular haemorrhage, periventricular leukomalacia
2. All infants: initial evaluation for suspected congenital anomaly, suspected congenital or post-natal intracranial infection, suspected hypoxic ischemic injury, increased or decreased head circumference, symptoms of central nervous system (CNS) disorder (e.g. seizures), follow-up of CNS abnormality seen at foetal US or MRI
3. Screening of infants at high risk for intracranial haemorrhage (e.g. those on extracorporeal membrane oxygenation support or therapeutic hypothermia)

Equipment

1. Small footprint curvilinear, high-frequency probe
2. Linear, high-frequency probe

Technique

1. The anterior fontanelle is located at the junction of the coronal and sagittal sutures. It is the largest fontanelle and is useful for both coronal and sagittal sonographic examination to get an overview of the neonatal brain. The anterior fontanelle closure occurs between 10 and 24 months. Palpation of the anterior fontanelle should be performed before head US at this age to ensure an adequate sonographic window.

2. Additional acoustic windows (e.g. posterior and mastoid fontanelles provide a better window for evaluating the posterior fossa structures and upper spinal canal)
3. Image the brain in both coronal and sagittal planes.
4. In the coronal plane, a minimum of six images are obtained by gently sweeping the probe from anterior to posterior. These images include:
   (a) Just anterior to the frontal horns of the lateral ventricles
   (b) At the level of the frontal horns of the lateral ventricles, anterior to the foramen of Monro (Fig. 3.12).
   (c) Body of lateral ventricles at the foramen of Monro, including the cingulate gyri and sylvian fissures
   (d) Body of lateral ventricles posterior to the foramen of Monro, including the pons and medulla
   (e) Posterior horn of the lateral ventricles
   (f) Parietal and occipital lobes and posterior interhemispheric fissure, posterior to the lateral ventricles
5. If there is ventricular dilation, measure the ventricular index in the coronal plane (Fig. 3.13). Capture an image showing both lateral and the third ventricles. Measure horizontally from the midline to

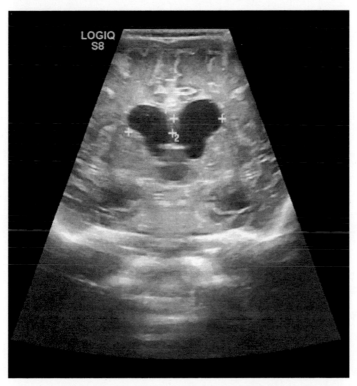

Fig. 3.12 Left (crosshairs labelled 1) and right ventricular (crosshairs labelled 2) indices on a coronal image taken at the level of the foramen of Monro. (Image courtesy of Birmingham Children's Hospital Referral and justification criteria for ultrasound of the neonatal head document.)

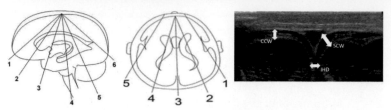

Fig. 3.13 Coronal *(left)* and sagittal *(middle)* imaging planes (1-5) through the anterior fontanelle. Measurements of the extraaxial spaces *(right)* at the calvarial vertex at the anterior fontanelle: Craniocortical width (*CCW*); Interhemispheric distance (*IHD*); Sinocortical width (*SCW*). (Images modified from the digital presentation by Richer EJ, et al. Review of Neonatal and Infant Cranial US. *Radiographics*. 2021;41(7):E206-E207.)

the most lateral aspect of the ventricles in the plane of the foramen of Munro.

6. In the sagittal plane, the transducer is placed longitudinally across the anterior fontanelle and angled to either side. The images to acquire include:

   (a) The midsagittal plane, at the interhemispheric fissure. At this level, the lateral ventricle (LV) is visualized with the caudate nucleus and thalamus housed within its course from anterior to posterior.

   (b) The caudothalamic groove, formed from the junction of caudate and thalamus, is the most common site of germinal matrix haemorrhage.

   (c) Right and left parasagittal images demonstrate a peripheral aspect of the ventricles and cerebral hemisphere including the temporal lobes.

7. Use the high-frequency linear probe to obtain targeted images of extraaxial spaces at the calvarial vertex at the anterior fontanelle.

8. Check patency and direction of flow in the superior sagittal sinus with colour Doppler.

9. Color Doppler US may also be used to evaluate bridging veins crossing normal subarachnoid space and identify flow in the superior sagittal sinus.

10. Measure sinocortical width (SCW), craniocortical width (CCW), and interhemispheric distance (IHD). Upper limit of normal values: SCW, 3 mm; CCW, 4 mm, IHD, 6 mm

Further Reading

Gupta P, Sodhi KS, Saxena AK, et al. Neonatal cranial sonography: a concise review for clinicians. *J Pediatr Neurosci*. 2016;11(1):7–13.

Maller VV, Cohen HL. Neonatal head ultrasound: a review and update—part 1: techniques and evaluation of the premature neonate. *Ultrasound Q*. 2019;35(3): 202–211.

Maller VV, Choudhri AF, Cohen HL. Neonatal head ultrasound: a review and update—part 2: the term neonate and analysis of brain anomalies. *Ultrasound Q*. 2019;35(3):212–223.

Richer EJ, Riedesel EL, Linam LE. Review of neonatal and infant cranial US. *Radiographics*. 2021;41(7):E206–E207.

Neonatal spine

Sonographic assessment of the neonatal spine should take place within the first 3 to 4 months of life, before ossification of the spinal processes. However, if there is delayed ossification or a defect in the vertebral column, US may still be possible even after 6 months of age. MRI is indicated when the infant is older than 4 months of age, when US is abnormal or equivocal, when there are neurological signs or when there is an anorectal malformation or discharging lesion.

Indications

1. Atypical sacral dimple such as large (>5 mm), high on the back (>2.5 cm from the anus) or appearing in combination with other lesions
2. Other stigmata of spinal dysraphism (e.g. hair tuff, skin tag, haemangioma, sinus tract, skin pigmentation)
3. Palpable sacral mass
4. Screening for associated anomalies (e.g. VACTERL screen, cloacal exstrophy, anorectal atresia)

Contraindications

Contraindications for US caused by the potential risk of infection include patients with spina bifida aperta, CSF-excreting lesions, discharging sinus or who are post spinal surgery

Equipment

Linear, high-frequency probe

Patient preparation

Position the infant prone on a soft pillow to assist positioning because spinal flexion allows a better acoustic window. Raise the patient's head to enable CSF to distend the distal thecal sac, aiding visualization of all structures.

Technique

1. The neonatal spine anatomy is examined in transverse and longitudinal planes. If sacral dimple present, assess for any dermal sinus tract.
2. Longitudinal (Fig. 3.14 and Fig. 3.15)
   (a) Sacral vertebral bodies and lumbosacral junction (standard: five sacral segments and a barely ossified coccyx)
   (b) Lumbar vertebral bodies (standard: five lumbar vertebrae).
   (c) Identify the conus medullaris and determine the termination point where it tapers. Normal level is at L2 vertebra (termination below the lower border of L2 is considered abnormal).
   (d) Evaluate the filum terminale; normal: less than 2 mm
3. Transverse
   (a) Conus medullaris surrounded by echogenic nerve roots
   (b) Nerve roots of the cauda equina; these should demonstrate oscillatory movements with respiration in dynamic imaging

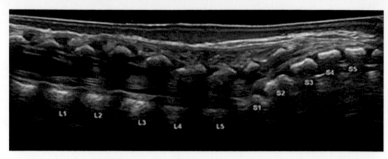

Fig. 3.14 Normal longitudinal view of the lumbosacral spine. (Image courtesy of the Birmingham Children's Hospital Referral and justification criteria for ultrasound of the neonatal spine document.)

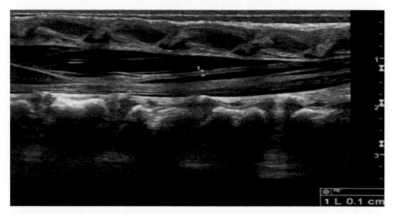

Fig. 3.15 Normal conus medullaris and filum terminale. (Image courtesy of the Birmingham Children's Hospital Referral and justification criteria for ultrasound of the neonatal spine document.)

Abnormalities to look for on neonatal spine USS include:

1. Any masses such as lipoma or thickening of the cauda equina
2. Thickening of the filum terminale greater than 2 mm
3. Low conus or tethered cord syndrome
4. Absent cauda equina nerve root movement: associated with a tethered cord
5. Dermal sinus tract: associated with sacral dimple or skin demarcation

Further Reading

Dick EA, Patel K, Owens CM, et al. Spinal ultrasound in infants. *Br J Radiol.* 2002;75(892):384–392.

Fitzgerald K. Ultrasound examination of the neonatal spine. *Australas J Ultrasound Med.* 2011;14(1):39–41.

Lowe LH, Johanek AJ, Moore CW. Sonography of the neonatal spine: part 1, normal anatomy, imaging pitfalls, and variations that may simulate disorders. *AJR Am J Roentgenol.* 2007;188(3):733–738.

Lowe LH, Johanek AJ, Moore CW. Sonography of the neonatal spine: part 2, spinal disorders. *AJR Am J Roentgenol.* 2007;188(3):739–744.

Robinson AJ, Russell S, Rimmer S. The value of ultrasonic examination of the lumbar spine in infants with specific reference to cutaneous markers of occult spinal dysraphism. *Clin Radiol.* 2005;60(1):72–77.

Szyszko TA, Watson M. The value of ultrasonographic examination of the lumbar spine in infants with specific reference to cutaneous markers of occult spinal dysraphism. *Clin Radiol.* 2005;60(8):935.

The Royal College of Radiologists. *iRefer: Making the Best Use of clinical Radiology,* 8th ed, Guidelines P19 and P08. <https://www.irefer.org.uk/guidelines/list/paediatrics>.

3

Radiography

Ventriculoperitoneal shunt series

The shunt series is a set of radiographs performed to assess the location and integrity of a ventriculoperitoneal shunt.

Indications

Shunt failure from mechanical malfunction: shunt breakage, disconnection, migration or obstruction; other shunt-related complications such as abdominal ileus or bowel perforation

Technique

1. The aim of the shunt series is to delineate the entire course of the shunt.
2. This includes frontal and lateral radiography of the head and neck and frontal radiography of the chest and abdomen and may vary according to local protocols.

Further Reading

Beattie G, Sinha S, Mason S, et al. Do children with suspected shunt failure also require a radiographic shunt series if head CT is going to be, or has been, performed? *Arch Dis Child.* 2021;106(6):609–611.

Pitetti R. Emergency department evaluation of ventricular shunt malfunction: is the shunt series really necessary? *Pediatr Emerg Care.* 2007;23(3):137–141.

Wallace AN, McConathy J, Menias CO, et al. Imaging evaluation of CSF shunts. *AJR Am J Roentgenol.* 2014;202(1):38–53.

BREAST

A breast mass in a young boy or girl may arise from normal and abnormal breast development. Other causes of breast masses include infection, trauma and cyst formation. After the onset of puberty, most cases of breast enlargement arise from benign fibroadenoma in girls and gynecomastia in boys. Malignant lesions of the breast in children are rare. In girls, diagnostic interventions may injure the developing breast and cause subsequent disfigurement. As such, a prudent course should be followed in the diagnosis of breast lesions. That said, biopsy or excision should still be considered for lesions with suspicious imaging findings or progressive growth.

Ultrasound

Indications

Unilateral gynaecomastia, chest wall asymmetry, breast and axillary lumps

Equipment

Linear, high-frequency probe

Patient preparation

Refer to the first section of this chapter.

Technique

1. Image any lesion two planes: radial and anti-radial or transverse and longitudinal.
2. Divide the breast into four quadrants: upper inner and outer; lower inner and outer quadrants. The area of the breast to be examined should extend superior to the clavicle, inferior to the inframammary fold, medial to midline and lateral to mid axillary line. The axilla should also be included as part of the breast examination.
3. Obtain at least one image in each quadrant to document that the area was scanned.
4. If a lesion is identified, record the size and position.
5. Consider examining the other breast for comparison (e.g. bilateral gynaecomastia).

Further Reading

Chung EM, Cube R, Hall GJ, et al. Breast masses in children and adolescents: radiologic-pathologic correlation. *Radiographics*. 2009;29(3):907–931.

Yang S, Leng Y, Chau CM, et al. The ins and outs of male breast and anterior chest wall lesions from childhood to adulthood. *Clin Radiol*. 2022;77(7): 503–513.

NON-ACCIDENTAL INJURIES

Child Protection and the Role of the Radiologist

Child protection is the responsibility of all health care professionals and members of the radiology department play a key role as they perform numerous in and outpatient investigations in young children. A measured approach is required, but practitioners should be alert to the presence of inappropriate bruising or scratches to the skin when a child is undressed for an investigation. There also needs to be a cognizance of unkempt children or inappropriate interactions (shouting or abusive language) between carers and children or their siblings.

Non-ambulant children rarely sustain fractures (of any sort), and a clear history of an accidental mechanism should be sought during consultation with emergency department or other referring colleagues. If there are concerns, these should be raised promptly via appropriate hospital pathways, typically via the local child safeguarding team.

There are clearly established radiology guidelines produced by the Royal College of Radiologists and endorsed by the Royal College of Paediatric and Child Health. These describe the imaging pathway in various scenarios based on age of child and whether there are features of a head injury.

Although we refer to the above document for detailed imaging protocols, the key points are:

3

1. A skeletal survey is performed to assess for fractures or injuries not apparent on clinical examination.
    (a) All children younger than 2 years of age should have a skeletal survey.
    (b) A skeletal survey is divided into parts 1 and 2, and the study should not be considered complete until both parts are performed and reported (unless there are extenuating circumstances).
    (c) Part 2 of the skeletal survey is performed 11–14 days after part 1 and assesses for healing fractures or evolving subperiosteal new bone formation. As a consequence, there is potentially increased accuracy of injury dating and greater sensitivity for subtle fracture detection.
2. All children younger than 1 year of age should have a non-contrast head CT.
3. Children between 1 year and 2 years of age should have a non-contrast head CT if there are concerns for a head injury (e.g. scalp swelling or neurological dysfunction).
4. Children with an abnormal head CT (or normal CT with ongoing neurology) should have a non-contrast brain and whole-spine MRI.
5. Children older than 2 years of age do not routinely have a full skeletal survey but rather discrete body parts guided by clinical concerns.

Other important components of the safeguarding process include:

1. Open and prompt communication with the referring and safeguarding teams is essential.
2. The skeletal survey should be double reported and a consensus agreement reached but with differing opinions noted.
3. In isolation, the radiologist cannot diagnose abusive injuries (many injuries can be classed as non-specific), and a multidisciplinary approach is always required.
4. There is an absolute requirement for high-quality imaging with well-trained and experienced radiographers.
5. It is essential for networks between smaller hospitals and tertiary centres to provide radiology and radiographer support and training.
6. Radiography is the mainstay of skeletal and body imaging; however, CT (e.g. chest) can be used for troubleshooting.
7. In children who are acutely unwell (e.g. haemodynamic instability secondary to intraabdominal bleeding), recognized paediatric trauma guidelines should be adhered to.

The vast majority of children are not subject to abusive injuries, but the radiology team should always be alert to those who are.

Further Reading

Royal College of Radiologists, The Society and College of Radiographers. *The Radiological Investigation of Suspected Physical Abuse in Children*, revised first edition—A joint publication from The Royal College of Radiologists and The Society and College of Radiographers, endorsed by the Royal College of Paediatrics and Child Health. <https://www.rcr.ac.uk/system/files/publication/field_publication_files/bfcr174_suspected_physical_abuse.pdf>.

Gastrointestinal system
Ravivarma Balasubramaniam

METHODS OF IMAGING THE GASTROINTESTINAL TRACT

1. Plain film
2. Barium swallow
3. Barium meal
4. Barium follow-through
5. Small bowel enema
6. Barium enema
7. Ultrasound (US):
   (a) Transabdominal
   (b) Endosonography
8. Computed tomography (CT)
9. Magnetic resonance imaging (MRI)
10. Angiography
11. Radionuclide imaging:
    (a) Inflammatory bowel disease
    (b) Gastro-oesophageal reflux
    (c) Gastric emptying
    (d) Bile reflux study
    (e) Meckel's scan
    (f) Gastrointestinal (GI) bleeding.

INTRODUCTION TO CONTRAST MEDIA

WATER-SOLUBLE CONTRAST AGENTS
(See Also Chapter 2)

Numerous water-soluble contrast agents are available. The two agents most widely used are Gastrografin and Gastromiro. Gastrografin is an aniseed-tasting, high-osmolarity contrast agent (sodium amidotrizoate and meglumine amidotrizoate), containing a wetting agent for oral or rectal use. Although primarily used in diagnosis, its high osmolarity is also exploited to help achieve bowel catharsis in CT colonography and to diagnose and treat patients with meconium ileus and adhesive small bowel obstruction. Its use should be monitored in frail and very young patients because of the risk of profound fluid and electrolyte disturbance. It is diluted one part Gastrografin to four parts water for rectal administration.

Low-osmolar contrast agents may be given orally, but the taste is unpleasant. Gastromiro, a low-osmolarity contrast agent containing iopamidol, is a more palatable orange-flavoured alternative.

Indications

1. Suspected perforation
2. Meconium ileus
3. To identify bowel lumen and communications with bowel lumen on CT. A dilute (c. 3%) solution of water-soluble contrast medium (e.g. 30 mL of Gastrografin in 1 L of flavoured drink) is used to minimize beam-hardening artefact.
4. Assessment for complications in the postoperative bowel
5. Low-osmolar contrast media (LOCM) is advised if the patient is vulnerable to aspiration.

Complications

1. Hyperosmolar contrast media (HOCM) can precipitate pulmonary oedema if aspirated (not LOCM)
2. HOCM can cause hypovolaemia and electrolyte disturbance caused by the hyperosmolality of the contrast media drawing fluid into the bowel (not LOCM)
3. May precipitate in hyperchlorhydric gastric acid (i.e. 0.1 M HCl).

GASES

1. **Oesophagus, stomach and duodenum:** The contrast agent should be palatable, produce an adequate volume of gas (200–400 mL) and not compromise the barium coating with bubbles, residue or by dilution. Carbon dioxide used in conjunction with barium achieves a 'double-contrast' effect. For the upper GI tract, CO_2 is administered orally in the form of gas-producing granules or powder (sodium bicarbonate) mixed with fluid (citric acid) Carbex. Alternative CO_2-producing drinks such as tonic water or ginger ale deliver less predictable volumes of gas and dilute the barium but may be used for functional studies in which barium coating and fine mucosal detail are not essential.
2. **Large bowel:** Pressure-regulated CO_2 insufflating pumps for the large bowel are widely available and produce optimal distension with continuous delivery of CO_2 at 15–25 mmHg.[1] Insufflation can also be administered by hand pump, but the carbon dioxide tends to resorb more quickly and produces inferior bowel distension compared with using air.[2] Room air administered per rectum via a hand pump attached to the enema tube is less desirable. Peaks and troughs in pressure associated with manual insufflation are more likely to cause discomfort and are associated with a higher risk of perforation.

Table 4.1   Barium Suspensions and Dilutions With Water to Give a Lower Density

Proprietary Name	Density (w/v): Use
EPI-C	150%: large bowel
E-Z-Cat	1%–2%: CT of the GI tract
E-Z HD	250%: oesophagus, stomach and duodenum
E-Z Paque	100%: small intestine
Micropaque DC	100%: oesophagus, stomach and duodenum
Micropaque liquid	100%: small and large bowel
Micropaque powder	76%: small and large bowel
Polibar	115%: large bowel
Polibar rapid	100%: large bowel

CT, Computed tomography; GI, gastrointestinal.

4

BARIUM

The use of barium has declined in the past decade, superseded by cross-sectional imaging; however, it still has a small number of indications as described in this chapter.

Barium suspension is made up of finely ground barium sulphate particles in the range of 0.3–1.0 μm. A non-ionic stabilizer creates a stable suspension and prevents clumping. The resulting solution has a pH of 5.3, which makes it stable in gastric acid.

There are many preparations of barium suspensions in use. Preparations are diluted with water to reduce the density (Table 4.1) and must be shaken well immediately before use.

Differing properties are required for optimal coating, which varies according to the anatomical site.

1. Barium swallow (e.g. E-Z HD 200%–250% 100–150 mL, as required).
2. Barium meal (e.g. E-Z HD 250% w/v). This is a high-density, low-viscosity barium that delivers a thin coating which is still sufficiently dense for satisfactory opacification in double-contrast studies. Simethicone and sorbitol provide antifoaming and coating properties.
3. Barium follow-through (e.g. E-Z Paque 60%–100% w/v 300 mL; can be reduced to 150 mL if performed after a barium meal). Sorbitol induces osmotic hyperperistalsis, especially when combined with metoclopramide and Gastrografin, and is partially resistant to flocculation.
4. Small bowel enema (e.g. two tubs of E-Z Paque, made up to 1500 mL; 60% w/v)

5. Barium enema (e.g. Polibar 115% w/v 500 mL or more, as required). Use reduced density between 20% and 40% w/v for single contrast examinations

Advantages

1. The main advantage of barium over water-soluble contrast agents is better coating, resulting in better mucosal detail.
2. Low cost

Disadvantages

1. Precludes accurate subsequent abdominal CT interpretation with potential delays of up to 2 weeks to allow satisfactory clearance of the barium
2. High morbidity associated with barium entering the peritoneal cavity (see later)

Complications

1. **Perforation:** Water-soluble contrast medium should be the initial agent used for any investigation in which there is a risk or suspicion of perforation. Barium leak into the peritoneal cavity is rare but extremely serious, resulting in pain and severe hypovolaemic shock. Treatment consists of intravenous fluid resuscitation, emergency surgery and washout with antibiotics. The mortality rate is in the order of 50%; of patients who survive, 30% will develop granulomata and peritoneal adhesions. Barium entering the mediastinal and pleural cavity also carries a significant mortality rate.
2. **Aspiration:** Aspirated barium is relatively harmless. Sequelae include pneumonitis and granuloma formation. Prompt physiotherapy is required (for both aspirated barium and LOCM) if the patient is unable to voluntarily clear the barium before leaving the hospital.
3. **Intravasation:** This very rare complication may result in a barium pulmonary embolus, which carries a mortality rate of 80%.

PHARMACOLOGICAL AGENTS

Hyoscine-N-Butylbromide (Buscopan)

This is an antimuscarinic agent and thus inhibits both intestinal motility and gastric secretion. It is not recommended in children.[1]

Indications

1. Reduce bowel spasm, which can cause diagnostic difficulty
2. To improve diagnostic accuracy in CT and MRI
3. Reduce patient distress of discomfort after bowel insufflation

Adult dose

20 mg IV may be repeated at 15-min intervals up to a dose of 40 mg in 1 h.

Advantages

1. Immediate onset of action
2. Short duration of action (~5–10 min)
3. Low cost

Side effects

1. Antimuscarinic blurring of vision, dry mouth, transient bradycardia followed by tachycardia; rare side effects of urinary retention and acute gastric dilatation
2. Precipitation of closed-angle glaucoma through pupillary dilation, which is an ophthalmological emergency

Contraindications

1. Cardiac, unstable angina or tachyarrhythmias
2. Closed-angle glaucoma (Buscopan can precipitate closed-angle glaucoma and result in related symptoms presenting in an undiagnosed patient. Therefore, the patient should be made aware of this eventuality during the procedure; see Aftercare section.)
3. Severe prostatism or bladder outflow obstruction

Aftercare

1. Patients should not drive until blurred vision has resolved.
2. A postprocedure patient information leaflet should explicitly state that in the rare event of sudden onset of a painful or painless red eye, the patient must attend A&E immediately.

Glucagon

This polypeptide hormone produced by the alpha cells of the islets of Langerhans in the pancreas has a predominantly hyperglycaemic effect but also causes smooth muscle relaxation. It is used in the United States as an alternative to hyoscine, which is not licensed there.

Indications

To decrease bowel motility as a diagnostic aid for GI studies.

Adult dose

- 0.2–0.5 mg IV over 1 min (or 1 mg intramuscular (IM)) for barium meal
- 0.5–0.75 mg IV over 1 min (1.0–2.0 mg IM) for barium enema
- 1 mg IM for CT or MRI small bowel imaging
- Bolus doses greater than 1 mg administered via IV may cause nausea and vomiting and are not recommended.

Advantages

1. More potent smooth muscle relaxant than hyoscine; arrests small bowel peristalsis more reliably and effect lasts longer compared with hyoscine[2]

2. Short duration of action (~15–20 min) similar in length to hyoscine
3. Does not interfere with small bowel transit time (SBTT)

Disadvantages

1. Relatively long onset of action (1 min), similar to hyoscine
2. Relatively high cost compared with hyoscine.

Side effects

1. Nausea (common), vomiting (uncommon) and abdominal pain (rare)
2. Paradoxically can cause hypoglycaemia, especially in those who have fasted
3. Hypersensitivity reactions (rare)

Contraindications

1. Phaeochromocytoma, precipitating a catecholamine crisis
2. Insulinoma (causes reactive hypoglycaemia)
3. Glucagonoma

Aftercare

No specific instructions

Metoclopramide (Maxolon)[3]

Indications

As a dopamine antagonist, metoclopramide stimulates gastric emptying, aids duodenal intubation and accelerates small-intestinal transit by coordinating peristalsis and dilating the duodenal bulb.

Contraindications

1. Parkinson's disease, epilepsy
2. Any suspicion of GI obstruction, bleeding or perforation

Adult dose

10–20 mg oral OR 10 mg IM OR 10 mg by slow IV injection

Advantages

1. Produces rapid gastric emptying and therefore increased jejunal peristalsis
2. Antiemetic effect

Side effects

Dystonic side effects with doses exceeding 0.5 mg kg^{-1}. This is more common in children and young adults. Side effects are usually self-limiting, but if hypotension or marked sedation occurs, then IM administration of an anticholinergic drug (e.g. biperiden 5 mg or procyclidine 5 mg)[4] is usually effective in relieving signs and symptoms within 20 min.

Aftercare

No specific instructions

References

Gases

1. *Guidelines for Use of Radiology in the Bowel Cancer Screening Programme.* 2nd ed. NHSBCSP Publication No 5; 09 November 2012.
2. Holemans JA, Matson MB, Hughes JA, et al. A comparison of air, carbon dioxide and air/carbon dioxide mixture as insufflation agents for double contrast barium enema. *Eur Radiol.* 1998;8:274–276.

Pharmacological Agents

1. Dyde R, Chapman AH, Gale R, et al. Precautions to be taken by radiologists and radiographers when prescribing hyoscine-N-butylbromide. *Clin Radiol.* 2008;63:739–743.
2. Froehlich JM, Daenzer M, von Weymarn C, et al. A peristaltic effect of hyoscine N-butylbromide versus glucagon on the small bowel assessed by magnetic resonance imaging. *Eur Radiol.* 2009;19:1387–1393.
3. Electronic Medicines Compendium. <http://www.medicines.org.uk>.
4. van Harten PN, Hoek HW, Kahn RS. Acute dystonia induced by drug treatment. *Br Med J.* 1999;319:623–626.

4

CONTRAST SWALLOW

Indication: Suspected Oesophageal Pathology

1. Endoscopy negative dysphagia or odynophagia (painful swallow)
2. Motility disorders
3. Globus sensation
4. Assessment of tracheo-oesophageal fistulae
5. Failed upper GI endoscopy
6. Timed barium swallow to monitor achalasia therapies[1]
7. Suspected primary or postoperative gastro-oesophageal perforation (though generally superseded by CT with oral prep)

Contraindications

None

Contrast Medium

1. E-Z HD 200%–250% 100 mL (or more, as required)
2. Water-soluble contrast agent if perforation is suspected (e.g. Conray, Gastrografin)
3. LOCM (~300 mg I mL^{-1}) is safest if there is a risk of aspiration
4. Gastrografin should NOT be used for the investigation of a tracheo-oesophageal fistula or when aspiration is a possibility. Use LOCM instead.
5. Barium should NOT be used initially if perforation is suspected. If perforation is not identified with a water-soluble contrast agent, then a barium examination should be considered.

Equipment

Rapid fluoroscopy images, rapid exposures (6 frames s^{-1}) or video recording may be required for assessment of the laryngopharynx and upper oesophagus during deglutition.

Patient Preparation

None (but as for barium meal if the stomach is also to be examined)

Technique

1. Start with the patient in the erect position, right anterior oblique (RAO) position to project the oesophagus clear of the spine. An ample mouthful of barium is swallowed, and the bolus is observed under fluoroscopy for dynamic assessment to assess the function of the oesophagus. Then further mouthfuls are swallowed with spot exposure(s) to include the whole oesophagus with dedicated anterior posterior (AP) views of the gastro-oesophageal junction.
2. Dynamic coned views of the hypopharynx with a frame rate of 3–4 s^{-1}, in AP and lateral, and views during patient swallowing
3. The patient is placed semiprone in a 'recovery position' in a left posterior oblique (LPO) position. A distended single-contrast view while drinking identifies hernias, subtle mucosal rings and varices.
4. Modifications may be required depending on the clinical indication.
   (a) If dysmotility is suspected, barium should be mixed with bread or a marshmallow bolus and observed under fluoroscopy to correlate symptoms with the passage of the bolus in the erect position.
   (b) If perforation is suspected, CT with quadruple strength oral contrast (100 mL Omnipaque 300 made up to 1 L with water) is more sensitive and provides improved anatomical localization of the site of perforation whilst also providing additional information on associated complications such as perioesophageal collections.[2]

Aftercare

Eat and drink as normal but with extra fluids.

Complications

1. Leakage of barium from an unsuspected perforation
2. Aspiration

References

1. Andersson M, Lundell L, Kostic S, et al. Evaluation of the response to treatment in patients with idiopathic achalasia by the timed barium esophagogram: results from a randomized clinical trial. *Dis Esophagus.* 2009;22(3):264–273.
2. Lantos JE, Levine MS, Rubesin SE, et al. Comparison between esophagography and chest computed tomography for evaluation of leaks after esophagectomy and gastric pull-through. *J Thorac Imaging.* 2013;28(2):121–128.

BARIUM MEAL

Methods

1. Double contrast is the method of choice to demonstrate mucosal pattern.

2. Single contrast uses include the following:
   (a) Children: because it usually is not necessary to demonstrate mucosal pattern
   (b) To demonstrate gross pathology only, typically very frail patients unable to swallow gas granules

Indications

1. Failed upper GI endoscopy or patient unwilling to undergo endoscopy
2. Gastro-oesophageal reflux disease when lifestyle changes and empirical therapies are ineffective
3. Partial obstruction

Contraindication

Complete large bowel obstruction

Contrast Medium

1. E-Z HD 250% w/v 135 mL
2. Carbex granules (double-contrast technique)

Patient Preparation

1. Nil orally for 6 h before the examination
2. Assess contraindications to the pharmacological agents used

Preliminary Image

None

Technique

The double-contrast method (Fig. 4.1):

1. A gas-producing agent is swallowed.
2. The patient then drinks the barium while lying on the left side, supported by their elbow. This position prevents the barium from reaching the duodenum too quickly, which can obscure the greater curve of the stomach.
3. The patient then lies supine and slightly on the right side to bring the barium up against the gastro-oesophageal junction. This manoeuvre is screened to assess for reflux, which may be revealed by asking the patient to cough or to swallow water while in this position (the 'water siphon' test). (Extreme provocation testing with the patient in a head-down position during swallowing is non-physiological.) If reflux is observed, images are taken to record the level to which it ascends. Clinically relevant reflux can be assessed by 24-h pH probe monitoring and by endoscopic evidence of oesophagitis.
4. An IV injection of a smooth muscle relaxant (Buscopan 20 mg or glucagon 250–500 mcg) may be given to better distend the stomach and to slow down the emptying of contrast into duodenum. (The administration of Buscopan has been shown to

not affect the detection of gastro-oesophageal reflux or hiatus hernia.)
5. The patient is asked to roll onto the right side and then quickly over in a complete circle, to finish in an RAO position. This roll is performed to coat the gastric mucosa with barium. Good coating has been achieved if the areae gastricae in the antrum are visible.

Images

Comprehensive documentation of the examination is provided by the following:

1. Spot exposures of the stomach (lying):
   (a) RAO to demonstrate the antrum and greater curve
   (b) Supine to demonstrate the antrum and body
   (c) LAO to demonstrate the lesser curve en face
   (d) Left lateral tilted, head up 45 degrees to demonstrate the fundus

From the left lateral position, the patient returns to a supine position and then rolls onto the left side and over into a prone position. This sequence of movements is required to avoid barium flooding into the duodenal loop, which would occur if the patient were to roll onto the right side to achieve a prone position.

2. Spot image of the duodenal loop (lying):
   (a) Prone: The patient lies on a compression pad to prevent barium from flooding into the duodenum.

An additional view to demonstrate the anterior wall of the duodenal loop may be taken in an RAO position.

3. Spot images of the duodenal cap (lying):
   (a) Prone
   (b) RAO: The patient attains this position from the prone position by rolling first onto the left side, for the reasons mentioned previously.
   (c) Supine
   (d) LAO
4. Additional views of the fundus in an erect position may be taken at this stage if there is suspicion of a fundal lesion.
5. Spot images of the oesophagus are taken, while barium is being swallowed, to complete the examination.

Complications

1. Leakage of barium from an unsuspected perforation
2. Aspiration
3. Conversion of a partial large bowel obstruction into a complete obstruction by the impaction of barium
4. Barium appendicitis if barium impacts in the appendix (exceedingly rare)
5. Side effects of the pharmacological agents used

Roll quickly in a complete circle 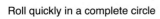 to coat the stomach with barium and finish in RAO position

Image	RAO	Supine	LAO	Left lateral tilted head up
Position				45°
Image				
Demonstrates	Antrum + greater curve	Antrum + body	Lesser curve en face	Fundus

A

Turn back from left lateral   to finish   Compression pad

Spot views of cap

Image	Prone	Prone	RAO	Supine	LAO
Position		(a)	(b)	(c)	(d)
Image		(a)	(b)		
		(c)	(d)		
Demonstrates	Duodenal loop	Caps			

B

Image	Erect	Erect caps		Swallow RAO
		RAO	Stoop LAO	
Position				
Image				
Demonstrates	Fundus	Caps		Oesophagus

C

Fig. 4.1 Barium meal sequence. Note that in **A, B** and **C** the patient position is depicted as if the operator were standing at the end of the screening table looking towards the patient's head. *LAO*, Left anterior oblique; *RAO*, right anterior oblique.

SMALL BOWEL FOLLOW-THROUGH

Methods

1. Single contrast
2. With the addition of an effervescent agent
3. With the addition of a pneumocolon technique[1]

Indications

Many of the indications for small bowel follow-through stated here have been superseded by CT or MRI. However, being a dynamic study, the investigation still gives functional information that can be of value.

1. Pain with weight loss
2. Diarrhoea
3. Transfusion-dependent anaemia or GI bleeding unexplained by colonic or gastric investigation[2]
4. Partial obstruction
5. Suspected abnormal small bowel transit time
6. Malabsorption
7. Small bowel adhesive obstruction (water-soluble contrast)[3,4]
8. Surgical treating planning, particularly in patients who have had previous GI resection.

Contraindications

1. Complete or high-grade obstruction is better evaluated by CT examination; without oral contrast as the intraluminal fluid caused by the obstruction functions as a natural contrast agent.
2. Suspected perforation is better evaluated by CT.

Contrast Medium

E-Z Paque 100% w/v 300 mL usually given divided over 20 min. The transit time through the small bowel is reduced by the addition of 10 mL of Gastrografin to the barium, improving distension and reducing flocculation.

Water-soluble small bowel contrast studies are rarely diagnostic because contrast becomes diluted in small bowel fluid, resulting in poor mucosal and anatomic detail. An exception is in adhesional small bowel obstruction, in which conservative investigation and 'treatment' with water-soluble contrast agents (frequently Gastrografin) may reduce the need for surgical intervention.[3,4] In this case, limited images are usually acquired at time intervals such as 1, 4 and 24 h, stopping when contrast is seen in the colon.

Patient Preparation

Metoclopramide 20 mg orally may be given before or during the examination to enhance gastric emptying.

Preliminary Image

If the patient is vomiting, a plain abdominal film should be performed to exclude high-grade small bowel obstruction.

Technique

The aim is to deliver a single continuous column of barium into the small bowel. This is achieved by the addition of 10 mL of Gastrografin to the barium solution and the patient lying on the right side to enhance gastric emptying. If a follow-through examination is combined with a barium meal, glucagon can be used for the duodenal cap views rather than Buscopan because it has a short length of action and does not interfere with the SBTT.

4

Images

1. Prone PA images of the abdomen are taken every 15–20 min during the first hour and subsequently every 20–30 min until the colon is reached. The prone position is used because the pressure on the abdomen helps separate the loops of the small bowel.
2. Each image should be reviewed, and spot supine fluoroscopic views, using a compression device or pad if appropriate, may be considered.
3. Dedicated spot views of the terminal ileum are routinely acquired.

Additional Images

1. To separate loops of the small bowel
   (a) Compression with fluoroscopy
   (b) With the x-ray tube angled into the pelvis
   (c) Obliques, in particular with the right side raised for terminal ileum views or occasionally with the patient tilted head down
   (d) Pneumocolon:[1] gaseous insufflation of the colon via a rectal tube after barium arrives in the caecum, which often results in good-quality double-contrast views of the terminal ileum
2. Erect image: occasionally used to reveal any fluid levels caused by contrast medium retained within diverticula

Aftercare

As for barium meal

Complications

As for barium meal

References

1. Pickhardt PJ. The peroral pneumocolon revisited: a valuable fluoroscopic and CT technique for ileocecal evaluation. *Abdom Imaging*. 2012;37(3):313–325.
2. Goddard AF, James MW, McIntyreet AS, et al. Guidelines for the management of iron deficiency anaemia. *Gut*. 2011;60:1309–1316.
3. Catena F, Di Saverio S, Kelly MD, et al. Bologna guidelines for diagnosis and management of Adhesive Small Bowel Obstruction (ASBO): 2010 evidence-based guidelines of the World Society of Emergency Surgery. *World J Emerg Surg*. 2011;6:5.

4. Abbas S, Bissett IP, Parry BR. Does the oral administration of water soluble contrast media followed by serial abdominal radiographs during the following 24 h predict the need for early operation or resolution? *Cochrane Database Syst Rev.* 2007;(3).

SMALL BOWEL ENEMA

This has been largely superseded by MRI of the small bowel.

Advantage

This procedure gives better distension and visualization of the proximal small bowel than that achieved by a barium follow-through because of the rapid infusion of a large continuous column of contrast medium directly into the jejunum. However, the degree of distal small bowel distension by small bowel enema and small bowel follow-through methods is usually sufficient.

Disadvantages

1. Nasal or oral intubation may be unpleasant for the patient and may prove difficult.
2. A longer room time and greater staff resources are required.
3. Potentially higher radiation dose to the patient (screening the tube into position)

Indications and Contraindications

These are the same as for a barium follow-through. In some departments, it is only performed in the case of an equivocal follow-through.

Contrast Medium

1. Single contrast: e.g. E-Z Paque 70% w/v diluted
2. 600 mL of 0.5% methylcellulose after 500 mL of 70% w/v barium[1]

Equipment

A choice of tubes is available:

1. Bilbao-Dotter tube (Cook Ltd) with a guidewire (the tube is blind ending). Comes in various sizes and modifications, including one variant with an inflatable balloon at the end to prevent reflux into the stomach.
2. Silk tube (E. Merck Ltd). This is a 10-Fr, 140-cm-long tube. It is made of polyurethane and the stylet, and the internal lumen of the tube are coated with a water-activated lubricant to facilitate the smooth removal of the stylet after insertion.

Patient Preparation

1. Nothing by mouth after midnight
2. Stop antispasmodic drugs 1 day before the examination.
3. Consider a tetracaine lozenge 30 mg 30 min before the examination.

Preliminary Image

If the patient is vomiting, a plain abdominal film to exclude small bowel obstruction.

Technique

1. The patient sits on the edge of the x-ray table. If a per-nasal approach is planned, the patency of the nasal passages is checked by asking the patient to sniff with one nostril occluded. The pharynx is anaesthetized with lidocaine spray or Xylocaine gel instilled into a nostril. The Silk tube should be passed with the guidewire prelubricated and fully within the tube; for the Bilbao-Dotter tube, the guidewire is introduced after the tube tip is in the stomach.

2. The tube is then passed through the nose or the mouth, and brief lateral screening of the neck may be helpful in negotiating the epiglottic region. The patient is asked to swallow with the neck flexed as the tube is passed through the pharynx. The tube is then advanced into the gastric antrum.

3. The patient then lies down, and the tube is advanced into the duodenum. Various manoeuvres may be used, alone or in combination, to help this part of the procedure, which can be difficult:

   (a) Leave the patient for 20 min with the guidewire removed and redundant tube in the stomach. Peristalsis will often pass the tube through the pylorus without further intervention. If this does not succeed, do the next step.

   (b) Put the patient on their left side so that the gastric air bubble rises to the antrum, thus straightening out the stomach.

   (c) Advance the tube whilst applying clockwise rotational motion (as viewed from the head of the patient looking towards the feet).

   (d) Get the patient to sit up to try to overcome the tendency of the tube to coil in the fundus of the stomach.

   (e) Metoclopramide (20 mg IV) may stimulate coordinated peristalsis and progress the tube.

   (f) Apply pressure to the epigastrium.

   (g) Squirt contrast down the tube to stimulate peristalsis.

4. When the tip of the tube has been passed through the pylorus, the guidewire tip is maintained at the pylorus as the tube is passed over it along the duodenum to the level of the ligament of Treitz. The tube is ideally passed beyond the duodenojejunal flexure to diminish the risk of aspiration caused by reflux of barium back into the stomach.

5. Barium is then run in, ideally with a controllable mechanical pump, or by gravity. Initially start at 50 mL min^{-1}, and with regular initial screening, aim to 'chase' the leading edge of the barium distally to maintain an unbroken column of contrast within the small bowel. The infusion can usually be increased rapidly to 100 mL min^{-1}, depending on the progress of the barium through the bowel. If

4

methylcellulose is used, administer an initial bolus of 500 mL of barium followed by a continuous infusion until the barium has reached the colon.

6. The tube is then withdrawn, aspirating any residual fluid in the stomach to decrease the risk of aspiration.

7. If the terminal ileum is obscured at the end of the examination, it can be helpful to further rescreen the patient after an interval once barium has emptied into the colon because better views may be then obtained. A pneumocolon, as per small bowel follow-through, may also help.

Images

Magnified views of each quadrant are recommended with at least one good view of the terminal ileum and an overall view of the abdomen. Fluoroscopic 'grab' images of the examination during the filling phase are also useful because they help record and assess motility.

Modification of Technique

In patients with malabsorption, especially if an excess of fluid has been shown on the preliminary image, the volume of barium should be increased (240–260 mL). Compression views of bowel loops should be obtained before obtaining double contrast. Flocculation is likely to occur early. If it is important to obtain images of the duodenum, the catheter tip should be sited proximal to the ligament of Treitz.

Aftercare

The patient should be warned that diarrhoea may occur as a result of the large volume of fluid given.

Complications

1. Aspiration
2. Perforation of the bowel owing to manipulation of the guidewire (very rare)

Reference

1. Ha HK, Park KB, Kim PN, et al. Use of methylcellulose in small bowel follow through examination: comparison with conventional series in normal subjects. *Abdom Imaging.* 1998;23(3):281–285.

Further Reading

Minordi LM, Vecchioli A, Guidi L, et al. Multidetector CT enteroclysis versus barium enteroclysis with methylcellulose in patients with suspected small bowel disease. *Eur Radiol.* 2006;16(7):1527–1536.

Nolan DJ. The true yield of the small intestinal barium study. *Endoscopy.* 1997;29(6):447–453.

BARIUM ENEMA

Methods

1. Double contrast: the method of choice to demonstrate mucosal pattern

2. Single contrast: uses:
   (a) Localization of an obstructing colonic lesion (use water-soluble contrast because surgery or stenting may be required shortly after the procedure)
   (b) Children: See Chapter 3.

Indication

For suspected large bowel pathology, colonoscopy is the investigation of choice allowing tissue diagnosis. Computed tomography colonography (CTC) is the alternative colon examination of choice and has superseded barium enema where facilities and expertise exist.[1–3]

If a tight stricture is demonstrated, run only a small volume of barium proximally to define the upper margin because otherwise the barium may impact. CTC avoids the risks of barium impaction.

Contraindications

Absolute

1. Toxic megacolon (CT is the radiological investigation of choice)
2. Pseudomembranous colitis
3. Recent biopsy[4] via:
   (a) Rigid endoscope within previous 5 days (the biopsy forceps used tend to be larger)
   (b) Flexible endoscope within previous 24 h (because the smaller biopsy forceps only allow superficial mucosal biopsies)

Relative

1. Incomplete bowel preparation. Consider if the patient can have extra preparation to return later that day or the next day.
2. Recent barium meal. It is advised to wait for 7–10 days.
3. Patient frailty

Contrast Medium

1. Polibar 115% w/v 500 mL (or more, as required)
2. Air

Equipment

Disposable enema tube and pump

Patient Preparation

Many regimens for bowel preparation exist. A suggested regimen is as follows:

For 3 days before examination

Low-residue diet

On the day before examination

1. Fluids only
2. Picolax at 08:00 and 18:00 h

Consider admitting frail older adults and those with social problems.

On the day of the examination

It is advisable to place patients with diabetes first on the list.

Technique

The double-contrast method:

1. The patient lies on their left side, and after initial digital rectal examination, the catheter is inserted gently into the rectum. It is taped firmly in position. The use of the retaining balloon is associated with a higher incidence of perforation. Connections are made to the barium reservoir and the hand pump for injecting air.
2. An IV injection of Buscopan (20 mg) or glucagon (1 mg) is given. Some radiologists choose to give the muscle relaxant halfway through the procedure instead of at this stage.[3]
3. The infusion of barium is commenced. Intermittent screening is required to check the progress of the barium, with a table tilt of 10 degrees head down. The barium is run to proximal sigmoid in the left lateral position. Repositioning from left lateral to prone may be required to navigate a tortuous sigmoid colon. The patient is returned to the left lateral position to fill the descending colon to the splenic flexure. Contrast is run to the hepatic flexure in the prone position until it tips into the right colon when barium administration should be paused. (Gentle puffs of air may be needed to encourage the barium to flow to the caecum.) The patient rolls onto the right and quickly onto the back. An adequate amount of barium in the right colon is confirmed with fluoroscopy. The column of barium within the distal colon is run back out by either lowering the infusion bag to the floor or tilting the table to the erect position.
4. The catheter tube is occluded, and air is gently pumped into the bowel to produce the double-contrast effect. The use of CO_2 gas has been shown to reduce the incidence of severe post-enema pain.

Exposures

There is great variation in views recommended. Fewer films may be taken to reduce the radiation dose. The sequence of positioning enables the barium to flow proximally to reach the caecal pole. Air is pumped in as required to distend the colon.

A suggested sequence of positioning and image acquisition using a standard over couch image intensifier includes the following:

Left lateral rectum; then roll the patient halfway back.

- RAO sigmoid; then roll the patient prone and insufflate to distend transverse colon. The patient lifts left side up to obtain.
- LPO sigmoid; then turn the patient supine
- AP view(s) of the whole colon.
- Raise the patient to the erect position. Further drainage of barium and reinflation of the colon may improve views of the sigmoid colon if initial images were flooded with barium. Obtain dedicated views of both flexures, with some LAO positioning for splenic flexure and

RAO positioning for hepatic flexure. Return the patient to the supine position.
- Over-couch views:
  - Left lateral decubitus
  - Right lateral decubitus
  - Prone angled view of rectosigmoid
- Dedicated views of the caecum and right colon, often with some RAO positioning (sometimes prior to the decubitus films)
- Dedicated views of any pathology encountered

Aftercare

1. The patient must not drive until any blurring of vision produced by Buscopan has resolved, usually within 30 min.
2. Patients should be warned that their bowel motions will be white for a few days after the examination. They may eat normally and should drink extra fluids to avoid barium impaction.

Antibiotic Prophylaxis in Barium Enema[5]

This is not routinely required, but barium enema is identified as the only lower GI intervention with a significant risk of endocarditis in patients with specific risk factors.

Offer antibiotic prophylaxis to those with:

- Previous infective endocarditis
- Acquired valvular heart disease with stenosis or regurgitation
- Valve replacement
- Structural congenital heart disease (but excluding isolated atrial septal defect, fully repaired ventricular septal defect or fully repaired patent ductus arteriosus)
- Hypertrophic cardiomyopathy

Complications (all are rare)

1. Cardiac arrhythmias induced by Buscopan or the procedure itself. This is the most frequent cause of death after barium enema.
2. Perforation of the bowel (often related to manipulation of the rectal catheter balloon) is the second most common cause of death after barium enema.
3. Transient bacteraemia
4. Side effects of the pharmacological agents used
5. Intramural barium
6. Venous intravasation. This may result in a barium pulmonary embolus, which carries an 80% mortality risk.

References
1. Halligan S, Wooldrage K, Dadswell E, et al. Computed tomographic colonography versus barium enema for diagnosis of colorectal cancer or large polyps in symptomatic patients (SIGGAR): a multicentre randomised trial. *Lancet.* 2013;381(9873):1185–1193.

2. Yee J, Kim DH, Rosen MP, et al. ACR Appropriateness Criteria colorectal cancer screening. *J Am Coll Radiol*. 2014;11(6):543–551.
3. Graser A, Stieber P, Nagel D, et al. Comparison of CT colonography, colonoscopy, sigmoidoscopy and faecal occult blood tests for the detection of advanced adenoma in an average risk population. *Gut*. 2009;58(2):241–248.
4. Low VH. What is the current recommended waiting time for performance of a gastrointestinal barium study after endoscopic biopsy of the upper or lower gastrointestinal tract? *AJR Am J Roentgenol*. 1998;170(4):1104–1105.
5. NICE. NICE Guidance. *Antimicrobial Prophylaxis Against Infective Endocarditis in Adults and Children Undergoing Interventional Procedures*. NICE Clinical Guidelines; 2008:64.

ENEMA VARIANTS

These variants have been superseded by CT but may provide extra information in selected cases.

THE 'INSTANT' ENEMA

Indications

1. To identify or confirm the level of suspected large bowel obstruction and to assess the degree of narrowing (e.g. sometimes helpful in stent planning)
2. Rarely, to show the extent and severity of mucosal lesions in active ulcerative colitis

Contraindications

1. Toxic megacolon
2. Rectal biopsy (as for barium enema)
3. Chronic ulcerative colitis: Optical colonoscopy to detect dysplasia and neoplasia in this high-risk group is preferred.
4. Crohn's colitis: Assessment in this situation is unreliable.

Contrast Medium

Water-soluble contrast (e.g. Urografin 150)

Preliminary Image

Plain abdominal film: to exclude:

1. Toxic megacolon
2. Perforation

Technique

1. The contrast medium is run until it flows into an obstructing lesion or dilated bowel loops.
2. Air insufflation is not required (i.e. single-contrast technique).

Images

Images are obtained as required, generally to include views of pathology encountered, but may include prone, left lateral decubitus and erect films as necessary.

AIR ENEMA

Very rarely used

Indication

Demonstrate the extent of ulcerative colitis

Technique

1. Insert a 14- to 16-Fr Foley catheter into rectum and inflate balloon (10–20 mL).
2. Take a preliminary overcouch AP film of abdomen.
3. View the film and without the patient moving, give relaxant (e.g. Buscopan) and then inflate air (gentle puffs) into catheter lumen.
4. Take an AP film of abdomen.

4

SINOGRAM

1. A water-soluble contrast medium should be used (e.g. Urografin 150).
2. A preliminary control film is taken to exclude the presence of a radio-opaque foreign body.
3. An appropriately sized Foley catheter is then inserted into the orifice of the sinus. The balloon may be inflated inside the sinus to prevent retrograde flow. Alternatively, the balloon may be inflated outside the sinus and pushed to the skin using Spencer-Wells forceps or similar to secure a seal.
4. The contrast medium is injected carefully under fluoroscopic control.
5. Fluoroscopic 'grab' images supplemented by proper exposures are taken as required, including tangential views.

RETROGRADE ILEOGRAM

Indication

To demonstrate anatomy of small bowel in patients with an ileostomy

Technique

1. Cannulate the ileostomy with an appropriate (16- to 22-Fr) Foley catheter. Carefully inflate the balloon at or just inside the stoma.
2. Inject contrast. Dilute barium (Baritop) or water-soluble contrast can be used as single contrast or as double contrast with either air or water/methyl cellulose (see the discussion on small bowel enemas).
3. Tangential views of the spout of the stoma may be obtained at the end of the examination upon deflation of the balloon.

COLOSTOMY ENEMA

Superseded by stoma CTC where available

Indication

To demonstrate proximal colon following resection of the rectum

Technique

1. Cannulate colostomy with a 22- to 26-Fr Foley catheter and gently inflate the balloon.
2. Infuse barium or water-soluble contrast as for a barium enema.

LOOPOGRAM

Indication

After bladder resection to demonstrate anatomy of ileal conduit, ureters and renal pelvicalyceal systems

Contrast

Low-concentration water-soluble contrast agent (150 mg I mL^{-1})

Technique

Cannulate ileal conduit with a 14- to 18-Fr Foley catheter and gently inflate the balloon. Inject contrast into the ileal conduit. Observe retrograde filling of the renal collecting systems. Stop injecting when adequately distended.

Images

- Plain AP of collecting systems
- Postfilling: AP of collecting systems, two obliques of the kidneys with an additional, often oblique, view of the ureteric–loop anastomosis

HERNIOGRAM

Superseded by cross-sectional CT and MRI where available

Indications

1. History suggestive of a hernia with a normal or inconclusive physical examination
2. Undiagnosed groin pain

Contraindications

1. Infancy
2. Pregnancy
3. Intestinal obstruction
4. Allergy to contrast medium

Patient Preparation

The patient is asked to empty their bladder just before the examination.

Contrast Medium

50–100 mL water-soluble medium (e.g. Omnipaque 300)

Technique
1. The patient lies supine on the x-ray table.
2. An aseptic technique is used.
3. 5–10 mL of 1% lidocaine is injected into the skin, subcutaneous tissues and peritoneum. The injection site varies between operators. The midline just below the umbilicus is most common, and the midpoint of the left lateral rectus muscle is one variation.
4. An 18- to 22-gauge spinal needle is introduced into the peritoneal cavity until a 'popping' sensation is felt (as the needle tip passes into peritoneal cavity). Contrast is injected. If the needle is in the correct position, a 'spider web' of intraperitoneal contrast outlining the outside of bowel loops is seen. If the needle tip is in an abdominal wall, a bleb is seen, and the needle requires repositioning.

4

Images
1. Prone view
2. Erect films: frontal, obliques, lateral views

The patient is asked to cough and perform the Valsalva manoeuvre while these are taken. The tube may be angled 25 degrees caudally.

Complications
These are uncommon, and patient admission for observation is all that is usually required:

1. Pain
2. Visceral puncture
3. Vascular puncture
4. Injection into the abdominal wall
5. Haematoma at the injection site
6. Allergy to contrast medium

Further Reading
Ekberg O. Inguinal herniography in adults: technique, normal anatomy, and diagnostic criteria for hernias. *Radiology*. 1981;138(1):31–36.
Hureibi KA, McLatchie GR, Kidambi AV. Is herniography useful and safe? *Eur J Radiol*. 2011;80(2):e86–e90.

EVACUATING PROCTOGRAM

Indications
1. Constipation
2. Suspected pelvic floor weakness: posterior (rectocele, enterocele or rectal intussusception)
3. Anorectal incontinence: anal manometry and anal US preferred.

Contraindication

Pregnancy

Contrast Medium

Baritop has been discontinued, and alternative barium sulfate formulations currently available are E-Z-Paque 96% w/w powder for oral suspension or E-Z-HD 98%. Neither of these agents is currently licensed for rectal administration; however, E-Z-Paque 96% has been used in some institutes off licence, a position currently endorsed by the British Society of Gastrointestinal and Abdominal Radiology.[1]

Thick barium paste consisting of 140–150 mL of barium sulfate solution mixed with around 15 to 20 g of oat meal or other alternative bulking agents such as mashed potatoes.

Technique

1. One can of barium sulphate solution (E-Z-Paque 96% w/w powder for oral suspension or E-Z-HD 98% w/w powder for oral suspension) orally 1 h before the examination to opacify the small bowel.
2. For female patients, approximately 20–30 mL of water-soluble contrast mixed with US gel is introduced into the vagina through a Foley catheter (not always required).
3. Approximately 120–250 mL of barium paste (or enough to fill the rectum) is instilled thorough a large-bore soft bore rectal catheter via a bladder syringe.

Films

1. These are taken in a lateral projection with the patient sitting on a commode.
2. Video recording at rest and during the Valsalva manoeuvre and during pelvic floor contractions
3. Video recording during defecation using a maximum of 1 min screening time to minimize patient dose

Reference

1. BSGAR guidance on withdrawal of Barium sulfate 100% w/v oral suspension (Baritop® 100) and Barium sulfate 94.6% w/w granules for suspension (Baritop® Plus) by Sanochemia Diagnostics UK Ltd- 10th Nov 2021. https://www.bsgar.org/media/BSGAR%20guidance%20on%20withdrawal%20of%20Baritop%20Barium%20sulfate%20November%202021%20final%20version_kdUK7sj.pdf.

Further Reading

Coeliac axis, superior mesenteric and inferior mesenteric arteriography: see Chapter 11.
Ganeshan A, Anderson EM, Upponi S, et al. Imaging of obstructed defecation. *Clin Radiol.* 2008;63(1):18–26.

ULTRASOUND OF THE GASTROINTESTINAL TRACT

ENDOLUMINAL EXAMINATION OF THE OESOPHAGUS AND STOMACH

Indications

1. Staging of primary malignant disease of the upper GI tract or mediastinal pathology, such as suspected lymphadenopathy or mass
2. US-guided biopsy of primary tumours (particularly submucosal lesions such as GI stromal tumours or suspected nodal disease

4

Equipment

1. 'Radial' echoendoscope with a 5.0- to 10-MHz 360 degrees transducer for diagnosis
2. 'Linear' echoendoscope with a 5.0- to 10-MHz transducer for diagnosis and to allow biopsies

Patient Preparation

Conscious sedation is usually required (e.g. with midazolam and/or fentanyl) and/or the throat anaesthetized with xylocaine spray.

Technique

Monitoring with a pulse oximeter is required. The patient is placed in the left lateral position. The echo-endoscope is passed during endoscopy, either combined with direct vision or blind by an experienced endoscopist. A 360-degree rotary transducer provides transverse scans with respect to the long axis of the tube.

Aftercare

The patient should be observed by experienced nursing staff until the effects of any sedation have worn off, in the same manner as for other endoscopic procedures.

TRANSABDOMINAL EXAMINATION OF THE LOWER OESOPHAGUS AND STOMACH

Indications

Not routinely indicated in adults

SMALL BOWEL

Indications

1. In expert hands, US has a useful role in the evaluation of small bowel Crohn's disease, including whether it is present and assessing disease activity. Contrast-enhanced US and Doppler flow US may help evaluate disease activity.

2. Malrotation of the small bowel may be suspected by alteration of the normal relationship between the superior mesenteric artery and vein. The vein should normally lie anterior and to the right of the artery.

Technique

1. The US examination should preferably be performed preprandial or after at least after 4 h fasting because this reduces bowel peristaltic movement and intraluminal air. The exception is in the acute emergency setting.
2. The patient is in the supine position.
3. Oral fluids and contrast agents may aid diagnostic interpretation by improving delineation of the bowel wall layers and lesion detection. The most frequently used agent is an iso-osmolar agent such as polyethylene glycol, which is ingested orally at a volume of 375–800 mL. The contrast is followed through the small bowel with images at 10-min intervals until seen flowing through the ileocaecal valve.
4. Graded compression of the ascending colon in the right lateral abdomen, transverse to the long axis of the colon, from distal to proximal, will locate the caecal pole and ileocaecal junction. Initially, a 3.5- to 5-MHz transducer is used to get an overview; then it is switched to a curved or linear transducer with frequencies in the range 7.5–17 MHz to evaluate the intestinal wall in greater detail.
5. Colour or power Doppler assessment may provide additional information regarding the vascularity of the bowel that can be of relevance particularly in assessing inflammatory bowel disease.

APPENDIX

Indication

Diagnosis of appendicitis and its complications

Equipment

5- to 7.5-MHz linear array transducer

Patient Preparation

None

Technique

The US transducer is used to apply graded compression to the right lower quadrant of the abdomen. This displaces bowel loops and compresses the caecum. The normal appendix should be compressible and have a maximum diameter of 6 mm. It should also exhibit peristalsis. Other features supportive of acute appendicitis, such as the presence of a faecolith or increased vascularity, can also be appreciated on US.

LARGE BOWEL

Indications

At present, colonoscopy, CT or barium examinations are first-line imaging investigations, but large bowel masses can be visualized by US during a routine abdominal scan.

ENDOLUMINAL EXAMINATION OF THE ANUS

Indications

1. Incontinence and suspected anal sphincter defects
2. Intersphincteric fistula

Patient Preparation

None

Equipment

5- to 7-MHz radial transducer. A linear transducer can be used but is less satisfactory.

Technique

1. The patient is placed in the left lateral position.
2. A careful digital rectal examination is carried out.
3. The probe is covered with a latex sheath containing contact jelly, and all air bubbles are expelled.
4. More jelly is placed over the latex sheath, and the probe is introduced into the rectum.

Aftercare

None

ENDOLUMINAL EXAMINATION OF THE RECTUM

Indication

1. Staging of early rectal cancers (suspected ≤T2)

Patient Preparation

None

Equipment

5- to 7-MHz radial transducer. A linear transducer can be used but is less satisfactory.

Technique

1. A review of the MRI is advised to roadmap the location and base of the tumour.
2. The patient is placed in the left lateral position.

4

3. A digital rectal examination is carried out.
4. The probe is covered with a latex balloon and sigmoidoscopy tube. Water is introduced into the balloon through a sealed unit and three-way tap, and all air is eliminated. The diameter of the balloon is restricted proximally by the constraint of the sigmoidoscopy tube.
5. The balloon is deflated, more jelly is placed over the latex sheath and the probe is introduced into the rectum. When the probe tip reaches the appropriate location indicated by the MRI, the balloon is inflated to achieve optimal contact.

Further Reading

Endoscopic Ultrasound

American Society for Gastrointestinal Endoscopy. Role of endoscopic ultrasonography. *Gastrointest Endosc.* 2000;52(6):852–859.
Weber WA, Ott K. Imaging of esophageal and gastric cancer. *Semin Oncol.* 2004;31(4):530–541.

Paediatric Gastrointestinal Ultrasound

King SJ. Ultrasound of the hollow gastrointestinal tract in children. *Eur Radiol.* 1997;7(4):559–565.
Misra D, Akhter A, Potts SR, et al. Pyloric stenosis. Is over reliance on ultrasound scans leading to negative explorations. *Eur J Pediatr Surg.* 1997;7(6):328–330.
Munden MM, Hill JG. Ultrasound of the acute abdomen in children. *Ultrasound Clin.* 2010;5(1):113–135.

Small Bowel Ultrasound

Calabrese E, Zorzi Pallone F. Ultrasound of the small bowel in Crohns disease. *Int J Inflamm.* 2012:964720.
Fraquelli M, Colli A, Casazza G, et al. Role of US in detection of Crohn disease: meta-analysis. *Radiology.* 2005;236(1):95–101.
Kuzmich Howlett DC, Andi A, et al. Transabdominal sonography in assessment of the bowel in adults. *AJR Am J Roentgenol.* 2009;191:197–212.
Nylund K, Ødegaard S, Hausken T, et al. Sonography of the small intestine. *World J Gastroenterol.* 2009;15(11):1319–1330.

Endorectal Ultrasound

Beynon J, Feifel GA, Hildebrandt U, et al. *An Atlas of Rectal Endosonography.* Springer-Verlag; 1991.

COMPUTED TOMOGRAPHY OF THE GASTROINTESTINAL TRACT

Indications

1. Abdominal mass
2. Suspected tumour and tumour staging
3. Appendicitis: focused appendiceal CT (FACT)
4. Acute abdomen
5. Altered bowel habit in older adult and infirm patients
6. Location of bleeding
7. Trauma

Intraluminal Contrast Agents

- Positive oral contrast:
  Positive oral contrast (e.g. 25 mL Omnipaque 300 made up to
  1 L with water, low in density to avoid beam hardening artifact)
  can be used in abdominal and pelvic CT to delineate the bowel
  from pathology, which is especially useful in the pelvis. In the
  small bowel, positive oral contrast is helpful in the postsurgical
  abdomen, improving conspicuity of abscess and fistulae and their
  communications (see postoperative section).
- Negative oral contrast:
  Multislice CT scanners have enabled the acquisition of thin slices
  (<3 mm), allowing multiplanar reformats such that the routine
  use of intraluminal contrast for all abdominal scanning (especially
  trauma and follow-up cancer imaging) is not usually necessary.
  The inherent negative properties of intraluminal contents can
  provide sufficient contrast in the setting of high-grade intestinal
  obstruction, with the fluid within dilated bowel acting as a
  negative contrast agent and allowing delineation of the transition
  point.
  Negative oral contrast is recommended for the evaluation of
  oesophageal and stomach, up to 1 L of water as tolerated, starting
  5–10 min before the scan. For the staging of oesophageal tumours,
  in patients who can tolerate the water despite dysphagia, the
  addition of 1 sachet of Carbex with prone scanning improves
  delineation of the tumour. The prone scanning allows gravity to
  separate the oesophageal tumour and aorta, reducing the false-
  positive rate of aortic serosal invasion. The distension by Carbex
  improves the gastro-oesophageal junction distension, more
  accurately categorizing the Siewert type and the length of the
  tumour.
- In specific disease patterns that involve serosal calcification such as
  ovarian cancer or primary peritoneal malignancy, water contrast is
  preferable because positive contrast obscures evaluation for these
  deposits.
- Full-fat milk:
  Alternatives preparations for the stomach include full-fat milk to
  take advantage of delayed gastric emptying of a fatty meal to
  distend the stomach and to provide low Hounsfield units contrast.
  This strategy needs caution in populations with a high incidence of
  lactose intolerance.
- Osmotic negative contrast agents:
  Distension of the small bowel by water is limited because it is rapidly
  resorbed. Agents with increased osmolality are therefore advised
  in the elective setting, including water–methylcellulose mixtures,
  polyethylene glycol (the osmotic laxative Klean-Prep), mannitol (e.g.
  250 mL of mannitol 10% and 750 mL of water), locust bean gum
  (a food additive) and Volumen (a low-density barium-based agent
  not available in the United Kingdom at present). In the majority of

patients, approximately 1½ L drunk gradually over 30–45 min will fill the small bowel adequately. Patient encouragement and supervision are important to achieve this.

- CT enteroclysis:
1.5–2 L of oral contrast agent may also be administered via an NJ tube and is termed 'enteroclysis'. The procedure is more invasive but can ensure good small bowel luminal distension, which can be of value in the assessment for mural abnormalities and intraluminal lesions.

- Faecal tagging:
Colonic pathology is best demonstrated on CT by a combination of catharsis, distension with gas and intraluminal contrast (see CT colonography). For patients who unable to tolerate full catharsis, oral contrast given at least 24 h before the examination (e.g. 30 mL of Omnipaque 300 given the evening before) 'tags' the faeces and enables obvious colonic pathology to be more easily identified. Divided doses given over 3 days achieve more uniform colon tagging.

Intravenous Contrast

Bolus timing

Scans of the colon are generally obtained in portal venous phase (70 s) after IV contrast. Modifications depend on the clinical question. In the case of suspected active GI bleeding precontrast, arterial (20–25 s), portal (70 s) and perhaps delayed (150 s) phase contrast should be considered. In the specific case of small bowel evaluation, peak mucosal enhancement is seen at 50 s, and this 'enteric' phase is recommended.

Positive Oral Preparations in the Postoperative Setting

Positive oral contrast can be used after GI surgery to clarify the presence of an anastomotic leak and assess for postoperative fistulas.

Indications

1. To confirm the presence of an anastomotic leak after oesophagectomy or gastrectomy
2. To confirm the presence of an anastomotic leak after colonic resection
3. To evaluate for a postoperative fistula such as an enterocutaneous
4. Clarification of interloop fluid collections

Technique

Water-soluble contrast is used with the volume, route of administration and timing of imaging after contrast administration, dependent on the area of clinical concern, for example,. 7.5% positive oral prep:25 mL Omnipaque 300 made up to 1 L with water (see Table 4.2). CT is routinely performed in the portal venous phase with thin sections (<3 mm) in multiplanar reformats.

Table 4.2 Positive Oral Contrast CT Protocol for Post-Operative Bowel Leak

Region of Concern for a Bowel Leak	Contrast	Time of Oral Preparation Before CT
Oesophagus	Oral: 500 mL of 5%–10% water-soluble contrast	15–30 min before scan
Upper GI (stomach, duodenum or small bowel)	Oral: 500 mL of 5%–10% water-soluble contrast	30–60 min before scan
Lower GI (distal small bowel or coalon)	Oral: 1000 mL of 5%–10% water-soluble contrast	>90 min before the scan

CT, Computed tomography; GI, gastrointestinal.

4

RECTAL CONTRAST

Indications

Confirm the presence of an anastomotic leak following an anterior resection.

Technique

A non-contrast CT through the pelvis from the pubic symphysis to the iliac crest should be initially performed. The patient is positioned prone or decubitus and a total of 500–1000 ml of 5%–10% of water-soluble contrast administered per rectum via a soft catheter inserted into the lower rectum without the balloon inflated. The patient is then reimaged supine with thin sections (<3 mm) in multi-planar reformats.

Contraindications

1. Concern for mesenteric bowel ischaemia
2. Suspected GI Bleed
3. CT abdominal angiography
4. Risk of aspiration with oral prep (relative contra-indication)

COMPUTED TOMOGRAPHIC COLONOGRAPHY

CTC, also known as 'virtual colonoscopy', is the radiological examination of choice for the detection of colonic neoplasia of the large bowel with superior sensitivity and better patient experience compared with barium enema. Where available, this supersedes barium enema.

Indications

1. Incomplete colonoscopy secondary to technical or pathological reasons. Proximal colon evaluation can be performed the same day if no biopsies have been taken. The patient should be given 30 mL of Gastrografin after recovery from sedation and 2 h before the

scan, which will deliver adequate tagging in a cleansed colon. If the patient has had a colonic biopsy, CTC can still be performed if the endoscopist confirms only superficial biopsies have been performed.

2. Comorbidities precluding colposcopy
3. Patient choice
4. Patients taking warfarin when the clinician preference is not to discontinue anticoagulants for colonoscopy
5. Alteration in bowel habit
6. Anaemia

Bowel Preparation

Full-bowel preparation with standard laxatives is used in many centres, but the benefits of faecal tagging are increasingly accepted. Three types of preparation may be considered:

1. 'Standard' purgative large-bowel preparation as for barium enema without tagging is no longer recommended.[1]
2. 'Faecal tagging' using water-soluble contrast (e.g. an additional 50 mL Gastrografin on the evening before the scan)
3. Faecal tagging alone with no formal bowel prep:
   (a) Low-residue diet for 2 days before the test
   (b) Light breakfast and light lunch on the day before the examination; then fasting until after the examination
   (c) 100 mL of Gastrografin or 150 mL of Omnipaque split in three divided doses on the day before the examination

Technique

1. The patient is instructed to go to the toilet immediately before the procedure.
2. 20 mg IV Buscopan is given (glucagon is not recommended).
3. The patient is positioned on the left side, and a thin (e.g. Foley) catheter is placed in the rectum and gas insufflated. The gas may be air, but CO_2 is better tolerated by patients. Gas is best administered by a dedicated pump. If a pump is available, then 1.5–2 L of CO_2 is initially administered, the patient is turned supine and further gas (typically ≤4–6 L) is administered. Pumps limit the administered pressure to 25 psi and deliver further gas to maintain this pressure. Manual inflation with a bulb-sized hand pump or alternatively an empty enema bag filled with air/CO_2 and gentle pressure on the enema bag have the disadvantage of surges of intraluminal pressure during insufflation and troughs during scanning with collapse of the lumen.
4. CT scout is performed to check satisfactory gaseous distension of large bowel.
5. CT parameters depend upon the type of CT scanner available, but collimation thickness should be 1–3 mm. IV contrast is commonly used in symptomatic patients when the extracolonic yield will be in the region of 4%–7%. Asymptomatic patients from cancer screening

programmes should not receive IV contrast. CT scan sequences without contrast should be performed using a low-dose technique (e.g. 80 mA).

6. The patient is turned prone during continued insufflations, and a further low-dose scanogram is performed. The retaining balloon should be deflated on the second scan position to avoid effacing low rectal pathology. If the patient is unable to turn prone, they can be scanned in the left lateral position. The supine and prone scans should be reviewed to ensure all areas of the colon are distended on at least one of the acquisitions. If segments remain collapsed, a further low-dose scan in a third position with continued insufflation and an additional dose of 20 mg of Buscopan IV can be considered. If a tumour is detected on the first position, the chest should be added to the field of scan for the second position for one-stop staging.

COMPLICATIONS

1. Perforations are rare (~1 in 3000 diagnostic CTC examinations in the United Kingdom). The operator needs to be trained to identify this at the time of scanning.
2. Discomfort
3. Adverse reaction to hyoscine or contrast

AFTERCARE

1. The patient should be advised that cramping sensations are normal for the subsequent 24 h and a mild analgesia should suffice but to contact the department if pain is severe.
2. The potential for acute closed angle glaucoma should be explicit in a written postcare leaflet, advising urgent attendance at A&E if a painful red eye or painless red eye develops.
3. The patient should be advised to consume additional fluids for the subsequent 24 h.

DUAL-ENERGY COMPUTED TOMOGRAPHY

Dual-energy computed tomography (DECT) can accentuate differences in the attenuation of structures and thereby improve contrast resolution. It achieves this by exploiting the differing x-ray absorption of each body composition through imaging at low energy (80–100 kVp) and compensating the image degradation from increased noise-to-signal ratio by combining scanning almost simultaneously at a higher-energy (140 kVp) X-ray. It is primary used to improve the conspicuousness of lesions and the visibility of vascular structures. It can also create a virtual noncontrast study on postcontrast CT acquisitions (Fig. 4.2)

Indications

1. GI tract lesion detection and characterization

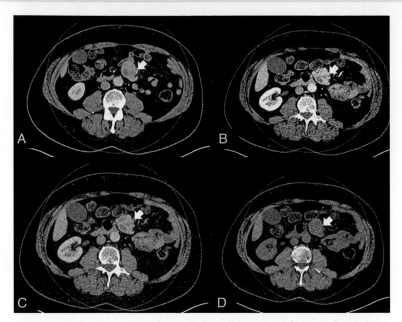

Fig. 4.2 Dual-energy computed tomography (CT) images. Axial images of an upper abdominal neuroendocrine tumour *(white arrow)* in the portal venous phase. **A,** Conventional CT (120 KeV). **B,** Lower energy (80 KeV). **C,** Fused images at both energy levels. **D,** Virtual noncontrast. Note the heterogeneity of the neuroendocrine lesion with areas of enhancement and cystic changes that are more conspicuous on both the lower energy and fused images compared to the conventional images.

2. Assessment for bowel ischemia
3. GI bleeding

Equipment

DECT images at both low energy (50–100 kVp) and higher-energy (140 kVp) x-rays. This is achieved either using

1. Two different X-ray tubes with matching detectors perpendicular to each other
2. A single X-ray source that can alternate between kVp combined with dual layer detectors

Technique

1. The postcontrast delays implemented are based on the specific protocol similar to conventional CT.
2. The inclusion of low-energy monochromatic images, iodine maps and virtual unenhanced images can be used to improve lesion detection and characterization
3. A low-energy (50–80 kVp) monochromatic series can be included for enterography protocols to improve bowel wall lesion conspicuity.

4. Virtual unenhanced and iodine maps should be considered as part of the series to aid in the characterization of incidental findings.

Limitations

- The low-energy component of DECT is suboptimal in patients with large body habitus because of photon starvation. Consideration should be given to omitting this technique in patients weighing more than 113 kg or if the body compartment to be imaged is unable to fit entirely within a field of view of 430 mm.

Reference

1. *Guidelines for the Use of Imaging in the NHS Bowel Cancer Screening Programme.* 2nd ed. NHS BCSP Publication No 5; November 2012.

Further Reading

Contrast Agents

Geffroy Y, Rodallec MH, Boulay-Coletta I, et al. Multidetector CT angiography in acute gastrointestinal bleeding: why, when, and how. *Radiographics.* 2011;31(3):E35–E46.

Graça BM, Freire PA, Brito JB, et al. Gastroenterologic and radiologic approach to obscure gastrointestinal bleeding: how, why, and when? *Radiographics.* 2010;30(1):235–252.

Ilangovan R, Burling D, George A, et al. CT enterography: review of technique and practical tips. *Br J Radiol.* 2012;85(1015):876–886.

Silva AC, Pimenta M, Guimarães LS. Small bowel obstruction: what to look for. *Radiographics.* 2009;29(2):423–439.

Slater A, Planner A, Bungay HK, et al. Three-day regimen improves faecal tagging for minimal preparation CT examination of the colon. *Br J Radiol.* 2009;82(979):545–548.

Wittenberg J, Harisinghani MG, Jhaveri K, et al. Algorithmic approach to CT diagnosis of the abnormal bowel wall. *Radiographics.* 2002;22(5):1093–1107.

Complications

Balthazar EJ. CT of the gastrointestinal tract: principles and interpretation. *AJR Am J Roentgenol.* 1991;156(1):23–32.

Burling D. International Collaboration for CT Colonography Standards. CT colonography standards. *Clin Radiol.* 2010;65(6):474–480.

Coursey CA, Nelson RC, Boll DI, et al. Dual-energy multidetector CT: how does it work, what can it tell us, and when can we use it in abdominopelvic imaging? *Radiographics.* 2010;30(4):1037–1055.

Fidler JL, Gunn ML, Soto JA, et al. Society of Abdominal Radiology Gastrointestinal Bleeding Disease-Focused Panel consensus recommendations for CTA technical parameters in the evaluation of acute overt gastrointestinal bleeding. *Abdom Radiol (NY).* 2019;44(9):2957–2962.

Fulwadhva UP, Wortman JR, Sodickson AD. Use of dual-energy CT and iodine maps in evaluation of bowel disease. *Radiographics.* 2016;36(2):393–406.

Marres CCM, Engelmann EWM, Buskens CJ, et al. The importance of rectal contrast in CT assessment to detect anastomotic leakage after colorectal surgery. *Colorectal Dis.* 2021;23(9):2466–2471.

Mileto A, Ananthakrishnan L, Morgan DE, et al. Clinical implementation of dual-energy CT for gastrointestinal imaging. *AJR Am J Roentgenol.* 2021;217(3):651–663.

Norton-Gregory AA, Kulkarni NM, O'Connor SD, et al. CT esophagography for evaluation of esophageal perforation. *Radiographics.* 2021;41(2):447–461.

Pickhardt PJ. Missed lesions at CT colonography: lessons learned. *Abdom Imaging*. 2013;38(1):82–97.

Power N, Atri M, Ryan S, et al. CT assessment of anastomotic bowel leak. *Clin Radiol*. 2007;62(1):37–42.

Tolan DJ, Armstrong EM, Chapman AH. Replacing barium enema with CT colonography in patients older than 70 years: the importance of detecting extracolonic abnormalities. *AJR Am J Roentgenol*. 2007;189(5):1104–1111.

Yonis G, Cabalag CS, Link E, et al. Utility of routine oral contrast study for detecting postesophagectomy anastomotic leak—a systematic review and meta-analysis. *Dis Esophagus*. 2019;32(7).

MAGNETIC RESONANCE IMAGING OF THE GASTROINTESTINAL TRACT

Indications

1. Suspected perianal fistula
2. Local staging of anal and rectal cancer
3. Evaluation of inflammatory bowel disease
4. Assessment for small bowel polyps and tumours

Contraindications

1. Standard MRI contraindications: see Chapter 1
2. Some gadolinium-based contrast agents are contraindicated in patients with known or suspected renal dysfunction: see Chapter 2

Contrast Agents

Contrast agents that can be used to alter the signal intensity within the bowel can be classified as positive contrast agents (high signal on T1 and T2 weighting) or negative agents (low signal on T1 and T2 weighting) but are usually biphasic (high signal on one sequence, low signal on the other). Water is a biphasic agent but is typically resorbed quickly, so a variety of formulations to increase osmolality are used, as discussed earlier. They include Klean-Prep or 250 mL of mannitol 10% solution made up to 1 L with water. Air within the bowel is a natural contrast agent and is usually sufficient for rectal and anal MRI.

Motion Artefacts

The time taken to obtain a scan can be in the order of several minutes if spin-echo (SE) sequences are used. Consequently, it is important to minimize peristalsis and respiration artefacts. Buscopan or glucagon may be used to try to minimize peristalsis. A prone position or a compression band can be used to help reduce respiratory motion of the anterior abdominal wall. The artefact, which is propagated from the anterior abdominal wall during respiration, is also caused by the high signal from fat. Consequently, fat suppression sequences can help minimize this and are particularly useful in assessing for acute inflammation.

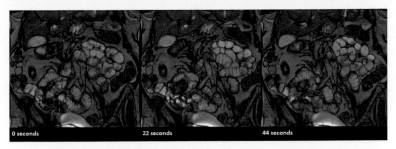

Fig. 4.3 Small bowel magnetic resonance images. Coronal T2 weighted true fast imaging with steady-state free precession acquired at 0, 22 s and 44 s. These images are amalgamated into a single sequence forming a continuous temporaneous cine loop, which can provide information on small bowel motility and luminal strictures.

4

Pulse Sequences

The sequences used for imaging the abdomen and GI tract depend on the nature of the clinical problem. Very fast sequences such as breath-hold gradient-echo (GE) and single-shot fast-SE sequences may be used to minimize any movement artefact. However, they do suffer from relatively poor contrast resolution. Standard fast-SE T1-weighted and T2-weighted sequences (with gadolinium and fat suppression added as necessary) are often used as baseline sequences, but on occasion, these suffer from movement artefact. The optimal plane of the sequences will be determined by the clinical problem, but axial scans are frequently used in the first instance with orthogonal planes (coronal or sagittal), as required.

Recently, motility assessment has emerged as another parameter for assessing small bowel disease. This is routinely performed using coronal single slice two-dimensional balanced fast-field echo sequences, positioned to include the terminal ileum, during an expiration breath-hold (Fig. 4.3). Quantitative and qualitative assessment of the small bowel motility is subsequently performed using specific software, sometimes with focus on specific regions of interest.

Techniques

Suspected perianal fistula

1. No special patient preparation required; the patient is scanned supine in the MRI scanner.
2. Buscopan is not routinely used.
3. The anal canal is angulated forward from the vertical by about 45 degrees. An initial midline sagittal T2 scan is used to identify the orientation of the canal. Oblique axial and coronal high-resolution scans at right angles, parallel to the anal canal complex, are obtained to facilitate interpretation. T2-weighted SE (with fat saturation) or short tau inversion recovery (STIR) are particularly useful sequences, but T1-weighted SE and scans following intravenous gadolinium using T1-weighted with fat saturation may also assist.

Local staging of anorectal cancer

1. Patient scanned supine; Buscopan not routinely used
2. Sagittal T2-weighted SE sequence of central pelvic structures. Large field of view axial T2-weighted scan of the whole pelvis. Use these scans to plan high-resolution 3-mm axial T2-weighted images perpendicular to and parallel to the long axis of the tumour. Coronal high-resolution scans are useful for low rectal tumours. Diffusion-weighted scans may also be useful.
3. Anal cancer staging needs to include the groins.

Small bowel magnetic resonance enteroclysis

1. Pass the Bilbao-Dotter tube to the duodenojejunal (DJ) flexure using fluoroscopy.
2. Transfer the patient to the MR scanner and obtain venous access.
3. Scan prone (though some centres scan supine) and obtain 'scout' localizer.
4. Connect the Bilbao-Dotter tube to the enteroclysis pump (situated in the control room if not MR compatible). Infuse (80–100 mL min^{-1}) oral contrast under MR fluoroscopy (coronal thick-slab single-shot sequence, e.g. half Fourier acquisition single-shot turbo spin echo (HASTE) to monitor filling of small bowel to ileocaecal valve). Check for reflux to stomach and slow or stop if significant. Stop the infusion when contrast reaches the colon.
5. Give Buscopan 20 mg IV.
6. Obtain sequences in coronal and transverse axial planes using HASTE and Fast Imaging with Steady state Precession (FISP) sequences to include one fat-saturated sequence.
7. Three-dimensional (3D) T1-weighted fat suppressed (e.g. volumetric interpolated breath-hold examination (VIBE) sequences before and after IV gadolinium administration).

Small bowel magnetic resonance enterography

1. The patient should steadily drink oral contrast (ideally 1.5 L) over 30–45 min and undergo scanning immediately.
2. Obtain venous access and give Buscopan 20 mg IV.
3. Obtain sequences in coronal and axial planes using HASTE and FISP sequences (or manufacturer's equivalent) to include one fat-saturated sequence. Obtain coronal precontrast 3D T1-weighted fat-suppressed (e.g. VIBE) images.
4. Give gadolinium-based contrast agent IV.
5. Obtain fast 3D T1-weighted fat-suppressed (e.g. VIBE) sequences in coronal and axial planes.
6. Diffusion-weighted imaging may be helpful.

Imaging during pregnancy for acute gastrointestinal pathology

MRI offers an alternative to the conventional assessment of the acute abdomen that is frequently undertaken using CT and thereby avoids the potential teratogenic and carcinogenic impact to the foetus of ionizing radiation. MRI is considered relatively safe in all trimesters of pregnancy provided contrast agents are not used. However, the heating effects of radiofrequency pulses have not been comprehensively acquitted of causing any harm to foetuses; therefore, it is strongly advised that the examination time is minimized and the sequences limited in the pregnant population.

Indications

1. Suspected acute appendicitis in pregnancy
2. Assessment for enteritis and colitis in pregnancy
3. Bowel obstruction in pregnancy

Contraindications

1. Standard MRI contraindications: see Chapter 1
2. Gadolinium-based contrast agents are contraindicated in pregnant patients.

Technique

Images are performed on a 1.5-T MRI system. There is some variance in the imaging protocol used as reducing sequences and scan time is of importance in the pregnant patient. The protocol is often tailored based on the clinical history and the initial findings if a real time image review is performed.

1. Breath-hold single-shot fast-spin echo (SSFSE) T2-weighted images in the axial plane through the abdomen and pelvis (images reviewed at the time of scanning ideally because this may negate the need for further sequences).
2. Breath-hold sagittal and coronal (SSFSE) T2-weighted images through the abdomen and pelvis
3. Axial T1-weighted GE images are optional and at the discretion of the radiologist, such as if there is concern for hemorrhage.
4. Diffusion-weighted images are optional and may be performed if indicated.
5. IV contrast and specifically gadolinium-based agents are not recommended.

Further Reading

Ali A, Beckett K, Flink C. Emergent MRI for acute abdominal pain in pregnancy-review of common pathology and imaging appearance. *Emerg Radiol.* 2020;27(2):205–214.

Amzallag-Bellenger E, Oudjit A, Ruiz A, et al. Effectiveness of MR enterography for the assessment of small-bowel diseases beyond Crohn disease. *Radiographics.* 2012;32:1423–1444.

Amzallag-Bellenger E, Soyer P, Barbe C, et al. Prospective evaluation of magnetic resonance enterography for the detection of mesenteric small bowel tumours. *Eur Radiol.* 2013;23:1901–1910.

de Jonge CS, Gollifer RM, Nederveen AJ, et al. Dynamic MRI for bowel motility imaging-how fast and how long? *Br J Radiol.* 2018;91(1088):20170845.

Halligan S, Stoker J. Imaging of fistula in ano. *Radiology.* 2006;239(1):18–33.

4

Masselli G, Brunelli R, Monti R, et al. Imaging for acute pelvic pain in pregnancy. *Insights Imaging.* 2014;5(2):165–181.

Shihab OC, Moran BJ, Heald RJ, et al. MRI staging of low rectal cancer. *Eur Radiol.* 2009;19(3):643–650.

Shin I, Chung YE, An C, et al. Optimisation of the MR protocol in pregnant women with suspected acute appendicitis. *Eur Radiol.* 2018;28(2):514–521.

Spalluto LB, Woodfield CA, DeBenedectis CM, et al. MR imaging evaluation of abdominal pain during pregnancy: appendicitis and other nonobstetric causes. *Radiographics.* 2012;32(2):317–334.

Tolan DJ, Greenhalgh R, Zealley IA, et al. MR enterographic manifestations of small bowel Crohn disease. *Radiographics.* 2010;30(2):367–384.

RADIONUCLIDE GASTRO-OESOPHAGEAL REFLUX STUDY

Indications

Diagnosis and quantification of suspected gastro-oesophageal reflux

Contraindications

None

Radiopharmaceuticals

^{99m}Tc-colloid (technetium) or ^{99m}Tc-DTPA (diethylenetriaminepentaacetic acid) mixed with:

1. Adults and older children: 150–300 mL of orange juice acidified with an equal volume of 0.1 M of hydrochloric acid
2. Infants and young children: normal milk feed

   Typical adult dose is 10–20 MBq, with a maximum of 40 MBq (0.9 mSv ED).

Equipment

1. Gamma camera
2. Low-energy general-purpose collimator
3. Abdominal binder for compression test

Patient Preparation

Nil by mouth for 4–6 h. Infants may be studied at normal feed times.

Technique

Physiological test : adults and older children

1. The liquid containing the tracer is given and washed down with unlabelled liquid to clear residual activity from the oesophagus.
2. The patient lies semirecumbent, with the camera centred over the stomach and lower oesophagus.
3. Dynamic imaging is commenced with 5-s 64 × 64 frames for 30–60 min.

Provocation with abdominal compression² : adults and older children

1. An abdominal binder is placed around the upper abdomen.
2. The radiolabelled liquid is given as previously.
3. The patient lies supine with the camera centred over the stomach and lower oesophagus.
4. An image is acquired at 30 s.
5. The pressure in the binder is increased in steps of 20 mmHg up to 100 mmHg, being maintained at each step for 30 s while an image is taken.
6. The test is terminated as soon as significant reflux is seen.

Analysis

1. For dynamic studies, regions are drawn round the stomach and lower, middle and upper oesophagus.
2. Time–activity curves of these regions are produced, from which may be calculated the size, extent, frequency, and duration of any reflux episodes.

Additional Technique: Oesophageal Transit

The reflux study may be combined with a bolus transport investigation by fast-frame (0.2–0.5 s) dynamic imaging during swallowing and the generation of a functional compressed image incorporating information from each frame.

Aftercare

None

Complications

None

References

1. Guillet J, Basse-Cathalinat B, Christophe E, et al. Routine studies of swallowed radionuclide transit in paediatrics: experience with 400 patients. *Eur J Nucl Med.* 1984;9:86–90.
2. Martins JC, Isaacs PE, Sladen GE, et al. Gastro-oesophageal reflux scintigraphy compared with pH probe monitoring. *Nucl Med Commun.* 1984;5:201–204.

Further Reading

Heyman S. Paediatric gastrointestinal motility studies. *Semin Nucl Med.* 1995;25:339–347.

Kjellén G, Brudin L, Håkansson HO. Is scintigraphy of value in the diagnosis of gastro-oesophageal reflux disease? *Scand J Gastroenterol.* 1991;26:425–430.

RADIONUCLIDE GASTRIC EMPTYING STUDY

Indications

1. Investigation of symptoms suggestive of gastroparesis
2. Before or after gastric surgery
3. Investigation of the effects of gastric motility–altering drugs

Contraindication

High probability of vomiting

Radiopharmaceuticals

Many radiolabelled meals have been designed for gastric emptying studies, but as yet, no standard has emerged. The emptying rate measured by radiolabelling is influenced by many factors—for example meal bulk, fat content, calorie content, patient position during imaging and labelling stability in vivo. For this reason, so-called normal emptying times need to be taken in the context of the particular meal and protocol used to generate them. It is important that the meal used is physiological and reproducible. For centres new to the technique, it is better to use a meal for which published data exist rather than create yet another formulation with inherently different behaviour.

Both liquid and solid studies may be performed, separately or simultaneously, as a dual isotope study. Liquids have generally shorter emptying times than solids and tend to follow an exponential emptying pattern. Solids tend to empty linearly after a lag phase. Prolonged solid emptying is highly correlated with prolonged liquid emptying, and thus there is debate as to whether both studies are routinely necessary.[1] Examples of meals used are the following:

1. Liquid meal: maximum of 12 MBq ^{99m}Tc-tin colloid (0.3 mSv ED) mixed with 200 mL of orange juice or with milk or formula feed for infants
2. Solid meal: scrambled egg prepared with a maximum of 12 MBq ^{99m}Tc-colloid (0.3 mSv ED) or ^{99m}Tc-DTPA. Bulk is made up with other nonlabelled foods such as bread and milk.
3. Dual-isotope combined liquid and solid meal:
   (a) Liquid: 12 MBq ^{99m}Tc-colloid (0.3 mSv ED) mixed with 200 mL of orange juice
   (b) Solid: 2 MBq ^{111}In-labelled resin beads (0.7 mSv ED) incorporated into a pancake containing 27 g of fat, 18 g of protein and 625 calories. Bulk is made up with other nonlabelled foods. Only 2 MBq of ^{111}In is suggested Administration of Radioactive Substances Advisory Committee (ARSAC maximum is 12 MBq, 4 mSv ED) to minimize the downscatter into the ^{99m}Tc energy window.

Equipment

1. Gamma camera, preferably dual headed
2. Low-energy general-purpose collimator for ^{99m}Tc; medium energy for ^{111}In/^{99m}Tc

Patient Preparation

1. Nil by mouth for 8 h
2. No smoking or alcohol from midnight before the test

3. When practical, stop medications affecting gastric motility such as dopaminergic agonists (e.g. metoclopramide, domperidone), cholinergic agonists (e.g. bethanechol), tricyclic antidepressants and anticholinergics for 24 h or more before the study, depending upon the medications' biological half-lives.

Technique

Imaging from a single projection can cause significant errors because of movement of the meal anteriorly as it transfers to the antrum, thereby altering the amount of tissue attenuation of gamma photons. The problem is likely to be exacerbated in obese patients. This can largely be overcome by taking pairs of opposing views and calculating the geometric, mean stomach activity in each pair:

4

1. The patient ingests the meal as quickly as they comfortably can. (If dumping syndrome is suspected, the meal should be eaten in front of the camera with a fast-frame dynamic acquisition running, or the dumping episode may be missed.)
2. The patient is positioned standing.
3. Every 5 min, a pair of 1-min anterior and posterior 128 × 128 images is obtained.
4. The patient sits and relaxes between images.
5. A liquid study should be continued for up to 60 min and a solid study for up to 90 min. If it can be seen that the majority of the meal has emptied within this time, the study may be terminated.
6. If emptying is very slow, later pairs of images may be acquired at intervals of 30–60 min.

Analysis

1. The stomach region of interest is drawn.
2. The stomach time–activity curve is produced, using geometric mean if anterior and posterior imaging performed.
3. The half-emptying time is calculated.
4. Other parameters may be calculated (e.g. lag-phase duration for solid studies or percentage left in the stomach at various time points).

Additional Techniques

1. The SBTT can be ascertained by continuing imaging at intervals until the caecum is seen. Because the position of the caecum is often not obvious and may be overlain by small bowel, a 12- to 24-h image can be useful to determine the position of the large bowel.
2. Frequency analysis of fast dynamic scans (1-s frame time) can be used to characterize antral contraction patterns.[2]

Aftercare

None

Complications

None

References

1. Siegel JA, Krevsky B, Maurer AH, et al. Scintigraphic evaluation of gastric emptying: are radiolabelled solids necessary. *Clin Nucl Med.* 1989;14:40–46.
2. Urbain J-L, Charkes ND. Recent advances in gastric emptying scintigraphy. *Semin Nucl Med.* 1995;25:318–325.

Further Reading

Maughan RJ, Leiper JB. Methods for the assessment of gastric emptying in humans: an overview. *Diabet Med.* 1996;13(suppl 5):S6–S10.

RADIONUCLIDE MECKEL'S DIVERTICULUM SCAN

Indications

Detection of a Meckel's diverticulum as a cause for GI bleeding, obstruction or abdominal pain

Contraindications

1. Barium study in previous 2–3 days (barium causes significant attenuation of gamma photons and may mask a diverticulum)
2. In vivo, labelled red blood cell study in previous few days (because of likelihood of pertechnetate adhering to red blood cells)
3. Precautions and contraindications to any preadministered drugs should be observed.

Radiopharmaceuticals

^{99m}Tc-pertechnetate, 200 MBq typical (2.5 mSv ED), 400 MBq maximum (5 mSv ED). Injected ^{99m}Tc-pertechnetate localizes in ectopic gastric mucosa within a diverticulum.

Equipment

1. Gamma camera
2. Low-energy general-purpose collimator

Patient Preparation

1. Nil by mouth for 6 h unless it is an emergency
2. It may be possible to enhance detection by prior administration of drugs (e.g. pentagastrin, cimetidine or ranitidine aimed at increasing the uptake of ^{99m}Tc-pertechnetate into gastric mucosa and inhibiting its release into the lumen of the stomach and progression into the bowel).

Technique

1. The bladder is emptied; a full bladder may obscure the diverticulum.
2. The patient lies supine with the camera over the abdomen and pelvis. The stomach must be included in the field of view because diagnosis is dependent on demonstrating uptake of radionuclide in the diverticulum concurrent with uptake by gastric mucosa.
3. Pertechnetate is administered IV.

4. Dynamic imaging is done.
5. Posterior and lateral images are acquired as required.

Aftercare
None

Complications
Preadministered drug sensitivity and side effects

Further Reading
Elsayes KM, Menias CO, Harvin HJ, et al. Imaging manifestations of Meckel's diverticulum. *AJR Am J Roentgenol.* 2007;189:81–88.
Ford PV, Bartold SP, Fink-Bennett DM, et al. Procedure guidelines for gastrointestinal bleeding and Meckel's diverticulum scintigraphy. *J Nucl Med.* 1999;40:1226–1232.

4

RADIONUCLIDE IMAGING OF GASTROINTESTINAL BLEEDING

Indication
GI bleeding of unknown origin[1]

Contraindications
1. No active bleeding at time scheduled for study
2. Slow bleeding of less than approximately 0.5 mL min^{-1}
3. Barium study in previous 2–3 days (Barium causes significant attenuation of gamma photons and may mask a bleeding site.)

Radiopharmaceuticals
1. ^{99m}Tc-labelled red blood cells, 400 MBq maximum (4 mSv ED). Red cells are pretreated with a stannous agent. ^{99m}Tc-pertechnetate is added and is reduced by the stannous ions, causing it to be retained intracellularly. Labelling efficiency is important because false-positive scans can result from accumulations of free pertechnetate. In vitro preparation gives the best labelling efficiency but is complex and time consuming. However, commercial kits are available that can reduce the preparation time to around 30 min. In vivo labelling is least efficient, and there is also a compromise in vivo–in vitro method in which the labelling occurs in the syringe as blood is withdrawn from the patient.[2]

Equipment
1. Gamma camera
2. Low-energy general-purpose collimator

Patient Preparation
1. In vivo or in vivo–invitro methods: A 'cold' stannous agent (15 g kg^{-1} tin) is administered directly into a vein 20–30 min before the ^{99m}Tc-

pertechnetate injection. (Injection via a plastic cannula will result in a poor label.)

2. The patient is asked to empty their bladder before each image is taken. Catheterization is ideal if appropriate.

Technique

1. The patient lies supine.
2. The camera is positioned over the anterior abdomen, with the symphysis pubis at the bottom of the field of view.
3. ^{99m}Tc-pertechnetate (in vivo method) or ^{99m}Tc-labelled red blood cells (in vitro or in vivo–in vitro methods) are injected IV.
4. A 128 × 128 dynamic acquisition is begun immediately with 2-s images for 1 min to help to demonstrate vascular blood pool anatomy followed by 1-min images up to 45 min. Dynamic imaging permits cinematic viewing of images to detect bleed sites and movement through the bowel.[3]
5. Further 15 × 1-min dynamic image sets are acquired at 1, 2, 4, 6, 8 and 24 h or until the bleeding site is detected (imaging much beyond 24 h is limited by radioactive decay).
6. Oblique and lateral views may help localize any abnormal collections of activity.

Aftercare

None

Complications

None

Alternative Investigative Imaging Modalities

1. Catheter angiography
2. Multidetector CT[4]

References
1. Bunker SR, Lull RJ, Tanasescu DE, et al. Scintigraphy of gastrointestinal hemorrhage: superiority of ^{99m}Tc red blood cells over 99mTc sulfur colloid. *AJR Am J Roentgenol.* 1984;143:543–548.
2. Chaudhuri TK. Radionuclide methods of detecting acute gastrointestinal bleeding. *Int J Rad Appl Instrum B.* 1991;18(6):655–661.
3. Maurer AH. Gastrointestinal bleeding and cine-scintigraphy. *Semin Nucl Med.* 1996;26:43–50.
4. Laing CJ, Tobias T, Rosenblum DI, et al. Acute gastrointestinal bleeding: emerging role of multidetector CT angiography and review of current imaging techniques. *Radiographics.* 2007;27:1055–1070.

LABELLED WHITE CELL SCANNING IN INFLAMMATORY BOWEL DISEASE

Described in Chapter 13.

Liver, biliary tract and pancreas

Raneem Albazaz

METHODS OF IMAGING THE HEPATOBILIARY SYSTEM

1. Plain film
2. Ultrasound (US):
   (a) Transabdominal (including contrast enhanced)
   (b) Endoscopic
   (c) Intraoperative
3. Computed tomography (CT), including:
   (a) Routine 'staging' (portal venous phase) CT
   (b) Triple phase 'characterization' CT
4. Magnetic resonance imaging (MRI)
5. Endoscopic retrograde cholangiopancreatography (ERCP)
6. Percutaneous transhepatic cholangiography (PTC)
7. Operative cholangiography
8. Postoperative (T-tube) cholangiography
9. Angiography—diagnostic and interventional
10. Radionuclide imaging:
    (a) Static, with colloid
    (b) Dynamic, with iminodiacetic acid derivatives

METHODS OF IMAGING THE PANCREAS

1. Plain abdominal films
2. US:
   (a) Transabdominal
   (b) Endoscopic
3. CT (dual or triple phase)
4. MRI
5. ERCP

PLAIN FILMS

Not a routine indication.[1] May incidentally demonstrate air within the biliary tree or portal venous system, opaque calculi or pancreatic calcification.

ULTRASOUND OF THE LIVER

Indications

1. Suspected focal or diffuse liver lesion
2. Jaundice
3. Abnormal liver function test results
4. Right upper quadrant pain or mass
5. Hepatomegaly
6. Suspected portal hypertension
7. Pyrexia of unknown origin, now superseded by CT for patients older than 30 years old
8. To provide real-time image guidance for the safe placement of needles for biopsy or drainage of collections
9. Doppler assessment of portal vein, hepatic artery or hepatic veins
10. Doppler assessment of patients with surgical shunts or transjugular intrahepatic portosystemic shunt (TIPSS) procedures
11. Follow-up after surgical resection or liver transplant

Contraindications

None

Patient Preparation

Fasting or restriction to clear fluids is only required if the gallbladder is also to be studied.

Equipment

Low-frequency 3- to 5-MHz curvilinear transducer and contact gel. Selection of the appropriate preset protocol and positioning of focal zone will depend upon the type of machine, manufacturer and patient habitus.

Technique

1. Patient supine
2. Time-gain compensation set to give uniform reflectivity throughout the right lobe of the liver
3. Suspended deep inspiration will be required intermittently to ensure entire liver thoroughly assessed
4. Longitudinal scans from epigastrium or left subcostal region across to right subcostal region. The transducer should be angled cephalad to include the whole of the left and right lobes.
5. Transverse scans, subcostally, to visualize the whole liver
6. If visualization is incomplete because of a small or high-positioned liver, then additional right intercostal, longitudinal, transverse and oblique scans may be useful. Suspended respiration without deep inspiration may allow useful intercostal scanning. In patients who are unable to hold their breath, real-time scanning during quiet respiration is often adequate. Upright or left lateral decubitus positions are alternatives if visualization is still incomplete.

7. Contrast-enhanced ultrasound (CEUS) of the liver uses microbubble agents to enable the contrast enhancement pattern of focal liver lesions, analogous to contrast-enhanced CT or MRI, to be assessed and thus to characterize them. It requires specific software on the US machine. The lesion to be interrogated is identified on conventional B-mode scanning, and then the scanner is switched to low mechanical index contrast-specific scanning mode (to avoid bursting the bubbles too quickly), with a split screen to allow the contrast-enhanced image to be simultaneously viewed with the B-mode image. The images are recorded after bolus injection of the contrast agent flushed with saline. Up to two boluses can be given during a single examination.

- Indications: Recommended as the first-line imaging technique for the characterization of incidentally detected, indeterminate liver lesions in low-risk patients with non-cirrhotic livers and without a history or clinical suspicion of malignancy. CEUS is also recommended for characterization of focal liver lesions in non-cirrhotic livers if both CT and MRI are contraindicated. In addition it can be very helpful in confirming or identifying an adequate biopsy site for US-guided liver biopsies.
- Contraindications: Right-to-left cardiac shunt, severe pulmonary hypertension, uncontrolled systemic hypertension, adult respiratory distress syndrome. Pregnancy is a relative contraindication (because of the paucity of data in this patient group).
- Advantages: Feasible even in the presence of impaired renal function
- Disadvantages: Limited to single-lesion visualization per pass and not possible to assess the whole liver in detail

Additional Views

Hepatic veins

These are best seen using a transverse intercostal or epigastric approach. During inspiration, in real time, these can be seen traversing the liver to enter the inferior vena cava (IVC). Hepatic vein walls do not have increased reflectivity in comparison with normal liver parenchyma. The normal hepatic vein waveform on Doppler is triphasic, reflecting right atrial pressures. Power Doppler may be useful to examine flow within the hepatic segment of the IVC because it is angle independent.

Portal vein

The longitudinal view of the portal vein is shown by an oblique subcostal or intercostal approach. Portal vein walls are of increased reflectivity in comparison with parenchyma. The normal portal vein blood flow is toward the liver. There is usually continuous flow, but the velocity may vary with respiration.

Hepatic artery

This may be traced from the coeliac axis, which is recognized by the 'seagull' appearance of the origins of the common hepatic artery and splenic artery. There is normally forward flow throughout systole and diastole, with a sharp systolic peak.

Common bile duct

See the discussion in the Ultrasound of the Gallbladder and Biliary System section.

Spleen

The spleen size should be measured in all cases of suspected liver disease or portal hypertension. The upper limit of the normal adult splenic length is typically cited at 12 cm, but lengths upwards of 14 cm can be seen in normal taller males. The spleen size is commonly assessed by 'eyeballing' and measuring the longest diameter. In children, splenomegaly should be suspected if the spleen is more than 1.25 times the length of the adjacent kidney; normal ranges have also been tabulated according to age and sex.[1–3]

References

1. iRefer. Guidelines: making the best use of clinical radiology. Version 8.0.1. <https://www.irefer.org.uk> for Members/Fellows of RCR via RCR website or via individual/organisation subscription: <https://www.irefer.org.uk/about/faqs#Q1>.
2. Chow KU, Luxembourg B, Seifried E, et al. Spleen size is significantly influenced by body height and sex: establishment of normal values for spleen size at US with a cohort of 1200 healthy individuals. *Radiology*. 2016;279(1):306–313.
3. Megremis SD, Vlachonikolis IG, Tsilimigaki AM. Spleen length in childhood with US: normal values based on age, sex, and somatometric parameters. *Radiology*. 2004;231(1):129–134.

Further Reading

Dietrich CF, Nolsøe CP, Barr RG, et al. Guidelines and Good Clinical Practice Recommendations for Contrast-Enhanced Ultrasound (CEUS) in the Liver-Update 2020 WFUMB in Cooperation with EFSUMB, AFSUMB, AIUM, and FLAUS. *Ultrasound Med Biol*. 2020;46(10):2579–2604.
Huang JX, Shi CG, Xu YF, et al. The benefit of contrast-enhanced ultrasound in biopsies for focal liver lesions: a retrospective study of 820 cases. *Eur Radiol*. 2022;32(10):6830–6839.

ULTRASOUND OF THE GALLBLADDER AND BILIARY SYSTEM

Indications

1. Suspected gallstones
2. Right upper quadrant pain
3. Jaundice
4. Fever of unknown origin
5. Acute pancreatitis
6. Guided percutaneous procedures

Contraindications

None

Patient Preparation

Fasting for at least 6 h, preferably overnight. Water is permitted.

Equipment

Low-frequency 3- to 5-MHz curvilinear transducer and contact gel. Selection of the appropriate preset protocol and positioning of focal zone will depend upon the type of machine, manufacturer and patient habitus.

Technique

1. The patient is supine.
2. The gallbladder can be located by following the reflective main lobar fissure from the right portal vein to the gallbladder fossa.
3. Developmental anomalies are rare, but the gallbladder may be intrahepatic or on a long mesentery. In the absence of a previous cholecystectomy, the commonest cause of a non-visualized gallbladder is when a gallbladder packed with stones is mistaken for gas-filled bowel (usually duodenal) loop.
4. The gallbladder is scanned slowly along its long axis and transversely from the fundus to the neck, leading to the cystic duct.
5. The gallbladder should then be rescanned in the left lateral decubitus or erect positions because stones may be missed if only supine scanning is performed.
6. Visualization of the neck and cystic ducts may be improved by head-down tilt.

Note: A normal gallbladder wall is never more than 3 mm thick.

Additional Views

Intrahepatic bile ducts

1. Left lobe: transverse epigastric scan
2. Right lobe: subcostal or intercostal longitudinal oblique

Normal intrahepatic ducts are visualized with modern scanners. Intrahepatic ducts are dilated if their diameter is more than 40% of the accompanying portal vein branch. There is normally acoustic enhancement posterior to dilated ducts but not portal veins (and portal veins typically have echogenic walls). Dilated ducts have a beaded branching appearance.

Extrahepatic bile ducts

1. The patient is supine or in a lateral position.
2. The upper common duct is demonstrated on a longitudinal oblique, subcostal or intercostal scan running anterior and parallel to the portal vein. The right hepatic artery is often seen crossing transversely between the two.

3. The common duct may be followed downward along its length through the head of the pancreas to the ampulla, and when visualized, transverse scans should also be performed to improve detection of intraductal stones. However, gas in the duodenum often impedes the view of the lower duct.

Distinction of the common hepatic duct from the common bile duct relies on identification of the junction with the cystic duct, with the common hepatic duct located above the junction. This is usually difficult with US, and often, it is the common hepatic duct size that is measured at the porta hepatis. Studies have reported variable normal size ranges for bile duct diameter, but it is generally accepted that a normal cut-off value is considered to be 6 mm (measured from inner wall to inner wall). Colour-flow Doppler enables quick distinction of bile duct from ectatic hepatic artery. In fewer than one-fifth of patients, the artery lies anterior to the bile duct.

Bile duct diameter with age and after cholecystectomy

There is general agreement that a small increase in bile duct diameter occurs with age and after cholecystectomy, but the exact values vary in the literature. Although the largest diameter of the common bile duct is considered up to 6 mm in most people, an upper limit of 8 mm is reasonable after the age of 50 years and an upper limit of 10 mm after cholecystectomy.[1] Symptomatic patients and those with abnormal liver function test results should have a lower threshold for further assessment of the bile duct.

Reference

1. Senturk S, Miroglu TC, Bilici A, et al. Diameters of the common bile duct in adults and postcholecystectomy patients: a study with 64-slice CT. *Eur J Radiol.* 2012;81(1):39–42.

Further Reading

Foley WD, Quiroz FA. The role of sonography in imaging of the biliary tract. *Ultrasound Q.* 2007;23(2):123–135.
Peng R, Zhang L, Zhang XM, et al. Common bile duct diameter in an asymptomatic population: a magnetic resonance imaging study. *World J Radiol.* 2015;7(12):501–508.

ULTRASOUND OF THE PANCREAS

Indications

1. Suspected pancreatic tumour (CT, MRI and endoscopic US are more sensitive for this indication)
2. Pancreatitis or its complications
3. Epigastric mass
4. Epigastric pain
5. Jaundice
6. To facilitate guided biopsy or drainage

Contraindications

None

Patient Preparation

Nil by mouth, preferably overnight

Equipment

Low-frequency 3- to 5-MHz curvilinear transducer and contact gel. Selection of the appropriate preset protocol and positioning of focal zone will depend upon the type of machine, manufacturer and patient habitus.

Technique

1. The patient is supine.
2. The body of the pancreas is located anterior to the splenic vein in a transverse epigastric scan.
3. The transducer is angled transversely and obliquely to visualize the head and tail.
4. The tail may be demonstrated from a left intercostal view using the spleen as an acoustic window.
5. Longitudinal epigastric scans may be useful.
6. The pancreatic parenchyma increases in reflectivity with age, being equal to liver reflectivity in young adults.
7. Gastric or colonic gas may prevent complete visualization. This may be overcome by left and right oblique decubitus scans or by scanning with the patient erect. Water may be drunk to improve the window through the stomach and the scans repeated in all positions. One cup is usually sufficient. Degassed water is preferable.

The pancreatic duct should not measure more than 3 mm in the head or 2 mm in the body.

Endoscopic US and intraoperative US are useful adjuncts to transabdominal US. Endoscopic US may be used to further characterize and biopsy pancreatic solid and cystic lesions. Intraoperative US is used to localize small lesions (e.g. neuroendocrine tumours before resection).

Further Reading

Dumonceau JM, Deprez PH, Jenssen C, et al. Indications, results, and clinical impact of endoscopic ultrasound (EUS)-guided sampling in gastroenterology: European Society of Gastrointestinal Endoscopy (ESGE) Clinical Guideline—Updated January 2017. *Endoscopy*. 2017;49(7):695–714.

COMPUTED TOMOGRAPHY OF THE LIVER AND BILIARY TREE

Indications

1. Suspected focal or diffuse liver lesion
2. Staging known primary or secondary malignancy
3. Abnormal liver function test results

4. Right upper quadrant pain or mass
5. Hepatomegaly
6. Suspected portal hypertension
7. Characterization of liver lesion
8. Pyrexia of unknown origin
9. To facilitate the placement of needles for biopsy or drainage
10. Assessment of portal vein, hepatic artery or hepatic veins
11. Assessment of patients with surgical shunts or TIPSS procedures
12. Follow-up after surgical resection or liver transplant

Contraindications

1. Pregnancy (particularly during the first trimester; can be performed in exceptional circumstances with appropriate consent if non-ionizing radiation techniques such as US and MRI have not provided sufficient information and CT will significantly impact management)
2. Allergy to iodinated contrast agents

Technique

Single-phase (portal phase) contrast-enhanced computed tomography

This is the technique for the majority of routine liver CT imaging. The liver is imaged during the peak of parenchymal enhancement—that is, when contrast-medium-laden portal venous blood has fully perfused the liver (~60–70 s after the start of a bolus injection). Oral contrast (usually negative contrast in the form of water) may be given but is not necessary if only the liver is being investigated. Slice thickness will depend upon the CT scanner specification but should be 3 mm or less.

Multiphasic contrast-enhanced computed tomography

The fast imaging times of helical or multislice CT enable the liver to be scanned multiple times after a single-bolus injection of contrast medium. Most primary liver tumours receive their blood supply from the hepatic artery, unlike normal hepatic parenchyma, which receives 70%–80% of its blood supply from the portal vein. Liver tumours (particularly hypervascular tumours such as hepatocellular carcinoma and neuroendocrine tumours) therefore enhance strongly during the arterial phase (usually late arterial phase beginning 35 s after the start of a bolus injection) but are of similar or lower density to enhanced normal parenchyma during the portal venous phase (lower density is termed *washout*). Thus, a patient who is likely to have hypervascular primary or secondary liver tumours should have a late arterial phase scan as well as a portal venous phase CT scan (discussed previously). Some centres also use a 'delayed' or 'equilibrium' phase scan at 180 s to help identify and characterize primary liver tumours. The addition of a non-contrast phase can be useful in patients with jaundice to help differentiate calcified stones in the CBD from enhancing soft tissue; it can also be useful in assessing response after locoregional therapy of a liver tumour to help differentiate residual enhancing tumour from posttreatment effect.

Further Reading

Francis IR, Cohan RH, McNulty NJ, et al. Multidetector CT of the liver and hepatic neoplasms: effect of multiphasic imaging on tumor conspicuity and vascular enhancement. *AJRAm J Roentgenol.* 2003;180(5):1217–1224. [Erratum in *AJR Am J Roentgenol.* 2003;181(1):283].

Oto A, Tamm EP, Szklaruk J. Multidetector row CT of the liver. *Radiol Clin North Am.* 2005;43(5):827–848.

The Royal College of Radiologists. *Recommendations for cross-sectional imaging in cancer management: liver metastases and primary liver cancer,* 3rd edition. BFCR(22)3 April 2022. https://www.rcr.ac.uk/system/files/publication/field_publication_files/recommendations_for_cross-sectional_imaging_in_cancer_-_liver_metastases_2022.pdf.

Vilgrain V. Tumour detection in the liver: role of multidetector-row CT. *Eur Radiol.* 2005;15(suppl 4):D85–D88.

5

COMPUTED TOMOGRAPHY OF THE PANCREAS

Indications

1. Epigastric pain
2. Obstructive jaundice
3. Suspected pancreatic malignancy
4. Acute pancreatitis and its complications
5. Chronic pancreatitis and its complications

Contraindications

1. Pregnancy (particularly during the first trimester; can be performed in exceptional circumstances with appropriate consent if non-ionizing radiation techniques such as US and MRI have not provided sufficient information and CT will significantly impact on management)
2. Allergy to iodinated contrast agents

Technique

1. Oral administration of 750 mL of water over 30 min to fill the stomach, duodenum and proximal small bowel is generally preferred for better delineation of anatomy.
2. 100–150 mL of intravenous (IV) iodinated contrast medium injected at 3–4 mL s^{-1} with a saline chaser (ideally using weight-based volume)
3. Dual-phase acquisition commenced at 35 s (pancreatic phase for optimum contrast differentiation between pancreatic lesions and normal pancreatic tissue) and 65–70 s after onset of injection (portal venous phase to show relationship of any tumour with the portal venous system and to investigate hepatic metastatic disease). If using bolus tracking, which is preferrable to optimize the vascular phases, then an 18-s delay in the abdomen followed by a further 25-s delay in the abdomen and pelvis is used to achieve these phases.
4. An initial non–contrast-enhanced examination to identify calcification is no longer routinely indicated because it will be evident on vascular phases.

5. Images should be acquired at 0.625-mm to 1.25-mm slice thickness in the pancreatic phase and 3-mm maximum slice thickness in the portal venous phase.
6. Coronal and sagittal reformatted CT images can be very useful to evaluate vascular involvement.
7. Neuroendocrine tumours and their metastases may show avid enhancement on arterial phase scans and become isodense with normal pancreatic tissue on portal phase scans.

Further Reading

NICE. Pancreatic cancer in adults: diagnosis and management. NICE guideline. February 2018. <http://www.nice.org.uk/guidance/ng85>.
Royal College of Radiologists. *The Royal College of Radiologists Recommendations for cross-sectional imaging in cancer management: pancreas.* 3rd edition; April 2022. https://www.rcr.ac.uk/system/files/publication/field_publication_files/recommendations_for_cross-sectional_imaging_in_cancer_-_pancrease_2022.pdf.

MAGNETIC RESONANCE IMAGING OF THE LIVER

Indications

1. Lesion characterization after detection by CT or US. Unenhanced MRI including heavily T2-weighted sequences and diffusion-weight imaging (DWI) can be considered the definitive protocol for detection and characterization of typical cystic and cystlike structures and haemangiomas.[1]
2. Lesion detection, particularly before hepatic resection for hepatic metastatic disease. Liver MRI is now widely accepted as the optimal imaging modality for detecting liver metastases, particularly subcentimetre lesions not visible on other forms of imaging.[2]

MRI is the imaging modality of choice for detection and characterization of liver lesions. There is high specificity with optimal lesion-to-liver contrast and characteristic appearances on differing sequences and after contrast agents. Focal lesions may be identified on most pulse sequences. Most metastases are hypo- to isointense on T1-weighted images and iso- to hyperintense on T2-weighted images. However, multiple sequences are usually necessary for confident tissue characterization. The timing, degree and nature of tumour vascularity form the basis for liver lesion characterization are based on enhancement properties. Liver metastases may be hypo- or hypervascular depending on the primary tumour site.

Magnetic Resonance Imaging Pulse Sequences

A minimum field strength of 1.5 T is required using a multichannel phased-array coil. Common pulse sequences are:

1. T1-weighted spoiled gradient echo (GRE). This has replaced the conventional spin-echo (SE) sequence. In- and out-of-phase scans

are used to investigate patients with suspected fatty liver or for identifying intracellular fat within focal lesions. The Dixon method of fat suppression has advantages over other techniques, including reduced susceptibility to artifacts and ability to quantify the amount of fat.

2. Magnetization-prepared T1-weighted GRE. This is a further breath-hold technique with very short sequential image acquisition.
3. T1-weighted GRE fat-suppressed volume acquisition. This sequence can be obtained rapidly after IV gadolinium.
4. T2-weighted SE. T2-weighted fast spin-echo (FSE) or turbo SE (TSE).

Compared with conventional T2-weighted SE images, FSE and TSE images show:

1. Fat with higher signal intensity
2. Reduced magnetic susceptibility effects, which are of advantage in patients with embolization coils, IVC filters and so on
3. Increased magnetization transfer, which may lower signal intensity for solid liver tumours. These sequences may be obtained with fat suppression.

5

Fat suppression:

1. Decreases the motion artifact from subcutaneous and intraabdominal fat
2. Increases the dynamic range of the image
3. Improves the signal-to-noise and contrast-to-noise ratios of focal liver lesions

Very heavily T2-weighted sequences can be used to show water content in bile ducts, cysts and some focal lesions. These may be obtained as:

1. GE breath-hold sequences (e.g. fast imaging with steady-state precession, fast imaging employing steady state acquisition)
2. Breath-hold very fast SE (e.g. half-Fourier acquisition single-shot turbo SE)
3. Non–breath-hold respiratory-gated sequences used for magnetic resonance cholangiopancreatography (MRCP)

Fat suppression is also used to allow better delineation of fluid-containing structures.

Short tau inversion recovery (STIR) also suppresses fat, which has a short T1 relaxation time. Other tissues with short T1 relaxation (e.g. haemorrhage and melanin) are also suppressed.

Because breathing artifacts are problematic for liver imaging, strategies to overcome this need to be used in all patients. The appropriate strategy depends on the MRI machine specifications but could include breath-holding and navigator assisted sequences.

Diffusion-Weighted Imaging

This sequence forms an image based on the random microscopic motion of water molecules (Brownian motion). Random water motion is more restricted in tissues with a high cellular density (e.g. tumour tissue). This sequence is now essential for lesion detection and characterisation and has excellent sensitivity for detection of even tiny liver lesions and for differentiating cysts and haemangiomas from other lesions.

Contrast-Enhanced Magnetic Resonance Liver Imaging

MRI contrast agents are broadly split into extracellular and hepatobiliary agents; the latter enable both extracellular and hepatobiliary phase imaging. Both gadoxetic acid (Primovist in Europe and Eovist in the United States) and gadobenate dimeglumine (MultiHance) may be used in hepatobiliary phase imaging, though MultiHance requires longer delays to reach the hepatobiliary phase (1–2 h for MultiHance vs ~20 min for Primovist).

Gadolinium-enhanced T1-weighted magnetic resonance imaging

Standard gadolinium extracellular agents are commonly used and probably do not increase sensitivity for focal abnormalities but help in tissue characterization. When used in conjunction with spoiled GRE sequences, it is possible to obtain images during the arterial phase (ideal for metastatic disease and hepatocellular carcinoma), portal phase (hypovascular malignancies and assessing washout) and equilibrium phase (cholangiocarcinoma, slow-flow haemangiomas and fibrosis). Hepatic arterial phase and diffusion-weighted sequences are the most sensitive sequences for the detection of hepatic metastases of neuroendocrine tumours. New technology has allowed the acquisition of multiple arterial phases in a single breath hold, which can further aid lesion characterization. Contrast should be administered at a rate of 1–2 mL s^{-1} followed by a 20-mL saline flush at 1–2 mL s^{-1} using a power injector. Bolus-triggered techniques are recommended for optimized arterial phase.

Liver-specific (hepatobiliary) contrast agents

Standard gadolinium extracellular agents are commonly used for liver MRI as described previously, but hepatobiliary agents enhance the distinction between normal liver and lesions, especially malignant lesions. These are mostly used in patients who are potentially suitable for major liver surgery (e.g. resection or transplantation) and for assessment of suspected hepatocellular lesions (focal nodular hyperplasia, hepatocellular adenoma and hepatocellular carcinoma).

Hepatobiliary agents are taken up by normal hepatocytes and excreted by normal liver into the bile. These contrast agents shorten T1 relaxation times, which results in normal liver showing increased signal on T1-weighted sequences. Metastases and other lesions not containing normal-functioning hepatocytes appear as a lower signal than the background liver. Lesions containing hepatocytes enhance to varying extents. High signal contrast can be seen in the bile ducts, which has clinical usefulness. These agents are also excreted by the kidneys. Further details can be found in Chapter 2.

The use of liver-specific contrast agents is recommended in all patients with liver metastases who are being considered for curative treatment. DWI should also be routinely performed because although less sensitive than the hepatobiliary phase for detecting liver metastases, the combination of both techniques has been shown to give the highest value of per-lesion sensitivity.[3]

References

1. Neri E, Bali MA, Ba-Ssalamah A, et al. ESGAR Consensus statement on MRI Imaging of the Liver. *Eur Radiol.* 2016;26(4):921–931.
2. Sivesgaard K, Larsen LP, Sørensen M, et al. Diagnostic accuracy of CE-CT, MRI and FDG PET/CT for detecting colorectal cancer liver metastases in patients considered eligible for hepatic resection and/or local ablation. *Eur Radiol.* 2018;28(11):4735–4747.
3. Vilgrain V, Esvan M, Ronot M, et al. A metaanalysis of diffusion-weighted and gadoxetic acid-enhanced MR imaging for the detection of liver metastases. *Eur Radiol.* 2016;26:4595–4615.

Further Reading

Donato H, França M, Candelária I, et al. Liver MRI: from basic protocol to advanced techniques. *Eur J Radiol.* 2017;93:30–39.

MAGNETIC RESONANCE CHOLANGIOPANCREATOGRAPHY

Indications

1. Investigation of obstructive jaundice
2. Suspected biliary colic or bile duct stones
3. Suspected chronic pancreatitis
4. Suspected sclerosing cholangitis
5. Investigation of jaundice or cholangitis in patients who have undergone biliary enteric anastomosis or after liver transplantation (to assess for biliary strictures)
6. Before ERCP or PTC for treatment planning

Contraindications

Those that apply to MRI (see Chapter 1)

Technique

MRCP is a non-invasive technique that uses heavily T2-weighted images to demonstrate the intra- and extrahepatic biliary tree and pancreatic duct. It is most commonly used to demonstrate the presence of stones and the level and cause of obstruction, especially combined with contrast-enhanced cross-sectional MRI, in cases of tumour or suspected tumour.

MAGNETIC RESONANCE IMAGING OF THE PANCREAS

Indications

1. Staging of pancreatic tumours when findings equivocal on CT
2. Surveillance in patients at high risk of developing neuroendocrine tumours (e.g. multiple endocrine neoplasia type 1
3. Surveillance of suspected intraductal papillary mucinous neoplasms of the pancreas
4. Other indications are similar to CT, although CT is generally preferred because of availability, cost and time implications.

Technique

Sequences are acquired in both axial and coronal oblique planes. The optimal plane depends on the location of the tumour. For pancreatic head tumours, the pancreatic and portal venous phase acquisitions are best acquired initially in an oblique coronal plane followed by axial to show relationship of the tumour with nearby vessels and the bile duct. The converse is true for tumours of the body and tail:

1. T1-weighted fat-suppressed GE: Normal pancreas hyperintense to normal liver
2. T1-weighted spoiled gradient-echo (SPGR fast low-angle shot, Siemens): Normal pancreas isointense to normal liver
3. T2-weighted turbo SE
4. Gadolinium-enhanced T1-weighted fat-suppressed spoiled GRE. Images are obtained immediately after the injection of contrast medium, after 45 s, after 90 s and after 10 min. Normal pancreas hyperintense to normal liver and adjacent fat on arterial phase, fading on later images. Neuroendocrine tumours can show early or delayed enhancement. Bolus-triggered techniques are recommended for an optimal arterial phase.

ENDOSCOPIC RETROGRADE CHOLANGIOPANCREATOGRAPHY

Diagnostic ERCP has been largely replaced by non-invasive investigations (e.g. CT, MRI supplemented by endoscopic US). With the advances in non-invasive imaging of the biliary tree and pancreas, more than 90% of ERCP procedures are performed with therapeutic (interventional) intent.

Indications

1. Management of bile duct stones
2. Management of benign and malignant biliary strictures
3. Evaluation of ampullary lesions

4. Diagnostic cholangiography in patients unsuitable or intolerant of MRCP and in whom endoscopic US is inconclusive or unavailable
5. Treatment and evaluation of patients with chronic pancreatitis
6. Investigation of diffuse biliary disease (e.g. sclerosing cholangitis)
7. Postcholecystectomy syndrome

Contraindications

1. Oesophageal obstruction; pyloric stenosis or gastric or duodenal obstruction
2. Previous gastric surgery that complicates access to the duodenum
3. Severe cardiac or respiratory disease

Contrast Medium

Pancreas

Low-osmolar contrast medium (LOCM) 240/300 mg I mL^{-1}

Bile Ducts

LOCM 150 mg I mL^{-1}; dilute contrast medium so that calculi will not be obscured

Equipment

1. Side-viewing endoscope
2. Polythene catheters
3. Fluoroscopic unit with spot image facilities

Patient Preparation

1. Nil orally for 4–6 h before the procedure
2. Premedication (see Chapter 21)
3. Antibiotic cover for patients with biliary obstruction or pseudocyst or at high risk of endocarditis

Preliminary Image

Prone anteroposterior and left anterior oblique (LAO) views of the upper abdomen to check for opaque gallstones and pancreatic calcification or calculi

Technique

The procedure is performed under conscious sedation. The pharynx may also be anaesthetized with 50–100 mg of xylocaine spray. The patient then lies in the left or prone position and the endoscope is introduced. The ampulla of Vater is located and intubated with a polythene catheter prefilled with contrast medium (after it is ensured that all air bubbles are excluded). A small test injection of contrast under fluoroscopic control is made to confirm the position of the cannula. It is important to avoid overfilling of the pancreatic duct. If it is desirable to opacify both the biliary tree and the pancreatic duct, the latter should be cannulated first. If there is evidence of biliary obstruction, a sample of bile should be sent for culture and sensitivity.

Images

Pancreas (using fine focal spot)

Prone; both posterior obliques

Bile ducts

1. Early filling images to show calculi
   (a) Prone: straight and posterior obliques
   (b) Supine: straight, both obliques; Trendelenburg to fill intrahepatic ducts; semierect to fill lower end of common bile duct and gallbladder
2. Images after removal of the endoscope, which may obscure the duct
3. Delayed images to assess the gallbladder and emptying of the common bile duct

Aftercare

1. Nil orally until conscious and sensation has returned to the pharynx (usually <1 h)
2. Pulse, temperature and blood pressure half-hourly for 6 h
3. Maintain antibiotics if there is biliary or pancreatic obstruction
4. Serum and urinary amylase if pancreatitis is suspected

Complications

Due to the contrast medium

1. Acute pancreatitis: more likely with large volumes, high-pressure injections
2. Acute cholangitis, particularly in sclerosing cholangitis with limited bile drainage
3. Allergic reactions: rare

Due to the technique

Local

Damage by the endoscope (e.g. rupture of the oesophagus, damage to the ampulla, proximal pancreatic duct and distal common duct or duodenal perforation (free gas))

Distant

Bacteraemia, septicaemia, aspiration pneumonitis, hyperamylasaemia (~70%); acute pancreatitis (0.7%–7.4%)

INTRAOPERATIVE CHOLANGIOGRAPHY

Indications

Performed during cholecystectomy or bile duct surgery to avoid the need for surgical exploration of the common bile duct (Preoperative MRCP or endoscopic US has replaced this technique in some centres, but some surgeons still perform it routinely to ensure no obstruction to bile flow such as caused by bile duct stones.)

Contraindications

None

Contrast Medium

High osmolar contrast media (HOCM) or LOCM 150 mg/mL, that is, low iodine content to avoid obscuring any calculi; 20 mL

Equipment

1. Operating table with Computed Radiography/Digital Radiography (CR/DR) available or a film cassette tunnel
2. Mobile x-ray machine

Patient Preparation

As for surgery

5

Technique

The surgeon cannulates the cystic duct with a fine catheter prefilled with contrast medium (with all air bubbles that might simulate calculi carefully excluded).

Images

1. After 5 mL have been injected, contrast medium should be seen within the bile duct.
2. After 20 mL have been injected, contrast medium should be seen to flow freely into the duodenum. Spasm of the sphincter of Oddi is a fairly frequent occurrence and may be caused by anaesthetic agents or surgical manipulation. It can be relieved by glucagon, propantheline or amyl nitrite.

The criteria for a normal operative choledochogram were given by Le Quesne[1] as the following:

1. Common bile duct width not greater than 12 mm
2. Free flow of contrast medium into the duodenum
3. The terminal narrow segment of the duct is clearly seen.
4. There are no filling defects.
5. There is no excess retrograde filling of the hepatic ducts.

POSTOPERATIVE (T-TUBE) CHOLANGIOGRAPHY

The technique is now less commonly performed because of decreasing use of T-tubes.

Indications

1. To exclude biliary tract calculi when (a) operative cholangiography was not performed, or (b) the results of operative cholangiography are not satisfactory or are suspect
2. Assessment of biliary leaks after biliary surgery

Contraindications

None

Contrast Medium

HOCM or LOCM 150 mg I mL^{-1}; 20–30 mL

Equipment

Fluoroscopy unit with spot image device.

Patient Preparation

Antibiotics may be considered if previous cholangitis or if immuno-suppressed (e.g. liver transplant)

Preliminary Image

Coned supine posteroanterior (PA) view of the right side of the abdomen

Technique

1. The examination is performed on or about the 10th postoperative day, before removal of the T-tube.
2. The patient lies supine on the x-ray table. The drainage tube is clamped off near to the patient and cleaned thoroughly with antiseptic.
3. A 23-gauge needle, extension tubing and 20-mL syringe are assembled and filled with contrast medium (e.g. a butterfly needle). After all air bubbles have been expelled, the needle is inserted into the tubing between the patient and the clamp. The injection is made under fluoroscopic control, the total volume depending on duct filling. In the case of recent biliary anastomosis (i.e. liver transplant), only a small volume of contrast (~10 mL), gently injected, is required.

Images

Intermittent fluoroscopic 'grab' images during filling are frequently useful. PA and oblique exposures are done when there is satisfactory opacification of the biliary system.

Aftercare

None

Complications

Due to the contrast medium

The biliary ducts do absorb contrast medium, and cholangiovenous reflux can occur with high injection pressures. Adverse reactions are therefore possible, but the incidence is small.

Due to the technique

Injection of contrast medium under high pressure into an obstructed biliary tract can produce septicaemia.

Reference
1. Le Quesne LP, Whiteside CG, Hand BH. The common bile duct after cholecystectomy. *Br Med J*. 1959;1:329–332.

PERCUTANEOUS TRANSHEPATIC CHOLANGIOGRAPHY

Indications

1. Before therapeutic intervention (e.g. biliary drainage procedure to relieve obstructive jaundice, or to drain infected bile)
2. Place a percutaneous biliary stent
3. Dilate a postoperative stricture
4. Stone removal (discussed later)
5. To facilitate ERCP by rendezvous technique
6. Rarely for diagnostic purposes only

Contraindications

1. Bleeding tendency:
   (a) Platelets less than 75×10^9 L^{-1} (the exact cut-off varies according to local practice)
   (b) Prothrombin time prolonged greater than 2 s more than control (again, varies as above)
   Vitamin K corrects abnormal prothrombin time caused by biliary obstruction if hepatocellular function is preserved; if it is not or the patient requires urgent intervention, then platelet transfusion and fresh-frozen plasma can be used (haematology advice helpful in this scenario).
2. Biliary tract sepsis except specifically to control the infection by drainage

Contrast Medium

LOCM 150 mg I mL^{-1}; 20–60 mL

Equipment

1. Fluoroscopy unit with digital spot film device (tilting table optional)
2. Chiba needle (a fine, flexible 22-gauge needle with stilette, 15–20 cm long)
3. Appropriate catheters and wire for drainage or interventional procedure planned

Patient Preparation

1. Haemoglobin, prothrombin time and platelets are checked and corrected if necessary.
2. Prophylactic antibiotics (e.g. ciprofloxacin 500–750 mg oral before and after procedure)
3. Nil by mouth or clear fluids only for 4 h before the procedure
4. Ensure patient well hydrated with IV fluids if necessary
5. Sedation (IV) and analgesia with oxygen and monitoring

Preliminary Imaging

US to confirm position of liver and dilated ducts

5

Technique

1. The patient lies supine. Using US, a spot is marked over the right or left lobe of the liver as appropriate. On the right side, this is usually intercostal between the mid and anterior axillary lines. For the left lobe, this is usually subcostal to the left side of the xiphisternum in the epigastrium.
2. Using aseptic technique, the skin, deeper tissues and liver capsule are anaesthetized at the site of the mark.
3. During suspended respiration, the Chiba needle is inserted into the liver; when it is within the liver parenchyma, the patient is allowed shallow respirations. The needle is advanced into the liver with real-time US or fluoroscopy control.
4. The stilette is withdrawn and the needle connected to a syringe and extension tubing prefilled with contrast medium. Contrast medium is injected under fluoroscopic control while the needle is slowly withdrawn. If a duct is not entered at the first attempt, the needle tip is withdrawn to approximately 2–3 cm from the liver capsule, and further passes are made, directing the needle tip more cranially, caudally, anteriorly or posteriorly, and contrast is injected until a duct is entered. The incidence of complications is not related to the number of passes within the liver itself, and the likelihood of success is directly related to the degree of duct dilatation and the number of passes made.
5. Excessive parenchymal injection should be avoided; when it does occur, it results in opacification of intrahepatic lymphatics. Injection of contrast medium into a vein or artery is followed by rapid dispersion.
6. If the intrahepatic ducts are seen to be dilated, bile should be aspirated and sent for microbiological examination. (The incidence of infected bile is high in such cases.)
7. Contrast medium is injected to outline the duct system and allow access for a guidewire or selection of an appropriate duct for drainage. When undertaken for diagnostic purposes only (PTC), the needle can be removed after suitable images have been obtained.
8. Care should be taken not to overfill an obstructed duct system because this may precipitate septic shock.

Images

Because contrast medium is denser than bile, the sequence of duct opacification is gravity dependent and determined by the site of injection and the position of the patient.

Using the undercouch tube with the patient horizontal:

1. PA
2. LAO
3. RAO
4. If on a non-tilting table, rolling the patient onto the left side will fill the left ducts and common duct above an obstruction.

When the previous images have shown an obstruction at the level of the porta hepatis, a further image after the patient has been tilted towards the erect position for 30 min may show the level of obstruction to be lower than originally thought.

Delayed Images

Images taken after several hours or the next day may show contrast medium in the gallbladder if this was not achieved during the initial part of the investigation.

Aftercare

Bed rest, pulse and blood pressure measurement half-hourly for 6 h.

Complications

The complication rate will depend on the level of experience at the treatment centre, but this is usually performed as a palliative procedure in most instances.[1]

Due to the contrast medium

Allergic or idiosyncratic reactions (very uncommon)

Due to the technique

Local

1. Puncture of extrahepatic structures (usually no serious sequelae)
2. Intrathoracic injection
3. Cholangitis
4. Bile leakage: may lead to biliary peritonitis. More likely if the ducts are under pressure and if there are multiple puncture attempts. Less likely if a drainage catheter is left in situ. (See the section on 'Biliary Drainage' later in the chapter.)
5. Subphrenic abscess
6. Haemorrhage
7. Shock owing to injection into the region of the coeliac plexus

Generalized

Bacteraemia, septicaemia and endotoxic shock. The likelihood of sepsis is greatest in the presence of choledocholithiasis because of the higher incidence of preexisting infected bile.

Reference

1. Duan F, Cui L, Bai Y, et al. Comparison of efficacy and complications of endoscopic and percutaneous biliary drainage in malignant obstructive jaundice: a systematic review and meta-analysis. *Cancer Imaging.* 2017;17(1):27.

Further Reading

Andriulli A, Loperfido S, Napolitano G, et al. Incidence rates of post-ERCP complications: a systematic survey of prospective studies. *Am J Gastroenterol.* 2007;102(8):1781–1788.

EXTERNAL BILIARY DRAINAGE

This is achieved after transhepatic cannulation of the biliary tree as described previously. The procedure may be performed to relieve jaundice or sepsis before surgery or more often as a palliative procedure to provide biliary drainage when internal drainage is not possible or has been unsuccessful.

INTERNAL BILIARY DRAINAGE

This can be achieved after transhepatic (as described previously) or endoscopic cannulation of the biliary tree. A percutaneous drainage catheter may allow internal or external drainage with side holes above and below the point of obstruction. At ERCP, an endoprosthesis or stent is placed to drain bile from above a stricture or to prevent obstruction by a stone in the duct.

Indications

1. Malignant biliary stricture
2. Benign stricture after balloon dilation

Contraindications

As for PTC

Contrast Media

LOCM 200 mg I mL^{-1}; 20–60 mL

Equipment

1. Wide-channelled endoscope for introduction of endoprosthesis by ERCP
2. A biplane fluoroscope facility is useful but not essential for transhepatic puncture.
3. Set including guidewires, dilators and endoprosthesis

Patient Preparation

See the discussion of PTC described previously.

Technique

Transhepatic

1. PTC is performed.
2. A duct in the right lobe of the liver that has a horizontal or caudal course to the porta hepatis is usually chosen. This duct is studied on US to judge its depth, and then a 22-gauge Chiba needle is inserted into the duct under US or fluoroscopic guidance. A coaxial introducer system is used over a 0.018-in guidewire to allow the 0.035-in wire and catheter access into the bile ducts. If the duct is not successfully punctured, the Chiba needle is withdrawn but remains within the liver capsule, allowing a further puncture attempt. After a 0.035-in wire is established in the bile duct, a sheath can be inserted (e.g.

7 Fr). Bile can be drained through the side arm of the sheath while a catheter is manipulated over the wire. For internal drainage or stent insertion, the wire and catheter must be passed through the stricture into the duodenum or postoperative jejunal loop. For external drainage, a suitable catheter can be inserted over the wire after the sheath is withdrawn. A variety of wires and catheters may be needed to cross difficult strictures. Failing this, external drainage is instituted, and a further attempt is made to pass the stricture a few days later.

3. An internal-external catheter may be placed across the stricture and secured to the skin with sutures.

4. A metal biliary stent may be positioned and deployed across a malignant stricture to facilitate internal drainage of bile. Balloon dilation may be required before or after stent deployment in some cases. A temporary external drainage tube may be left in place for 24–48 h.

Endoscopic

1. Cholangiography after cannulation of the biliary tree
2. Endoscopic sphincterotomy
3. A guidewire is placed via the channel of the endoscope through the sphincter and pushed past the stricture using fluoroscopy to monitor progress.
4. After dilation of the stricture, the endoprosthesis (plastic stent) is pushed over the guidewire and sited with its side holes above and below the stricture. Metal biliary stents can also be placed at ERCP when appropriate.

Aftercare

1. As for PTC
2. Antibiotics for at least 3 days
3. An externally draining catheter should be regularly flushed through with normal saline and exchanged at 3-month intervals. (It is rare to leave a drain in situ for such a long period.)

Complications

1. As for PTC, ERCP and sphincterotomy
2. Sepsis: particularly common with long-term, externally draining catheters
3. Dislodgement of catheters or endoprostheses
4. Blockage of catheters or endoprostheses
5. Perforation of bile duct above the stricture on the passage of guidewires.

PERCUTANEOUS EXTRACTION OF RETAINED BILIARY CALCULI (BURHENNE TECHNIQUE)

Indications

Retained biliary calculi seen on the T-tube cholangiogram (incidence, 3%)

Contraindications

1. Small T-tube (<12 Fr)
2. Tortuous T-tube course in soft tissues
3. Acute pancreatitis
4. Drain in situ (cross connections exist between the drain tract and the T-tube tract)

Contrast Medium

HOCM or LOCM 150 mg I mL^{-1} (Low-density contrast medium is used to avoid obscuring the calculus.)

Equipment

1. Fluoroscopy unit with spot film device
2. Steerable catheter system with wire baskets

Patient Preparation

1. Prophylactic antibiotics and premedication 1 hour before the procedure
2. Analgesia during the procedure

Technique

1. The patient lies supine on the x-ray table. PTC is performed if a biliary drainage catheter is not already in situ.
2. The drainage catheter is removed over a guidewire, and a sheath is inserted into the ducts (7 or 8 Fr).
3. Contrast is injected to identify presence and location of stones and strictures.
4. If there is a stricture, advance a biliary manipulation catheter and guidewire (0.035 in) across it. Commence balloon dilatation over the guidewire (e.g. 8, 10 and possibly 12 mm).
5. Attempt to dislodge stones with balloons into the Roux loop.
6. If this is unsuccessful, pass the Dormier basket through the sheath and attempt to catch the stone in the basket.
7. Advance the basket into the Roux loop and release the stone into the loop.
8. Remove the basket.
9. Pass the guidewire, remove the sheath and place the biliary drainage catheter.
10. Intermittently inject the contrast media to clarify the position of the stones.

Aftercare

1. Pulse and blood pressure half-hourly for 6 h
2. Bed rest for 4–6 h

Complications

Due to the contrast medium

1. Allergic reactions (rare)
2. Pancreatitis

Due to the technique

1. Fever
2. Perforation of the T-tube tract

Further Reading

Uberoi R, Das N, Moss J, et al. British Society of Interventional Radiology: Biliary Drainage and Stenting Registry (BDSR). *Cardiovasc Intervent Radiol.* 2012;35(1):127–138.

ANGIOGRAPHY

COELIAC AXIS, SUPERIOR MESENTERIC AND INFERIOR MESENTERIC ARTERIOGRAPHY

5

Indications

1. Suspected haemorrhage or haemobilia before intervention (embolization of bleeding point or aneurysm usually identified initially on CT)
2. Gastrointestinal (GI) ischaemia
3. Before embolization and intervention (e.g. embolization, chemoembolization, radioembolization of tumours)
4. Suspected polyarteritis nodosa

Contrast Medium

LOCM 280–370 mg I mL^{-1}

Equipment

1. Digital fluoroscopy with C-arm angiography facility
2. Pump injector
3. Catheter—selection of both forward- and reverse-facing catheters

Technique

1. Femoral artery puncture: See Chapter 11 for more details.
2. Bowel movement causing subtraction artefact can be reduced by using a smooth muscle relaxant (e.g. Buscopan 10–20 mg IV) and abdominal compression.
3. When performed for GI bleeding, provided that the patient is actively bleeding at the time, a blood loss of 0.5–0.6 mL min^{-1} can be demonstrated. The site of active bleeding is revealed by extravasated contrast medium remaining in the bowel on the late films, when intravascular contrast has cleared. Vascular malformations, tumours and varices may be demonstrated.
4. Catheter angiography is now rarely used for diagnosis alone and instead is reserved for guiding endovascular intervention. The volume and rate of contrast to be injected should reflect the size and flow rate of the vessel in question.

RADIONUCLIDE IMAGING OF THE LIVER, GALLBLADDER AND SPLEEN

The widespread availability of MRI (with hepatobiliary-specific agents, e.g. gadoxetate disodium, Primovist) has replaced radionuclide imaging for characterization of liver and spleen lesions and can be used to determine functional and structural abnormalities such as bile leaks and choledochal cysts. Functional assessment of the gallbladder cannot be easily achieved with MRI; therefore, radionuclide imaging remains in routine use for specific indications.

LIVER AND GALLBLADDER

Indications

1. Assessment of gallbladder, common bile duct and sphincter of Oddi function[1,2]
2. Assessment of neonatal jaundice when biliary atresia is considered
3. Suspected bile leaks after trauma or surgery[3] (with single-photon emission computed tomography (SPECT)–CT)
4. Assessment of choledochal cysts
5. Investigation of biliary drainage (after Kasai procedure)
6. Staging of gallbladder cancer and cholangiocarcinoma (fluorodeoxyglucose (FDG) positron emission tomography (PET) CT; see Chapter 13).
7. Staging of neuroendocrine tumours (somatostatin receptor imaging; see Chapter 13).

Contraindications

None

Radiopharmaceuticals

^{99m}Tc-disofenin or ^{99m}Tc-mebrofenin (iminodiacetic acid (IDA) derivatives); 110–185 MBq typical for adults (1–2 mSv estimated dose (ED)); 1.8 MBq kg^{-1} for children and infants (minimum dose, 18.5 MBq)

These ^{99m}Tc-labelled IDA derivatives are rapidly cleared from the circulation by hepatocytes and secreted into bile in a similar way to bilirubin[4]; this allows the assessment of biliary drainage and gallbladder function. Modern tracers have high hepatic uptake and low urinary excretion, giving better visualization of the biliary tract at high bilirubin levels than the earlier agents.

Equipment

1. Gamma camera
2. Low-energy general-purpose collimator

Patient Preparation

1. Nil by mouth for 4–6 h for adults, 2–4 h for children and 2 h for infants

2. For the investigation of biliary atresia, infants are given phenobarbital orally 5 mg kg^{-1} day^{-1} in two divided doses for 3–5 days before the study to enhance hepatic excretion of the radiopharmaceutical.

Technique

The imaging protocol depends upon the clinical question being asked. A dynamic study should be performed where it is important to visualize the progress of the bile in detail (e.g. after surgery).

1. The patient lies supine with the camera anterior and liver at the top of the field of view.
2. The radiopharmaceutical is injected IV.

Images

1. 1 minute 128 × 128 dynamic images are acquired for 45–60 min after injection.
2. If gallbladder or choledochal cyst visualization is the reason for the study, the study can be stopped early when activity is seen within these structures
3. If not, 30–45 min postinjection when the gallbladder is well visualized, a liquid fatty meal (e.g. 300 mL full-cream milk) is given through a straw to stimulate gallbladder contraction, and imaging is continued for a further 45 min. A gallbladder ejection fraction can be calculated.
4. If the gallbladder and duodenum are not seen, static images are obtained at intervals of up to 4–6 h.
5. If images are suggestive of reflux, 100–200 mL of water is given through a straw to diffuse any activity in the stomach and thereby differentiate it from nearby bowel activity.
6. If no bowel activity is seen by 4–6 h and it is important to detect any flow of bile at all (e.g. in suspected biliary atresia), a 24-hour image should be taken.

Additional Techniques

Cholecystokinin and morphine provocation

Pharmacological intervention can be used in combination with IDA scanning to improve diagnosis of diseases affecting the gallbladder, common bile duct or sphincter of Oddi.[1] Synthetic cholecystokinin (i.e. Sincalide) causes gallbladder contraction and sphincter of Oddi relaxation. A pretest IV infusion of Sincalide is administered.

Quantitative measures of gallbladder ejection fraction and emptying rate can be calculated. It has been suggested that a slow cholecystokinin (i.e. Sincalide) infusion over 30–60 min may improve specificity.[5]

Morphine causes sphincter of Oddi contraction. In a clinical setting of suspected acute cholecystitis, if the gallbladder is not observed by 60 min, an infusion of 0.04 mg kg^{-1} over 1 minute can be given, and imaging is continued for a further 30 min. Continued non-visualization of the gallbladder up to 90 min is considered to confirm the diagnosis. Morphine provocation has also found success in diagnosis of elevated sphincter of Oddi basal pressure.[2]

Quantitative analysis

Some investigators have calculated liver function parameters from dynamic studies (e.g. to attempt to differentiate between transplant rejection and hepatocyte dysfunction).

Aftercare

None

Complications

Monitor for adverse reactions to CCK analogues and morphine.

SPLEEN

Indication

1. To detect splenunculi (ectopic splenic tissue)

Contraindications

None

Radiopharmaceuticals

^{99m}Tc sulphur colloid 150–220 MBq (ED 1.5–2 mSv). Cleared by phagocytosis into the reticuloendothelial cells, where it is retained. The spleen is demonstrated as well as the liver.

Equipment

1. Gamma camera
2. Low-energy general-purpose collimator

Patient Preparation

None

Technique

1. The patient lies supine.
2. Image at 20 min after injection.
3. Images anterior with costal margin markers, posterior, and both left and right laterals

   500 kilocounts are used for each view. SPECT or SPECT-CT can be used when necessary.

Aftercare

None

Complications

None

Alternative Investigative Imaging Modalities

1. Multidetector CT
2. MRI with reticuloendothelial contrast agent
3. 18FDG-PET for investigation of primary or secondary malignancy (see Chapter 13)
4. Platelet or denatured red blood cell scan for splenunculi

References

1. Krishnamurthy S, Krishnamurthy GT. Cholecystokinin and morphine pharmacological intervention during ^{99m}Tc-HIDA cholescintigraphy: a rational approach. *Semin Nucl Med.* 1996;26(1):16–24.
2. Thomas PD, Turner JG, Dobbs BR, et al. Use of ^{99m}Tc-DISIDA biliary scanning with morphine provocation for the detection of elevated sphincter of Oddi basal pressure. *Gut.* 2000;46(6):838–841.
3. Rayter Z, Tonge C, Bennett C, et al. Ultrasound and HIDA: scanning in evaluating bile leaks after cholecystectomy. *Nucl Med Commun.* 1991;12(3):197–202.
4. Krishnamurthy GT, Turner FE. Pharmacokinetics and clinical application of technetium 99m-labeled hepatobiliary agents. *Semin Nucl Med.* 1990;20(2):130–149.
5. Tulchinsky M, Ciak BW, Delbeke D, et al. SNM Practice Guideline for Hepatobiliary Scintigraphy. *J Nucl Med Tech.* 2010;38(4):210–218.

Further Reading

Harding LK, Notghi A. Gastrointestinal tract and liver. In: Sharp PF, Gemmell HG, Murray AD, eds. *Practical Nuclear Medicine.* 3rd ed. London: Springer-Verlag; 2005:273–304.

INVESTIGATION OF SPECIFIC CLINICAL PROBLEMS

INVESTIGATION OF LIVER TUMOURS

Investigation

This falls into three stages:

1. Detection
2. Characterization of the tumour
3. Assessment for surgical resection or staging for chemotherapy

The clinical context and proposed management course usually determine the extent of investigation. Liver metastases are much commoner than primary liver cancers. Benign haemangiomas are also common, being present in 5%–10% of the population. Other benign liver lesions, except cysts, are less common.

The clinical data correlated with the radiological investigations usually enable the character of a liver tumour to be determined with a high degree of probability. This can be confirmed with image-guided or surgical biopsy when appropriate. Many surgeons are averse to preoperative biopsy in a patient with a potentially resectable or curable lesion because of the small risk of seeding and disseminating malignant cells and the possibility of misleading sampling error. If biopsy is performed, it is sometimes important to sample the 'normal' liver as well as the lesion. The presence of cirrhosis may have a major impact on management and on narrowing the differential diagnosis given the high incidence of hepatocellular carcinoma (and to a lesser degree cholangiocarcinoma) in this setting. Hepatic resection is an established procedure for the management of selected hepatic metastases and primary liver tumours. Imaging is used to assess the number and location of tumours.

Unlike most other cancers, hepatocellular carcinoma can be diagnosed non-invasively in the setting of cirrhosis with imaging without mandatory pathology confirmation given the high pretest probability. This can be performed with multiphasic CT, dynamic contrast-enhanced MRI or CEUS. CT or MRI should be used first given their higher sensitivity and ability to analyze the whole liver. Most recently, a group of experts supported by the American College of Radiology developed and revised the Liver Imaging Reporting and Data System (LI-RADS) version 2018, a system in which features of liver nodules are used to give a score as an indicator of the probability of a particular nodule being a HCC.[1]

Ultrasound

Often the first modality to detect an unsuspected focal liver lesion or lesions but no longer appropriate for screening or surveillance of liver metastases. US does have a role in screening patients at high risk of developing hepatocellular carcinoma (e.g. those with cirrhosis), with 6-month surveillance US examinations.

CEUS is a very useful technique for characterizing some liver lesions, particularly solitary lesions in low-risk patients, which are likely to be benign such as haemangiomas, focal nodular hyperplasia or uneven fat. It is cheaper and quicker to perform than MRI and avoids any claustrophobia issues, but lesion selection is important and depends on local practice and expertise.

Computed Tomography

Widely used for general screening, staging and follow-up, with the benefits of screening the extra hepatic structures in the thorax, abdomen and pelvis.

Magnetic Resonance Imaging

Very useful for determining the nature of an unknown liver lesion and for characterizing and staging patients who are considered to be suitable for surgical resection based on CT findings.

INVESTIGATION OF JAUNDICE

The aim is to separate haemolytic causes of jaundice from obstructive jaundice or hepatocellular jaundice. Clinical history and examination are followed by biochemical tests of blood and urine and haematological tests.

Investigations

Obstructive jaundice

US is the primary imaging investigation. The presence of dilated ducts suggests obstructive jaundice. MRI or CT examination of the bile ducts, gallbladder and pancreas should be performed to determine the level and cause of obstruction and the stage if it is a tumour. MRCP is a non-invasive method of imaging the ducts to demonstrate the presence of stones and the level and cause of obstruction, especially combined with cross-sectional contrast-enhanced MRI in cases of tumour or suspected tumour. Endoscopic US also can be very helpful in cases when the diagnosis is in doubt after cross-sectional imaging, to confirm or exclude small tumours or small stones and to obtain histology.

ERCP or PTC for higher-level obstruction should be reserved for cases when a non-operative management strategy has been determined or in cases with severe jaundice requiring drainage before definitive treatment.

Non-obstructive jaundice

When US shows no dilated ducts and hepatocellular jaundice is suspected, liver biopsy is considered. There may be other US evidence of parenchymal liver disease or signs of portal hypertension.

If obstructive jaundice is still suspected despite the US result, then MRCP is required. Extrahepatic obstruction may be present in the absence of duct dilation, and patients with primary sclerosing cholangitis or widespread intrahepatic metastases may have intrahepatic obstruction without duct dilatation.

INVESTIGATION OF PANCREATITIS

US can be the first investigation, but in acute pancreatitis, the presence of a sentinel loop of bowel often obscures the pancreas and prevents good visualization. Even if the pancreas is seen, it can appear normal in acute pancreatitis. US to establish whether gallstones are responsible is indicated in the first 24 h of presentation.

CT is indicated for a late presentation of pancreatitis, to look for suspected complications of pancreatitis and to diagnose chronic pancreatitis. In the acute setting, a dual-phase (arterial and portal venous) scan around day 7 is optimal to identify a non-viable pancreas and to characterize peripancreatic collections and vascular complications such as splenic venous thrombosis or pseudoaneurysm formation.

PANCREATITIS-ASSOCIATED COLLECTIONS

Acute pancreatitis is now divided into two distinct subtypes, necrotizing pancreatitis and interstitial oedematous pancreatitis, based on the presence or absence of necrosis, respectively.[2] Four distinct collection subtypes are identified on the basis of the presence of pancreatic necrosis and time elapsed since the onset of pancreatitis. Acute peripancreatic fluid collections (APFCs) and pseudocysts occur in interstitial oedematous pancreatitis and contain fluid only. Acute necrotic collections (ANCs) and walled-off necrosis (WON) occur only in necrotizing pancreatitis and contain variable amounts of fluid and necrotic debris. APFCs and ANCs occur within 4 weeks of disease onset. After this time, APFCs or ANCs may either resolve or persist, developing a mature wall to become a pseudocyst or a WON, respectively.

Initial investigation can be done with US. Collections can occur anywhere in the abdomen or pelvis (or even the thorax). The spleen and left kidney may provide useful acoustic windows to visualize the region of the tail of the pancreas.

CT scanning is now more frequently performed for this indication and should always be performed before radiologically guided intervention to prevent drainage of a pseudoaneurysm. (During US, supposed fluid collections can be interrogated with colour or duplex Doppler.) Pseudocysts can also be drained by endoscopic US.

References

1. The American College of Radiology. CT/MRI LI-RADS v2018 CORE. <http://www.acr.org/-/media/ACR/Files/RADS/LI-RADS/LI-RADS-2018-Core.pdf?la=en>.
2. Foster BR, Jensen KK, Bakis G, et al. Revised Atlanta Classification for Acute Pancreatitis: a pictorial essay. *Radiographics*. 2016;36(3):675–687 Erratum in: *Radiographics*. 2019;39(3):912.

Further Reading

Galea N, Cantisani V, Taouli B. Liver lesion detection and characterization: role of diffusion-weighted imaging. *J Magn Reson Imaging*. 2013;37(6):1260–1276.
Silva AC, Evans JM, McCullough AE, et al. MR imaging of hypervascular liver masses: a review of current techniques. *Radiographics*. 2009;29(2):385–402.

Urinary tract
Douglas Pendse

6

METHODS OF IMAGING THE URINARY TRACT

1. Plain radiography
2. Excretion urography (intravenous urogram
3. Ultrasound (US)
4. Computed tomography (CT):
   (a) CT for urological diagnosis and urological cancer staging
   (b) CT for characterization of renal lesion
   (c) CT of the adrenals
   (d) CT of the KUB (kidneys, ureters, bladder)
   (e) CT urography (CTU)
   (f) CT angiography (see Chapter 11 for angiographic principles)
5. Magnetic resonance imaging (MRI):
   (a) MR of the kidneys
   (b) MR of the prostate
   (c) MR urography
   (d) MR of the adrenals
   (e) MR angiography (see Chapter 11)
6. Micturating cystography and cystourethrography (paediatrics)
7. Urethrogram (male)
8. Conduitogram or loopogram
9. Percutaneous urological procedures:
   (a) Renal biopsy
   (b) Percutaneous nephrostomy
   (c) Percutaneous nephrolithotomy
   (d) Suprapubic catheter insertion
10. Arteriography (see Chapter 11)
11. Venography (see Chapter 12)
12. Radionuclide imaging:
    (a) Static renography
    (b) Dynamic renography
    (c) Radionuclide cystography: direct and indirect

PLAIN FILM RADIOGRAPHY

Indications

Plain film abdominal (or KUB) radiography is seldom used for evaluation of the renal tract. It is a poorly sensitive technique for renal stone detection and not indicated as a first-line test in the evaluation of suspected renal colic. There are some instances when plain film radiographs may be used for follow-up of renal stone disease, although dose savings compared with modern ultra-low-dose CT KUB are marginal.

Further Reading

Kanno T, Kubota M, Funada S, et al. The utility of the kidneys-ureters-bladder radiograph as the sole imaging modality and its combination with ultrasonography for the detection of renal stones. *Urology.* 2017;104:40–44.

Shim YS, Park SH, Choi SJ, et al. Comparison of submillisievert CT with standard-dose CT for urolithiasis. *Acta Radiol.* 2020;61(8):1105–1115.

INTRAVENOUS EXCRETION UROGRAPHY

The technique is less frequently used than in the past and has now been very largely replaced by US, CT, MRI or a combination.

Indications

1. Haematuria
2. Renal colic (see section on technique variation below)
3. Recurrent urinary tract infection (UTI)
4. Loin pain
5. Suspected urinary tract pathology

Contraindications

See Chapter 2 for general contraindications to intravenous (IV) water-soluble contrast media and ionizing radiation. In patients with contrast medium allergies, alternative modalities such as US or MR can be considered. Patients with impaired renal function, particularly those with diabetes, should be prepared with oral or IV hydration, or an alternative imaging modality should be considered. See Chapter 2.

Contrast Medium

Low-osmolar contrast material (LOCM) 300–370 mg I mL^{-1}

Adult dose

50–100 mL

Paediatric dose

1 mL kg^{-1}

Patient Preparation

1. No food for 5 h before the examination. Dehydration is not necessary and does not improve image quality.
2. The routine administration of bowel preparation has been shown not to improve the diagnostic quality of the examination.

Preliminary Images

Supine, full-length anteroposterior (AP) of the abdomen in inspiration. The lower border of the cassette is at the level of the symphysis pubis, and the x-ray beam is centred in the midline at the level of the iliac crests.

If necessary, the location of overlying opacities may be further determined by:

- Supine AP film of the renal areas in expiration. The x-ray beam is centred in the midline at the level of the lower costal margin.
- 35-degree posterior oblique views (side of interest towards the film)
- Tomography of the kidneys

6

The examination should not proceed further until these images have been reviewed by the radiologist or radiographer and deemed satisfactory.

Technique

Venous access is established. The gauge of the cannula or needle should allow the injection to be given rapidly as a bolus to maximize the density of the nephrogram.

Images

1. **Immediate film:** AP view of the renal areas. This film is taken 10–14 s after the injection (approximate 'arm-to-kidney' time). It aims to show the nephrogram at its most dense (i.e. the renal parenchyma opacified by contrast medium in the renal tubules). Tomography may assist in evaluation of the renal outline or possible masses (or US if subsequently available).
2. **5-min film:** AP view of the renal areas. This film gives an initial assessment of pathology, specifically the presence or absence of obstruction before administering compression. A compression band is then applied positioned midway between the anterior superior iliac spines (i.e. over the ureters as they cross the pelvic brim). The aim is to produce pelvicalyceal distension. Compression is, however, contraindicated:
   (a) After recent abdominal surgery
   (b) After renal trauma
   (c) If there is a large abdominal mass or aortic aneurysm
   (d) When the 5-min film shows already distended calyces indicative of obstruction

3. **10-min film:** AP view of the renal areas. There is usually adequate distension of the pelvicalyceal systems with opaque urine by this time. Compression is released when satisfactory demonstration of the pelvicalyceal system has been achieved. If the compression film is inadequate, the compression should be checked and repositioned if necessary, a further 50 mL of contrast medium administered and a repeat film taken after 5 min.

4. **Release film:** Supine AP view of the abdomen taken immediately after the release of compression. This film is taken to show the ureters. If this film is satisfactory, the patient is asked to empty the bladder.

5. **After micturition film:** Full-length supine AP view of the abdomen. The aims of this film are to assess bladder emptying, to demonstrate drainage of the upper tracts, to aid the diagnosis of bladder tumours, to confirm ureterovesical junction calculi and, uncommonly, to demonstrate a urethral diverticulum in female patients.

Additional Images

1. 35-degree posterior oblique view of the kidneys, ureters or bladder for equivocal collecting system lesions or localization of calculi
2. Tomography if renal outlines are not well seen
3. Prone abdomen after the release film: may improve visualization of distal ureters
4. Delayed films at increasing (doubling of time intervals) up to 24 h after injection in renal obstruction

Variation

Renal colic: a limited study may be performed: preliminary films; 20-min full length (no compression); postmicturition full length; delayed films up to 24 hours as required to show level and cause of obstruction

Further Reading

Amis ES. Epitaph for the urogram. *Radiology*. 1999;213:639–640.
Becker JA, Pollack HM, McClennan BL. Urography survives. *Radiology*. 2001;218:299–300.
Webb JAW. Imaging in haematuria. *Clin Radiol*. 1997;52:167–171.

ULTRASOUND OF THE URINARY TRACT

Indications

1. Acute or chronic kidney injury
2. Renal mass
3. Renal parenchymal disease
4. Suspected ureteric colic (in children)
5. Haematuria
6. Hypertension (if MR or CT angiography is contraindicated)
7. Renal cystic disease
8. Renal size measurement
9. Bladder outflow obstruction
10. UTI

11. Bladder tumour
12. After renal transplant:
    (a) Obstruction
    (b) Patency of vessels
    (c) Perirenal collections
13. Renal vascular studies

Contraindications

None

Patient Preparation

Kidneys only: none
    Kidneys and bladder: prehydrate with oral fluids (e.g. 500–1000 mL 1 h before scan); patient attends with a full bladder. This may have the disadvantage of making the collecting systems appear mildly hydronephrotic premicturition.

Equipment

3.5- to 5-MHz curvilinear transducer

Technique

Kidney Ultrasound

1. Patient supine, right anterior oblique (RAO) and left anterior oblique (LAO) positions or lateral for the kidneys. The kidneys are scanned longitudinally in an oblique coronal plane supplemented by transverse sections perpendicular to the axis. The right kidney may be scanned through the liver and posteriorly in the right loin. The left kidney is often more difficult to visualize anteriorly but can be visualized from a lateral approach. In difficult cases, the patient should lie on their side with a pillow under the loin to widen the space between the rib cage and pelvis.
2. With US measurement, care must be taken to ensure that the true longitudinal length (rather than oblique) measurement is obtained. The range of lengths of the normal kidneys is 9–12 cm, and the difference between each kidney should be less than 1–2 cm.
3. Examination should evaluate the renal parenchyma, collecting system and renal sinus. In a normal kidney, the parenchyma of the renal cortex should appear slightly echogenic compared with the renal medulla. Focal scarring and parenchymal thinning or atrophy should be recorded, and renal masses and cysts should be characterized. The collecting system is normally decompressed, although a small amount of fluid in the renal pelvis may be seen. If hydronephrosis is present, a repeat scan after micturition should be obtained. Mild pelvicalyceal dilation in the presence of a very full bladder can be a normal finding, but this should decompress after voiding.
4. Renal stones are often detected, although US may miss small calculi. Renal stones are hyperechoic foci in the collecting system that often demonstrate posterior acoustic shadowing and twinkle artefact on Doppler. Comet-tail artefact may also be present.

Bladder Ultrasound

1. The bladder is scanned with the probe in a suprapubic position in both transverse and longitudinal planes. The gain should be set to make urine appear anechoic and the time-gain compensation adjusted to take account of acoustic enhancement of urine within the bladder lumen.
2. Examination should aim to detect focal urothelial or bladder wall lesions. Diffuse changes secondary to bladder outflow obstruction should also be evaluated, including wall thickening, trabeculation, calculi and the presence of diverticulum.
3. Ureteric 'jets' are seen on Doppler US representing urine entering the bladder as a result of normal ureteric peristalsis.
4. Measurements taken of the three orthogonal diameters before and after micturition enable an approximate volume to be calculated by multiplying the three diameters and applying a conversion coefficient. Although most machines use the ellipsoid formula for generic volume estimation (~0.52), many have a specific bladder calculation function with a bladder-specific volume estimation (using a coefficient of 0.7).
5. A postvoid residual estimation is often necessary. A residual greater than 50 mL is considered significant in adult patients.

Renal Transplant Ultrasound

1. Renal transplants are usually located in the right or left iliac fossa. These lie superficially and are easy to evaluate using oblique planes and gentle pressure to displace overlying bowel loops. It is often possible to use a medium- or high-frequency transducer to evaluation the transplant kidney.
2. Transplant renal artery stenosis (TRAS) is diagnosed by direct Doppler interrogation of the main renal arteries from a transabdominal approach. Elevated peak systolic velocities in the transplant renal artery greater than 200 cm s^{-1} and an acceleration time of 0.1 s or more are suggestive of TRAS. Renal vein thrombosis is diagnosed by absent colour Doppler venous flow, direct visualization of thrombus within the distended vein, and a raised resistive index with reversal of arterial diastolic flow within the intrarenal arteries.

Further Reading

Bih L-I, Ho C-C, Tsai S-J, et al. Bladder shape impact on the accuracy of ultrasonic estimation of bladder volume. *Arch Phys Med Rehabil.* 1998;79:1553–1556.

de Morais RH, Muglia VF, Mamere AE, et al. Duplex Doppler sonography of transplant renal artery stenosis. *J Clin Ultrasound.* 2003;31:135–141.

iRefer: Making the best use of Radiology. RCR guidelines. 8th edition. 2017. <https://www.irefer.org.uk/guidelines>.

Kotval PS. Doppler waveform parvus and tardus. A sign of proximal flow obstruction. *Ultrasound Med.* 1989;8(8):435–440.

NICE guidelines. Renal or ureteric colic-acute-last revised August 2020. <http://cks.nice.org.uk/renal-or-ureteric-colic-acute>.

Sidhu R, Lockhart ME. Imaging of renovascular disease. *Semin Ultrasound CT MRI.* 2009;30(4):271–288.

COMPUTED TOMOGRAPHY OF THE URINARY TRACT

Indications

1. Renal stone disease and suspected renal colic
2. Renal mass characterization and local staging of renal cancer
3. Renal abscess, perirenal collection or urine leak
4. Staging of urinary tract cancers
5. Investigation of renal tract obstruction or hydronephrosis
6. Urinary tract trauma
7. Characterization of adrenal mass
8. Renal artery angiography

Techniques

Computed tomography of the abdomen and pelvis

This technique is used to stage and follow up known renal tract malignancy and to investigate non-specific signs attributed to the renal tract. Examination of the thorax may also be performed in addition to the abdomen and pelvis, where pulmonary metastatic disease or mediastinal nodal spread is a possibility:

Position: supine; arms above the head
Scan planning: above the diaphragm to below the symphysis pubis
Contrast administration: IV only
Breathing: breath-hold, inspiration
Contrast delay: 70 s (portal venous)

Technical notes: It is often necessary to perform CT of the chest. This can be done as a separate volume or as part of a single-volume chest, abdomen and pelvis technique according to local protocol.

Computed tomography of renal mass

This is used to assess lesions such as solid masses or renal cystic masses. These are often identified on US or as incidental findings on a non-dedicated abdominal CT or MRI.

Non-contrast and postcontrast scans are required to assess lesion attenuation and subsequent enhancement patterns. The nephrographic phase is optimal for assessing renal parenchymal masses because early postcontrast imaging may result in small intraparenchymal lesions being obscured by corticomedullary differentiation.

Position: supine; arms above the head
Scan planning: above the diaphragm to below the symphysis pubis
Contrast administration: IV at high flow rates (3–5 mL s^{-1})
Breathing: breath-hold, inspiration
Contrast delay: non-contrast, nephrographic (100 s)

Technical notes: A corticomedullary phase (20–30 s) of the kidneys is often added. This is useful for evaluation of renal vessels and to assess for arterial enhancement within renal tumours. Excretory phase imaging at 5 mins postcontrast can be included if pelvicalyceal opacification is necessary.

Computed tomography of the adrenals

Technique used for characterization of adrenal lesions:

Position: supine; arms above the head
Scan planning: above the diaphragm to the iliac crests
Contrast administration: IV
Breathing: breath-hold, inspiration
Contrast delay: non-contrast, venous (70–80 s), delayed (15 min)

Technical notes: An ideal protocol and workflow would allow for review of the study after the non-contrast phase has been acquired. If adrenal mass lesion density is less than 10 HU (highly specific for a benign lipid-rich adenoma), no further imaging is required.

In cases in which lesion density on non-contrast CT exceeds 10 HU, it is necessary to administer contrast and acquire venous and delayed phase imaging to calculate absolute washout of the adrenal lesion. It should be noted that utility of calculating washout may be limited in small adrenal 'incidentalomas'.

Further Reading

Corwin M, Badawy M, Caoili E, et al. Incidental adrenal nodules in patients without known malignancy: prevalence of malignancy and utility of washout CT for characterization—a multi-institutional study. *AJR Am J Roentgenol.* 2022;219(5):804–812.

LOW-DOSE COMPUTED TOMOGRAPHY OF THE KIDNEYS, URETERS AND BLADDER

Low-dose CT KUB is the primary investigation for suspected renal colic (replacing plain KUB radiograph) and renal stone evaluation.

Position: supine; arms above the head
Scan planning: above upper pole of kidneys to below bladder base
Contrast administration: none
Breathing: breath-hold, inspiration

Technical notes: Some authorities advise prone scanning to differentiate if stones are impacted at the vesicoureteric junction or have passed into the bladder lumen. A low radiation dose protocol should be used. Multidetector CT should acquire thin-slice (1–1.25 mm) data to allow for multiplanar reformats. Scans should be acquired from above the upper pole of the kidneys to below the bladder base. Iterative recontraction and spectral filtering techniques may be used to limit noise and radiation dose. Ultra-low-dose protocols may be used in the follow-up of renal stone disease.

COMPUTED TOMOGRAPHY UROGRAM

This technique uses a combination of unenhanced, nephrographic and delayed scans after IV contrast to sequentially allow examination of renal parenchyma and collecting systems. Initial low-dose unenhanced scans of urinary tract (CT KUB) are performed to determine if renal tract calculus disease is present. Multiple techniques have been described, and the choice of technique depends on the clinical indication.

Position: supine; arms above the head
Scan planning: above the diaphragm to below the symphysis pubis
Contrast administration: IV contrast ± diuretic or oral water
Breathing: breath-hold, inspiration
Contrast delay: three phase: non-contrast, venous or nephrographic
    (70–100 s), delayed or excretory (7–10 min)

Technical notes: Non-contrast phase is excluded as a dose-saving measure in some protocols. The nephrographic phase may be omitted if the scan is specifically for assessment of the collecting system or ureteric anatomy.

Many protocols use diuretics (10–20 mg furosemide) before contrast administration to improve distension of the pelvicalyceal systems and ureters on the excretory phase. An alternative is to prehydrate with oral water load 45–60 min before the examination.

It is possible to acquire both the nephrographic and excretory phase scans simultaneously with a single-bolus technique. Split-bolus protocols confer significant dose savings but eliminate the possibility of detecting enhancing urothelial tumours because of the presence of opacified urine in the upper tracts.

Renal Computed Tomography Angiography

See Chapter 11 for angiography principles.

Indications

1. Renal artery stenosis
2. Renal artery aneurysm, arteriovenous malformation, dissection or thrombosis
3. Delineation of vascular anatomy before laparoscopic surgery, e.g. nephrectomy, pyeloplasty

Technique

Position: supine; arms above the head
Scan planning: above the upper pole of the kidneys to the aortic bifurcation
Contrast administration: IV contrast at 3–5 mL/s
Breathing: breath-hold, inspiration
Contrast delay: arterial

Technical notes: Use of bolus tracking/triggering or timing test injections is recommended to ensure appropriate timing. Otherwise scans are initiated after a preset empiric delay of 20–25 s from start of contrast material injection.

Further Reading

Johnson PT, Horton KM, Fishman EK. Adrenal imaging with multidetector CT: evidence-based protocol optimization and interpretive practice. *Radiographics.* 2009;29:1319–1331.

Johnson PT, Horton KM, Fishman EK. Optimizing detectability of renal pathology with MDCT: protocols, pearls, and pitfalls. *AJR Am J Roentgenol.* 2010;194(4):1001–1012.

Low G, Dhliwayo H, Lomas DJ. Adrenal neoplasms. *Clin Radiol.* 2012;67(10): 988–1000.

O'Connor OJ, Fitzgerald E, Maher MM. Imaging of hematuria. *AJR Am J Roentgenol.* 2010;195(4):W263–W267.

O'Connor OJ, Maher MM. CT urography. *AJR Am J Roentgenol.* 2010;195(5): W320–W324.

O'Regan KN, O'Connor OJ, McLoughlin P, et al. The role of imaging in the investigation of painless hematuria in adults. *Semin Ultrasound CT MRI.* 2009;30(4):258–270.

MAGNETIC RESONANCE IMAGING OF THE URINARY TRACT

MULTIPARAMETRIC PROSTATE MAGNETIC RESONANCE IMAGING

Indications

1. Detection and local staging of prostate cancer
2. Follow-up of prostate cancer as part of active surveillance
3. Follow-up of prostate ablation (e.g. High-Intensity Focused Ultrasound [HIFU] or cryotherapy)

Technique and Example Protocol

1. Prostate MRI should be performed before prostate biopsy. Haemorrhage in the prostate as a result of biopsy significantly decreases the accuracy of multiparametric (mp) MRI and may persist for 3–6 months.
2. Field strength of either 1.5 or 3 T may be used. 3-T scanners afford better signal-to-noise ratio but may be subject to more artefacts, notably susceptibility. Generally, the advantages of increased spatial or temporal resolution at 3 T makes it the preferable choice for mpMRI of the prostate if available.
3. Patient supine with a phased-array body coil
4. Antiperistaltic drugs (hyoscine butyl-bromide or glucagon) are recommended to reduce artefact from bowel motion.
5. T2-weighted Rapid Acquisition with Relaxation Enhancement (TSE and FSE) scans in transverse, coronal or sagittal planes. These should be 3-mm slice thickness with a small field of view (≤20 cm) to encompass the whole prostate and seminal vesicles.

6. Diffusion-weighted imaging (DWI) with a free-breathing spin-echo Echo planar imaging (EPI) technique. Choice of B values should include both low (0–100) and intermediate (800–1000) for generation of ADC map, with the same small field of view and axial imaging plane as the T2 weighted if possible. In addition, a separate acquisition of a long b-value (≥1400) sequence that may need different geometry to allow adequate Signal-to-Noise Ration (SNR). Calculated long b-value images can be used as an alternative time-saving step.

7. Dynamic contrast-enhanced T1-weighted fat-saturated imaging with either a two- or three-dimensional (3D) gradient echo (GE) technique. The slice thickness, plane and geometry should match the T2-weighted imaging.

Further Reading
American College of Radiology. Prostate Imaging-Reporting and Data System version 2.1. <http://www.acr.org/-/media/ACR/Files/RADS/Pi-RADS/PIRADS-V2-1.pdf?la=en>.

6

MAGNETIC RESONANCE IMAGING OF THE KIDNEYS

Indications

1. Renal mass characterization and local staging or renal tumours
2. Investigation and follow-up of benign renal lesions (e.g. angiomyolipoma, renal abscess)

Technique

1. Supine position, body coil
2. Renal imaging is often limited by breathing artefacts. Respiratory-triggering or breath-hold techniques should be used.
3. True-axial and coronal-oblique to the long axis of the kidneys should be used. If available, 3D techniques and the Dixon method can be used.
4. T2-weighted TSE axial and coronal-oblique planes
5. T1 GE in/opposed phase, axial breath hold (or 3D Dixon technique)
6. DWI in axial plane; 5 mm slice thickness. B-values should include up to 800–1000.
7. Dynamic 3D T1-weighted fat-saturated imaging. Timings of 0, 30–45, 90, and 180 s.

MAGNETIC RESONANCE UROGRAPHY

Indications

1. Urinary tract stricture or upper tract dilation or obstruction
2. Urography in patients with allergy to iodinated contrast media
3. Congenital renal tract anomalies

CTU is the preferred in the investigation of haematuria and upper tract cancers.

Technique

1. Oral hydration before scan, particularly if diuretics are not used
2. Supine position; moderately full bladder if possible
3. Antiperistaltic drugs (hyoscine butyl-bromide or glucagon) are recommended to reduce artefact from bowel motion
4. T2-weighted imaging of the whole abdomen and pelvis in axial and coronal planes. A single-shot TSE and FSE technique is often preferred.
5. T1-weighted imaging of the whole abdomen and pelvis
6. Administration of diuretic if used
7. Static MRI urography: Axial and coronal or coronal-oblique T2-weighted fat-saturated imaging of the whole abdomen and pelvis. This should include a heavily T2-weighted MRI technique to visualize fluid-filled structures (equivalent to magnetic resonance cholangiopancreatography). This may include 3D respiratory-triggered sequences to obtain thin-section data sets, which can be processed into thick-slab maximum intensity projection images.
8. Excretory MR urography: A gadolinium-based contrast agent is administered. The collecting systems are imaged during the excretory phase using a breath-hold or respiratory-triggered, 3D GE, T1-weighted sequence. Fat suppression should be used. T2* effects from a high concentration of contrast agent may reduce the signal intensity of urine and potentially obscure small masses within the collecting system. This can be overcome by using a lower volume of IV contrast but may compromise soft tissue imaging. Precontrast imaging is mandatory. Various timing strategies can be used, which are dependent on the use of diuretics and the clinical indication. Early dynamic imaging of the kidneys in the arterial and venous phases is usual with excretory imaging of the whole urinary tract at 5 and 10 or 15 m.
9. The excretory urography may be avoided if the injection of gadolinium is contraindicated such as in pregnancy or end-stage renal failure.

Further Reading

O'Connor O, McLaughlin P, Maher M. MR urography. *AJR Am J Roentgenol.* 2010;195(3):W201–W206.

MAGNETIC RESONANCE IMAGING OF THE ADRENALS

Indications

1. Characterization of adrenal mass
2. Investigation of refractory or early-onset hypertension (with MR renal angiography)

Adrenal MRI relies on chemical shift imaging. Intracellular lipid causes alteration of the local magnetic environment within the voxel and hence resonant frequency of protons. Lipid-rich benign adenomas can be shown to lose signal on opposed phase T1-weighted imaging compared with in-phase studies.

Technique

1. No specific patient preparation is necessary.
2. Supine position
3. T1- and T2-weighted imaging of kidneys and adrenals in axial and coronal planes. Breath-hold techniques are often preferred.
4. T1 in and opposed-phase imaging in axial plane. GE technique during breath-hold.
5. Use of dynamic contrast-enhanced MRI and DWI is not well established in adrenal imaging.

Further Reading

Low G, Dhliwayo H, Lomas DJ. Adrenal neoplasms. *Clin Radiol*. 2012;67(10):988–1000.

MAGNETIC RESONANCE RENAL ANGIOGRAPHY

See Chapter 11 for principles of MR angiography.

6

URETHROGRAM (MALE)

Indications

1. Urethral stricture
2. Urethral trauma
3. Fistula or false passage
4. Congenital abnormalities

Contraindications

1. Acute UTI
2. Recent instrumentation

Contrast Medium

LOCM 200–300 mg I mL^{-1} 50 mL

Equipment

1. 10-Fr urethral catheter without a balloon (6–8 Fr may be necessary in some cases)

Patient Preparation

Patient consent is obtained.
    The patient washes his hands and is given non-sterile gloves.

Technique

Ascending or retrograde urethrogram (for anterior urethra)

1. In LAO position (towards operator) 20–30 degrees
2. A catheter is connected to a 50-mL syringe containing contrast medium and flushed to eliminate air bubbles.
3. Using aseptic technique, the tip of the catheter is inserted to the penile urethra so the tip lies below the level of the glans penis. The

patient is asked to place the thumb and index finger of his right hand circumferentially around the penis at the level of the coronal sulcus so he can prevent contrast from escaping and keeping the catheter in place. The patient should gently pull the penis away from the body to stretch out the urethra to avoid kinks or foreshortening from obscuring pathology.

4. The explorator is centred at the penoscrotal junction, and a collimated view from the penile tip to the bladder neck (level of femoral head) is obtained.

5. As the patient is asked to 'squeeze hard' with his hand, contrast medium is gently injected under fluoroscopic control until contrast enters the bladder. An exposure image of the whole distended urethra and bladder neck is obtained. The fluoro capture or loop is often useful, but the single exposure image is sufficient.

6. The ascending study should be repeated with a different view, particularly in case of an abnormality. This may include a true lateral RAO or supine position. (If supine, the penis should be orientated toward the feet.)

7. Views of the meatus and fossa navicularis are obtained in the same LAO position. Contrast should be instilled whilst screening and the patient asked quickly to let go and remove his hand. This distends the urethra, and contrast flows through the meatus.

Descending or micturating urethrogram (posterior urethra)

1. The bladder is catheterized (6- to 10-Fr catheter), and the catheter is connected to contrast media via a giving set. Contrast is slowly dripped into the bladder with intermittent spot images taken of the bladder until the patient feels that he can void.

2. The catheter is removed, and the patient is moved from supine to a standing position. The patient should be in an oblique position, but care should be taken so the bladder neck and posterior urethra do not overlap with the projection of the pelvic bones (especially the ischium).

3. Oblique views of the entire urethra are obtained whilst the patient is voiding, including an exposure image.

Complications Due to the Technique

1. Acute UTI
2. Urethral trauma or a small amount of bleeding from meatus can occur rarely.
3. Intravasation of contrast medium, especially if excessive pressure is used to overcome a stricture

Consider prophylactic antibiotics in case of trauma (blood at meatus) or contrast intravasation.

Further Reading

Kawashima A, Sandler CM, Wasserman NF, et al. Imaging of urethral disease: a pictorial review. *Radiographics*. 2004;24(suppl):S195–S216.

RETROGRADE PYELOURETEROGRAPHY

In many departments, this test has been superseded by CTU but is sometimes still performed.

Indications

1. Demonstration of the site and nature of an obstructive lesion
2. Demonstration of the pelvicalyceal system and potential urothelial abnormalities after previous indeterminate imaging

Contraindication

Acute UTI

Contrast Medium

High-osmolar contrast media (HOCM) or LOCM 150–200 mg I mL^{-1} (i.e. not too dense to obscure small lesions): 10 mL

Equipment

Fluoroscopy unit

Patient Preparation

As for surgery

Preliminary Image

Full-length supine AP abdomen when the examination is performed in the x-ray department

Technique

In the operating theatre

The surgeon catheterizes the ureter via a cystoscope and advances the ureteric catheter to the desired level. Contrast medium is injected under fluoroscopic control, and spot films are exposed. Some form of hard copy or soft copy recording is recommended, ideally to the hospital PACS (picture archiving and communication system).

In the x-ray department

1. With ureteric catheter(s) in situ, the patient is transferred from the operating theatre to the x-ray department.
2. Urine is aspirated, and under fluoroscopic control, contrast medium is slowly injected. Care should be taken to eliminate air bubbles before injection (because these may mimic pathology such as tumour or calculus). About 3–5 mL is usually enough to fill the pelvis, but if the patient complains of pain or fullness in the loin, the injection should be terminated before this.
3. Images are taken as the catheter is withdrawn. These should include frontal and oblique projections.

6

Aftercare

1. Postanaesthetic observations
2. Prophylactic antibiotics may be used.

Complications

1. Pyelosinus extravasation and pyelotubular reflux caused by overfilling may result in pain, fever and rigors.
2. Introduction of infection
3. Damage or perforation of the ureters or renal pelvis

CONDUITOGRAM OR LOOPOGRAM (IN PATIENTS WITH ILEAL CONDUIT)

Indications

1. Investigation of urinary tract obstruction or hydronephrosis
2. Suspected stricture at anastomosis of ureter and ileal urinary conduit
3. Suspected narrowing of conduit

CT is the preferred investigation for detection of upper tract tumours.

Contrast

LOCM or HOCM 150 mg I mL^{-1}

Technique

1. The patient should be advised to bring a spare stoma bag, or one should be available.
2. A urinary catheter is chosen tailored to the size of the stoma. (Although larger catheters may pass more easily, a smaller catheter may be needed.)
3. The catheter is flushed with contrast medium, and a syringe or giving set with contrast medium is connected. It is very important to exclude air bubbles, which can be confused for upper tract tumours.
4. The conduit is then catheterized using a sterile technique.
5. Opacify the loop with a small amount of contrast to check catheter position, confirming tip of catheter and balloon are deep to the abdominal wall and rectus sheath.
6. The catheter balloon is inflated with 5–10 mL of air, allowing it to be easily identified as a negative contrast structure.
7. Contrast is instilled under fluoroscopic control into the lumen of the conduit. The aim is to opacify both upper tracts.
8. Supine position. AP and oblique views are taken as appropriate, of sufficient number to demonstrate the whole pelvicalyceal systems, ureters and ureteric anastomoses.
9. With the patient in an oblique or lateral position, views of the distal part of the conduit and stoma are obtained showing the conduit through the abdominal wall (a potential site of narrowing).
10. An AP view of the kidneys should be taken at the end of the study to ensure upper tract drainage. If residual contrast remains, a 15-min delayed view after patient has been upright is recommended.

PERCUTANEOUS RENAL BIOPSY

Indications
1. Characterization of focal renal lesion
2. Non-targeted biopsy for assessment of renal disease

Contraindication
Uncorrectable bleeding diathesis

Equipment
US or CT guidance

Patient Preparation
Anaesthetic support and sedation may be necessary in some circumstances.

Technique
Insertion of the needle can be controlled by either US or CT:

6

1. The patient is placed in the prone position or as appropriate depending on patient habitus and the position of the lesion. For CT-guided biopsies, a lateral position may be needed depending on the location of the lesion.
2. The kidney is located directly with US or CT, and the biopsy path is planned.
3. The skin and subcutaneous tissues are infiltrated with 1% lidocaine.
4. The needle is passed directly into the lesion during suspended respiration. US or CT is used to monitor the path of the needle. Coaxial systems are available that allow for fewer passes of the needle through the parenchyma.
5. For biopsy, the biopsy needle is deployed after confirmation of needle position with imaging.

Complications
- Perinephric or retroperitoneal haemorrhage
- Haematuria
- Arteriovenous fistula or pseudoaneurysm
- Pneumothorax or visceral injury.

PERCUTANEOUS NEPHROSTOMY

This is the introduction of a drainage catheter into the collecting system of the kidney.

Indications
1. Renal tract obstruction
2. Pyonephrosis
3. Before percutaneous nephrolithotomy or antegrade ureteric stent insertion
4. For urinary diversion (often in the postsurgical setting for urinary leak)

Contraindication

Uncontrolled bleeding diathesis

Equipment

1. Puncturing needle: coaxial needle and catheter set or sheathed 18-gauge needle
2. Drainage catheter: usually an 8-Fr locking pigtail catheter with multiple side holes
3. Guidewires: hydrophilic angled and stiff wires (0.035 in)
4. US and fluoroscopy

Patient Preparation

1. Anaesthetic support and sedation are often required.
2. Prophylactic antibiotic

Technique

Patient position

The patient lies prone or prone oblique with a foam pad or pillow under the abdomen to present the kidney optimally.

Identifying the collecting system before the definitive procedure

1. US guidance is the most common method for localizing the kidney and guiding the initial needle puncture into the collecting system.
2. In a non-dilated system, the calyces may be difficult to delineate and target on US. Fluid challenges with or without diuretic may result in sufficient pelvicalyceal dilation to allow direct puncture with US.
3. IV contrast medium may be given, allowing direct puncture of the opacified system under fluoroscopic control using a parallax or 'bull's eye' technique, with US as an adjunct to establish safe point of needle entry to skin.
4. Occasionally, retrograde injection through an ileal conduit or a ureteric catheter may be used to demonstrate the target collecting system. This may require assistance from a urologist.

Site and plane of puncture

A point on the posterior axillary line is chosen below the 12th rib. Having identified the mid or lower pole calyces with US or contrast, the plane of puncture is determined. This will be via the soft tissues and renal parenchyma, avoiding direct puncture of the renal pelvis, so vessels around the renal pelvis are avoided and the drainage catheter gains some purchase on the renal parenchyma. There is a relatively avascular plane between the ventral and dorsal parts of the kidney, which affords the ideal access.

Techniques of puncture and catheterization

The skin and soft tissues are infiltrated with local anaesthetic using a spinal needle.

Puncture may then be made using one of the following systems (depending on preference):

1. An 18-gauge sheathed needle or Kellett needle using the Seldinger technique for catheterization. After the system is punctured, the needle should be removed, leaving the sheath in situ. A hydrophilic angled wire should be advanced to the proximal ureter (or renal pelvis) under fluoroscopic control, allowing the sheath to safely be advanced into the collecting system. Urine should be aspirated and a sample obtained if possible. Contrast injection is used to confirm successful siting of the needle and for preliminary demonstration of the pelvicalyceal system. Care should be taken not to overdistend the collecting system, particularly in the case of an infected or obstructed system. The hydrophilic wire should be exchanged for a stiff wire at this point. Dilation is then performed to the size of the drainage catheter, which is then inserted. Care must be taken not to kink the guidewire within the soft tissues. Sufficient guidewire should be maintained within the collecting system, ideally with the wire in the upper ureter to maintain position, and if kinking does occur, the kinked portion of the wire can be withdrawn outside the skin.

2. Coaxial needle puncture systems using a 22- or 21-guage puncturing needle that takes a 0.018-in guidewire. This affords a single puncture with a fine needle, with insertion of a three-part coaxial system to allow insertion of 0.035-in guidewire and then proceeding as above.

6

After the catheter has been successfully introduced, it is securely fixed to the skin, and drainage commences.

Aftercare

1. Bed rest for 4 h
2. Pulse, blood pressure and temperature half-hourly for 6 h
3. Analgesia
4. Urine samples sent for culture and sensitivity

Complications

1. Sepsis, UTI
2. Haemorrhage (haematuria, retroperitoneal perinephric haemorrhage)
3. Renal pseudoaneurysm
4. Perforation of the collecting system with urine leak
5. Unsuccessful drainage
6. Injury to adjacent organs such as the lung, pleura, spleen or colon
7. Later catheter dislodgement

Further Reading
Dyer RB, Regan JD, Kavanagh PV, et al. Percutaneous nephrostomy with extensions of the technique: step by step. *Radiographics*. 2002;22:503–525.

PERCUTANEOUS NEPHROLITHOTOMY

This is the removal of renal calculi through a nephrostomy track. It is often reserved for large, complicated calculi, which are unsuitable for extracorporeal shock-wave lithotripsy.

Indications

1. Removal of renal calculi
2. Disintegration of large renal calculi

Contraindication

Uncontrolled bleeding diathesis

Contrast Medium

As for percutaneous renal puncture

Equipment

1. Puncturing needle (18 gauge): Kellett (15–20 cm length) or equivalent
2. Guidewires, including hydrophilic and superstiff
3. Track dilating equipment: Metal coaxial dilators or high-pressure nephrostomy balloon catheter systems may be used.
4. US machine
5. Fluoroscopy facilities with rotating C-arm

Patient Preparation

1. Preoperative CT to demonstrate position of calculus and relationship to calyces
2. Preoperative workup, including full-blood count and clotting studies
3. Joint case with urology team under general anaesthetic
4. Antibiotic cover
5. Bladder catheterization

Technique

Patient position

As for a percutaneous nephrostomy; usually prone

Puncture of the collecting system

US-guided puncture of the collecting system is usually possible, as per the technique described earlier. The approach and choice of calyx depend on the position of the stone and agreed surgical plan. Often cystoscopy and retrograde ureteric catheterization by the urologist allows for distension or opacification of the collecting system.

Upon successful puncture, angled hydrophilic guidewire is guided into the collecting system and manipulated into the distal ureter (if possible). Track dilation is performed using metal or balloon dilators. A sheath is inserted over the largest dilator or balloon, through which the nephroscope is passed to allow endoscopic removal or fragmentation of the stone.

Complications

1. Failure of access, dilatation or stone removal
2. Infection or sepsis
3. Perforation of the renal pelvis

4. Haemorrhage, vascular injury, pseudoaneurysm, arteriovenous fistula
5. Damage to surrounding structures (i.e. diaphragm, colon, spleen, liver and lung)

Radiopharmaceuticals

^{99m}Tc-dimercaptosuccinic acid (DMSA), 80 MBq max (0.7 mSv estimated dose). DMSA undergoes tubular reabsorption and binds to the intracellular proteins in the proximal convoluted tubule of the nephron and is retained in the renal cortex with no significant excretion during the imaging period. Hence, DMSA gives the best morphological images of any renal radiopharmaceutical and is used for assessment of cortical scarring. It also gives the most accurate assessment of differential renal function.

Equipment

Gamma camera with a low-energy, high-resolution collimator

Patient Preparation

None

6

Technique

1. The radiopharmaceutical is administered IV.
2. Images are acquired at any time 2–3 h later. Imaging in the first hour is to be avoided because of free ^{99m}Tc in the urine.

Images

1. Posterior, right and left posterior oblique views with camera head close to the patient. Anterior images only in cases of suspected pelvic or horseshoe kidney and severe scoliosis or if relative function is to be calculated by geometric mean method.
2. Zoomed or pinhole views may be useful in children.

Analysis

Posterior views are generally used for analysis unless anatomical variation indicates anterior acquisition with geometric mean calculation. Background corrected activity using the region of interest on posterior views.

Additional Techniques

1. Single-photon emission computed tomography (SPECT) in the assessment of scarring and renal masses or 'pseudotumours'. But SPECT is not widely used.
2. ^{99m}Tc-mercaptoacetyltriglycine (MAG-3; maximum, 100 MBq, 0.7 mSv ED) can be used to estimate relative renal function but is inferior in terms of assessment of cortical scarring.
3. Fast dynamic frames with motion correction may be useful to reduce movement artefact, particularly in young children.

Aftercare

None

Complications

None

Further Reading
Blaufox MD. Procedures of choice in renal nuclear medicine. *J Nucl Med.* 1991;32:1301–1309.
Hilson AJ. Functional renal imaging with nuclear medicine. *Abdom Imaging.* 2003;28:176–179.

DYNAMIC RENAL RADIONUCLIDE SCINTIGRAPHY

Indications

1. Evaluation of obstruction
2. Assessment of renal function after drainage procedures to the urinary tract
3. Assessment of perfusion in acute native or transplant kidney failure
4. Demonstration of vesicoureteric reflux
5. Assessment of renal transplantation
6. Renal trauma
7. Diagnosis of renal artery stenosis (RAS)

Contraindications

None

Radiopharmaceuticals

1. ^{99m}Tc-MAG-3 (mercaptoacetyltriglycine), 100 MBq maximum (0.7 mSv ED); 200 MBq maximum (1 mSv ED) for first-pass blood flow imaging. Highly protein bound, it is mainly cleared by tubular secretion (80%) but with around 20% glomerular filtration. It is now the radiopharmaceutical of choice, owing to better image quality, particularly in patients with impaired renal function (compared with ^{99m}Tc-DTPA).
2. ^{99m}Tc-DTPA, 150 MBq typical (1 mSv ED), 300 MBq maximum (2 mSv ED); 800 MBq maximum (5 mSv ED) for first-pass blood flow imaging. This is cleared by glomerular filtration. There is a lower kidney-to-background ratio than for MAG-3, resulting in poorer image quality and noisier clearance curves.
3. ^{123}I-orthoiodohippurate (hippuran). This is almost entirely cleared by tubular secretion. It has high radiation dose and is not in clinical use now.

Equipment

Gamma camera with a low-energy general purpose collimator

Patient Preparation

1. The patient should be well hydrated with around 500 mL of fluid immediately before administration of tracer.
2. The bladder should be voided before injection.

Technique

1. The patient lies supine or sits reclining with the back against the camera.
2. The radiopharmaceutical is injected IV, and image acquisition is started simultaneously.
3. Perform dynamic acquisition with 10–15 s frames for 30–40 min. (For quantitative perfusion studies, e.g. in a transplanted kidney, 1–2 s frames over the first minute are acquired.)
4. There are different protocols for diuretic use, but in general, a diuretic (furosemide 40 mg IV or weight based in paediatrics) is administered along with or 10 min after radiotracer injection. Preadministration of diuretic (i.e. so-called F-15 or F-20 protocols) is used in dilated collecting systems with equivocal imaging on conventional protocol because maximum diuretic effect occurs 15 min after furosemide.
5. If significant tracer retention in the collecting system is apparent at the end of the imaging period, the patient is asked to stand up, void and walk around for 1 min; then a further short acquisition is taken. Postmicturition images can be analysed with quantification if required.

6

Images

1. All posterior
2. 2- to 5-min images for duration of study (~30 min)

Analysis

The following information is produced using standard computer analysis:

1. Kidney time–activity ('renogram') curves (background subtracted)
2. Relative function figures: additional figures are sometimes calculated:
3. Perfusion index, especially in renal transplant assessment
4. Parenchymal and whole kidney transit times, excretion indices and so on

Additional techniques

1. Pre- and 1 h postcaptopril (25–50 mg) study for diagnosis of RAS. Radionuclide techniques have the advantage of showing the functional effect of a stenotic renal artery, as opposed to the anatomical demonstration as provided by angiographic techniques. Thus, this helps identify patients in whom RAS is the cause of hypertension (renovascular). The patient should, ideally, stop diuretics and angiotensin-converting enzyme inhibitors 3–5 days before the test. The renogram curves after captopril are compared with the baseline study to look for a deterioration.
2. Indirect micturating cystography after renography to demonstrate vesicoureteric reflux. The bladder must not have been emptied, and the kidneys should be reasonably clear of activity. Continuous

dynamic 5-s images are acquired for 2 min before and up to 3 min after micturition, with generation of bladder and kidney time–activity curves.

3. Glomerular filtration rate (GFR) measurement and individual kidney GFR can be performed with ^{99m}Tc-DTPA or ^{51}Cr EDTA (not available at the time of writing this article) by taking blood samples for counting.

Aftercare

1. The patient should be warned that the effects of diuresis may last a couple of hours. The patient may experience postural hypotension when standing erect at the end of the procedure.
2. If captopril has been administered, blood pressure should be monitored until it has returned to baseline level.
3. Normal radiation safety precautions (see Chapter 1)

Complications

None, except after captopril, when care must be taken in patients with severe vascular disease to avoid hypotension and renal failure.

Further Reading

Blaufox MD. Procedures of choice in renal nuclear medicine. *J Nucl Med.* 1991;32:1301–1309.

Hilson AJ. Functional renal imaging with nuclear medicine. *Abdom Imaging.* 2003;28:176–179.

Taylor A, Nally J, Aurell M, et al. Consensus report on ACE inhibitor renography for detecting renovascular hypertension. *J Nucl Med.* 1996;37:1876–1882.

Woolfson RG, Neild GH. The true clinical significance of renography in nephro-urology. *Eur J Nucl Med.* 1997;24(5):557–570.

DIRECT RADIONUCLIDE MICTURATING CYSTOGRAPHY

Indications

Vesicoureteric reflux

Contraindication

Acute UTI

Radiopharmaceuticals

^{99m}Tc-pertechnetate, 25 MBq maximum (0.3 mSv ED), administered into the bladder

Equipment

Gamma camera with a low-energy general purpose collimator

Technique

This examination is most frequently performed on children.

The technique requires catheterization and is similar to that for Micturating Cystourethrography (MCU) but enables continuous imaging and is a lower-dose investigation. It is not commonly used.

Aftercare

As for conventional cystography

Complications

As for conventional cystography

Alternative

Direct radionuclide cystography is less commonly performed in most UK centres compared with fluoroscopic micturating cystography and provides less anatomical detail. However, it is purported to be more sensitive in the detection of vesicoureteral reflux and has a much less radiation dose penalty. Indirect radionuclide cystography may be performed after conventional radionuclide renography (see the section on dynamic renal scintigraphy) or fluoroscopic cystography (see previous discussion).

6

Further Reading

Jana S, Blaufox MD. Nuclear medicine studies of the prostate, testes, and bladder. *Semin Nucl Med.* 2006;36(1):51–72.

Mandell GA, Eggli DF, Gilday DL, et al. Procedure guideline for radionuclide cystography in children. *J Nucl Med.* 1997;38:1650–1654.

7

Ablation techniques

Pavan Najran

Minimally invasive image-guided percutaneous ablation is commonly used by interventional radiologists specializing in oncological treatment of a range of malignancies such as cancers of the liver, renal, lung, bone, pancreas, adrenals and spleen. This technology uses both thermal and non-thermal ablative techniques. Thermal ablative technology includes using heat-based energy from the electromagnetic spectrum, such as radiofrequency ablation (RFA) and microwave ablation (MWA), as well as cold-based energy, such as cryoablation. More recently, non-thermal ablative techniques, such as irreversible electroporation (IRE), have been developed, most commonly used in the treatment of patients with pancreatic cancers.

TYPES OF ABLATIVE TECHNOLOGY

1. Thermal ablative technology:
   (a) Heat-based energy:
      (i) RFA
      (ii) MWA
   (b) Cold-based energy: cryoablation
2. Non-thermal ablative technology: IRE

RADIOFREQUENCY ABLATION

Background Information

The radiofrequency (RF) generator produces a high-frequency (461,000 Hz) alternating current within the targeted cancerous tissue to cause ionic agitation, generating frictional heat and leading to cancer cell destruction or desiccation when the temperatures exceed 60°C.

Indications

1. Small cancers (typically <2 cm) and non-central location (not close to vital structures; e.g. liver, lung and renal cancers)
2. Non-surgical candidate because of the need to preserve the organ (e.g. multiple previous resections, nephron sparing in solitary kidney)
3. Patient choice

Contraindications

1. Poor life expectancy (<1 year)
2. Multiple metastases (relative)
3. Technically unsuitable because of the size or location of the tumour

Patient Preparation

1. Pre-assessment to check for fitness for general anaesthesia (GA)
2. Baseline bloods (e.g. clotting parameters, full blood count, liver function test and renal function test)
3. GA preparation, including starvation 6 h before the procedure

Equipment

Many types of RFA generators are available, such as the impedance-controlled and temperature-controlled generators.

Imaging Guidance Technique

The cancer can be targeted under ultrasound (US), computed tomography (CT) or magnetic resonance imaging (MRI) guidance.

Postprocedural Care, Imaging and Follow-up

After RFA, the imaging follow-up depends on the organ site.

1. Liver: CT or MRI
2. Renal: CT or MRI
3. Lung: CT

The frequency of follow-up is dependent on the local policy and the operator's experience, usually at 1, 3, 6 and 12 months for the first year and subsequent follow-up determined by the tumour type.[1]

MICROWAVE ABLATION

Background Information

MWA is an electromagnetic radiation that lies in the electromagnetic spectrum between the infrared and the RF wave, and it typically oscillates at 2.45 GHz (2.45 billion cycles s^{-1}). Water molecules (H_2O) are strongly polar, and when in a field that oscillates between a positive and negative charge the water molecules heat dielectrically. Using ultrathin needles, MWA produces a faster and larger zone of ablation with no charring effect as seen in RFA. It is becoming popular when a larger zone of ablation is desirable for the 'surgical' treatment margin.

Indications

1. Liver cancer: non-central location and especially when size is larger than 2 cm
2. Lung cancer: non-central location and especially when size is larger than 2 cm

3. Renal cancer: depends on the operator's experience and preference, because MWA can produce a larger zone of ablation, balanced against the need for nephron sparing.

Contraindications

1. Poor life expectancy (<1 year)
2. Multiple metastases (relative)
3. Technically unsuitable because of the size or location of the tumour

Patient Preparation

1. Pre-assessment to check for fitness for GA
2. Baseline bloods (e.g. clotting parameters, full blood count, liver function test and renal function test)
3. GA preparation, including starvation 6 h before the procedure

Equipment

There are several types of MWA generator available, and operator familiarity and availability determine the choice.

Imaging Guidance Technique

The cancer can be targeted under US, CT or MRI guidance.

Postprocedural Care, Imaging and Follow-up

After RFA, the modality follow-up depends on the organ site.

1. Liver: CT or MRI
2. Renal: CT or MRI
3. Lung: CT

The frequency of follow-up is dependent on the local policy and operator's experience, usually at 1, 3, 6 and 12 months for the first year, with subsequent follow-up depending on the tumour type.

CRYOABLATION

Background Information

In cryoablation, the ice ball is created using the Joule Thomson effect. This is a process whereby high pressurized gas is allowed to undergo expansion through a valve or restrictive orifice, resulting in a massive change in temperature (i.e. cooling and leading to ice formation in the cryoablation setting).[2,3] In renal cryoablation, argon gas is used for this purpose, and this causes tumour cell destruction by forming intracellular and extracellular ice in the cells as well as cellular ischemia.[4,5]

Indications

1. Renal cancer: commonly used in the treatment of renal cancer because of the ability to visualize the ice ball and be more certain of

the treatment margin and confident of nephron sparing given the precision.

2. Lung cancers, especially those close to soft tissues.

3. Liver cancer: rarely used in the liver because of the potential of *cryoshock syndrome*, especially in larger liver lesions.

Contraindications

1. Poor life expectancy (<1 year)
2. Multiple metastases (relative)
3. Technically unsuitable because of the size or location of the tumour

Patient Preparation

1. Pre-assessment to check for fitness for GA
2. Baseline bloods (e.g. clotting parameters, full blood count, liver function test and renal function test)
3. GA preparation, including starvation 6 h before the procedure

Equipment

There are a few commercially available cryoablation generators. Typically, in Europe, Galil Medical is the one commonly used.

Imaging Guidance Technique

The cancer can be targeted under US, CT or MRI guidance.

Postprocedural Care, Imaging and Follow-up

After cryoablation, the imaging follow-up depends on the organ site.

1. Liver: CT or MRI
2. Renal: CT or MRI
3. Lung: CT

The frequency of follow-up is dependent on the local policy and operator's experience, usually at 1, 3, 6 and 12 months for the first year, with subsequent follow-up depending on the tumour type.[1]

IRREVERSIBLE ELECTROPORATION

Background Information

IRE is non-thermal ablative energy (electrical field) using short high-voltage pulses of DC current, creating permanent nanopores in the cell membrane. This initiates apoptosis, leading to permanent cell death.[6] This particular non-thermal ablative energy preserves the vital structures, and non-cellular tissue is not affected because there is no lipid bilayer structure. All collagen structures (e.g. blood vessels and bile ducts) are preserved.

Indications

1. Liver cancer:
   (a) Central lesions (portal vein and bile ducts)

(b) Lesions enveloping hepatic vein confluence
(c) Lesions close to vital structures that cannot be moved by hydrodissection
2. Renal cancer: centrally located lesions close to blood vessels or ureter or tumour close to other vital structures (e.g. colon)
3. Pancreatic cancer

Contraindications

1. Poor life expectancy (<1 year)
2. Multiple metastases (relative)
3. Technically unsuitable because of the size or location of the tumour

Patient Preparation

1. Preassessment to check for fitness for GA
2. Baseline bloods (e.g. clotting parameters, full blood count, liver function test and renal function test)
3. GA preparation, including starvation 6 h before the procedure

Equipment

The only IRE generator currently available is the NanoKnife generator (AngioDynamics).

Imaging Guidance Technique

The cancer can be targeted under US or CT guidance.

Postprocedural Care, Imaging and Follow-up

After IRE, the imaging follow-up depends on the organ site.

1. Liver: CT or MRI
2. Renal: CT or MRI
3. Pancreatic: CT or positron emission tomography (PET)

The frequency of follow-up is dependent on the local policy and operator's experience, usually at 1, 3, 6 and 12 months for the first year, with subsequent follow-up depending on the tumour type.[1] The post-IRE pancreatic cancer follow-up depends on local policy; typically a combination of CT and PET is used.

References

1. Matin SF, Ahrar K, Cadeddu JA, et al. Residual and recurrent disease following renal energy ablative therapy: a multi-institutional study. *J Urol.* 2006;176(5):1973–1977.
2. Adamson AW. *Chemical Thermodynamics. The First Law of Thermodynamics. A Textbook of Physical Chemistry.* 1st ed. Academic Press; 1973.
3. Castellan GW. *Energy and the First Law of Thermodynamics; Thermochemistry. Physical Chemistry.* 2nd ed. Addison-Wesley; 1971.
4. Sprenkle PC, Mirabile G, Durak E, et al. The effect of argon gas pressure on ice ball size and rate of formation. *J Endourol.* 2010;24(9):1503–1507.
5. Weber SM, Lee FT. Cryoablation: history, mechanism of action, and guidance modality. In: van Sonnenberg E, McMullen W, Solbiati L, eds. *Tumour Ablation.* Springer; 2005:250–265.

7

6. Lee EW, Thai S, ST Kee. Irreversible electroporation: a novel image-guided cancer therapy. *Gut Liver.* 2010;4(suppl):S99–S104.

GENERAL PROCEDURAL TECHNIQUE

1. Imaging assessment is essential; depending on the target organ anterior, a posterior or lateral approach may be adopted.
2. Hepatic ablation traditionally uses a microwave or RF method of ablation as noted earlier. An anterior or posterior approach is most frequently used, although the lateral approach can be adopted for lesions located within the posterior segments.
3. For optimum analgesic control and stability of the patient through the procedure, GA is desirable. This also allows controlled breath hold, which is optimal for hepatic dome target lesions. Jet ventilation is also a useful method of ventilating the patient with minimal disturbance of the diaphragm. This reduces the movement of the liver during procedures, allowing for more accurate targeting and treatment.
4. Liver lesions within segment 5 or 6 can be challenging because of the proximity of the hepatic flexure. In addition, the colon may obscure the treatment field or impede the needle insertion; therefore, a hydrodissection technique can be adopted to open the treatment field, allowing a clear margin between the target lesions and adjacent at risk structures. This is more commonly required in the renal ablation because of the proximity of the colon and exophytic nature of the target renal lesions. A spinal needle is inserted between the target lesion and adjacent structure, normal saline is subsequently injected and reimaging is then performed to confirm a safe target approach.
5. Liver ablation is most often performed under US guidance, allowing for dynamic needle guidance. Lesions within the dome of the liver may require a combination of US and CT guidance to ensure the pleura is not traversed.
6. After the needle position is confirmed, ablation is performed. Before ablation, a biopsy can be performed for histological confirmation if required. In the case of liver ablation, most manufactures have a preset ablation protocol that is activated. When it is complete, the needle entry tract is embolized to the liver capsule, reducing periprocedural complications, including bleeding and biliary leak.
7. In the case of renal cryoablation, a surrounding ice ball can be seen extending approximately 1 cm from the target lesion.
8. Follow-up imaging varies depending on the target lesions; typically, 3-, 6- and 9-month surveillance imaging is performed.

KEY CHALLENGES & TIPS

Adjacent vascular structures can conduct heat away from the ablation zone with RFA, and consideration should be made to the potential for incomplete ablation when using RFA. Hydro- and gas dissection to mitigate this effect can be successful but lengthen the time of procedure and potential for additional complications. As with all ablative techniques, the operator must balance the risk of complications, from considerations such as ablation zone sizing to number of ablations, with the risk of not achieving a complete tumour lysis.

If there is a concern regarding the proximity of important adjacent structures, techniques to either protect or displace these away from the area of ablation can be used.

In the lung, the intentional creation of a pneumothorax, after the needle placement and fixation of the pulmonary tumour, controlled via a small pleural catheter, can displace the pleura away from the zone of ablation and create a relatively thermally insulated barrier with air. At the end of the procedure, the intrapleural air may be removed and the drain occluded until resolution of the pneumothorax has been confirmed. There always remains a risk of residual pneumothorax, which increases with gauge of needle, depth of lesion, presence of adjacent emphysema and number of passes.[1] Tract ablation, in which additional ablation of the parenchymal path of the needle is undertaken, also increases the risk of postprocedural pneumothorax, and a postprocedural chest radiography at 2–4 h is therefore necessary.

A similar technique can be adopted when ablating spinal tumours, the spinal cord can be displaced and insulated with either epidural gas or fluid via a spinal needle. CO_2 is thought to be a better insulator than air and mitigates the risk of air embolus. Saline should be avoided with RFA because of its high electrical conductivity, which is not an issue with MWA, but generally, gas dissection is thought to be superior to fluid dissection in thermal ablative techniques.[2-3] Fluid dissection should not be used with cryoablation because it will also freeze.

Close proximity of important structures in renal and hepatic tumours is more challenging, but the same techniques may be used to displace and protect. Some thermal ablative systems have trialled using saline injection intratumourally to increase the thermal effects of the ablation, however as there is a greater heat sink effect, particularly near fast-flowing or large vessels in the liver and kidney, non-thermal techniques should also be considered.

References

1. Khan MF, Straub R, Moghaddam SR, et al. Variables affecting the risk of pneumothorax and intrapulmonary haemorrhage in CT-guided transthoracic biopsy. *Eur Radiol*. 2008;18:1356–1363.
2. Tsoumakidou G, Buy X, Garnon J, et al. Percutaneous thermal ablation: how to protect the surrounding organs. *Tech Vasc Interv Radiol*. 2011;14(3):170–176.
3. Fillippadis DK, Tutton S, Mazioti A, et al. Percutaneous image-guided ablation of bone and soft-tissue tumours: a review of available techniques and protective measures. *Insights Imaging*. 2014;5:339–346.

Reproductive system

Balashanmugam Rajashanker

TECHNIQUES IN IMAGING THE FEMALE REPRODUCTIVE SYSTEM

1. Plain abdominal film
2. Hysterosalpingography
3. Ultrasound (US): transabdominal/transvaginal
4. Computed tomography (CT)
5. Magnetic resonance imaging (MRI)
6. Minimally invasive procedures including biopsies, cyst drainage, angiography, fibroid embolization.
7. Positron emission tomography (PET)–CT

Techniques in Imaging the Male Reproductive System (Scrotum and Testes)

1. US
2. MRI
3. Radionuclide imaging
4. Venography (including embolization of varices) and angiography

Further Reading

Barakat RR, Hricak H. What do we expect from imaging? *Radiol Clin North Am.* 2002;40(3):521–526, vii.

Cao L, Wei M, Liu Y, et al. Validation of American College of Radiology Ovarian-Adnexal Reporting and Data System Ultrasound (O-RADS US): analysis on 1054 adnexal masses. *Gynecol Oncol.* 2021;162(1):107–112.

Maciel C, Bharwani N, Kubik-Huch RA, et al. MRI of female genital tract congenital anomalies: European Society of Urogenital Radiology (ESUR) guidelines. *Eur Radiol.* 2020;30(8):4272–4283.

HYSTEROSALPINGOGRAPHY

Indications

1. Infertility
2. Recurrent miscarriages: investigation of suspected incompetent cervix, suspected congenital anomaly

209

3. After tubal surgery, after sterilization to confirm obstruction and before reversal of sterilisation
4. Assessment of the integrity of a caesarean uterine scar (rare)

Contraindications

1. Pregnancy or unprotected intercourse during the cycle
2. Active menstruation, recent uterine or tubal surgery
3. A purulent discharge on inspection of the vulva or cervix or recent diagnosis of pelvic inflammatory disease in the preceding 6 months
4. Contrast sensitivity (relative).

Contrast Medium

Low-osmolar iodinated contrast material (LOCM) 270/300 mg I mL^{-1}; volume 10–20 mL

Equipment

1. Fluoroscopy unit with spot film device
2. Disposable vaginal speculum
3. Vulsellum forceps
4. Hysterosalpingography balloon catheter (5–7 Fr). In patients with narrow cervix or stenosis of cervical os, a Margolin HSG cannula may be used. It has silicone tip and provides tight occlusion of the cervix for contrast injection.
5. Appropriate connecting tubes

Patient preparation

1. The examination is performed in the proliferative phase of menstrual cycle and can be booked between the 4th and 10th days in a patient with a regular 28-day cycle.
2. The patient should also abstain from intercourse between booking the appointment and the time of the examination unless she uses a reliable method of contraception.
3. A patient leaflet should be provided.
4. Apprehensive patients may need premedication.
5. Consent should be obtained.[1]

Technique

1. A sliding sheet placed below the patient sheet at the beginning will be useful to move the patient after insertion of the speculum. The patient lies supine on the table with the knees flexed and the legs abducted. The buttock is placed at the edge of the table for easy visualization of the cervix.
2. The vulva can be cleaned with chlorhexidine or saline. A disposable speculum is then placed using sterile jelly, and the cervix is exposed.
3. The cervical os is identified using a bright light. The cervix is examined for significant discharge or inflammation. If satisfactory, the HSG catheter is inserted into the cervical canal using the plastic guide provided. It is usually not necessary to use a Vulsellum forceps to hold the cervix with a forceps, but occasionally this may be necessary.

The catheter should be left within the lower cervical canal if cervical incompetence is suspected.

4. The catheter and connecting tubes should be primed with contrast. Care must be taken to expel all air bubbles from the syringe and cannula because these would otherwise cause confusion in interpretation. Contrast medium is injected slowly into the uterine cavity under intermittent fluoroscopic control.

5. Contrast should be injected until the uterine cavity shows satisfactory filling and all portions of the fallopian tube are visualized up to the infundibulum and fimbrial end. Spilling will usually occur at this point. Sometimes spill into the peritoneal cavity may be delayed by muscle spam. Spasm of the uterine cornu may be relieved by 20-mg intravenous (IV) glucagon if there is no tubal spill bilaterally. Please check for contraindications to Buscopan.

Note: Opiates increase pain by stimulating smooth muscle contraction.

Films

The radiation dose should be kept as low as possible. Intermittent screening should be performed to the minimal requirement. Images should demonstrate:

1. The endometrial cavity, demonstrating or excluding congenital abnormalities or filling defects

8

2. Full view of the tubes demonstrating spill. If occluded, show the extent and level of block.

3. If there is abnormal loculation of contrast, a delayed view may be useful.

Aftercare

1. It must be ensured that the patient is in no serious discomfort nor has significant bleeding before she leaves.

2. The patient must be advised that she may have spotting or occasionally bleeding per vagina for 1–2 days, and pain may persist for up to 2 weeks.

3. Prophylactic antibiotics are routinely given in some centres and is a good practice to prevent the risk of pelvic infections.

Complications

Due to the contrast medium

Allergic phenomena, especially if contrast medium is forced into the circulation

Due to the technique

1. Pain may occur at the following times:
   (a) While the speculum is being used
   (b) During insertion of the cannula or inflation of balloon; some patients may have a cervical shock

   (c) With tubal distension proximal to a block
   (d) With distension of the uterus if there is tubal spasm
   (e) With peritoneal irritation during the following day and for up to 2 weeks
2. Bleeding from trauma to the uterus or cervix
3. Transient nausea, vomiting and headache
4. Intravasation of contrast medium into the venous system of the uterus results in a fine lacelike pattern within the uterine wall. When more extensive, intravasation outlines larger veins. It is of little significance when water-soluble contrast media are used. Intravasation may be precipitated by direct trauma to the endometrium, timing of the procedure near menstruation or curettage, tubal occlusion or congenital abnormalities.[2]
5. Infection, which may be delayed. Occurs in up to 2% of patients and is more likely with a previous history of pelvic infection. Using prophylactic antibiotics is useful to prevent this complication.

Detectable Pathology

1. Congenital uterine anomalies
2. Intrauterine lesions such as polyps, submucosal fibroids or uterine malignancy
3. Intrauterine adhesions and synechiae (Asherman's syndrome)
4. Blocked tubes
5. Hydrosalpinx
6. Mass within fallopian tubes

References

1. Onwuchekwa CR, Oriji VK. Hysterosalpingographic (HSG) pattern of infertility in women of reproductive age. *J Hum Reprod Sci.* 2017;10(3):178–184.
2. Úbeda B, Paraira M, Alert E, et al. Hysterosalpingography spectrum of normal variants and nonpathologic findings. *AJR Am J Roentgenol.* 2001;177:131–135.

PELVIC ULTRASOUND OF THE FEMALE REPRODUCTIVE SYSTEM

Indications

1. Pelvic mass
2. Pregnancy: normal and suspected ectopic
3. Precocious puberty or delayed puberty
4. Pelvic pain
5. Assessment of tubal patency
6. In assisted fertilization techniques
7. Postmenopausal bleeding
8. Menstrual problems, location of IUD
9. Ovarian cancer screening

Contraindications

None

Patient Preparation

1. Transabdominal: full bladder
   Transvaginal: empty bladder
2. Patient consent[1]
   It is always advisable to have a chaperone.

Equipment

Transabdominal: 4- to 10-MHz curvilinear transducers
Transvaginal: 9 to 13 endovaginal transducers

Reporting Gynaecological Ultrasound

The following format may be useful to assess the female reproductive system.

1. Uterine size in three dimensions; note any congenital anomalies
2. Comment on the endometrium thickness, presence of polyps and the junctional zone to evaluate for adenomyosis. The endometrium has a physiological trilaminar (three-layered) appearance during midcycle.
3. Comment on the presence of fibroids. Size, number and location of fibroids. Comment on the cervix.
4. Three-dimensional (3D) ovarian measurements and volume. Presence of features such as polycystic ovaries, significant cysts or mass lesions. Colour Doppler is useful in the assessment of complex adnexal mass lesions, helping to differentiate retracted clot from solid components with blood supply.
5. Comment on adnexa for extraovarian lesions.
6. Examine the cul-de-sac for the presence of endometriotic deposits or mass lesions. Note the presence of free fluid or ascites.
7. If bowel gas interferes with visualization of ovaries, hand compression and bimanual examination may be helpful.

Several software programs are available to improve resolution. Tissue harmonic imaging is useful for interrogation of difficult patients. Three- and four-dimensional US are also widely available currently and mainly used in obstetric imaging. In gynaecology, 3D endometrial imaging may be useful in patients with congenital anomalies, although MRI may be more conclusive.

Contrast Medium

Galactose monosaccharide microparticles (Echovist) can be used as a specific contrast agent in the assessment of tubal patency; contrast is administered via an intrauterine catheter and the spillage of the microparticles into the peritoneal cavity infers patency.

Reference
1. *Guidance on Professional Standards and Ethics for Doctors: Decision Making and Consent.* General Medical Council; 2020.

Further Reading

Ascher SM, Reinhold C. Imaging of cancer of the endometrium. *Radiol Clin North Am.* 2002;40(3):563–576.

Bates J. *Practical Gynaecological Ultrasound.* 2nd ed. Cambridge University Press; 2006.

Bhatt S, Ghazale H, Dogra VS. Sonographic evaluation of ectopic pregnancy. *Radiol Clin North Am.* 2007;45(3):549–560.

Funt SA, Hann LE. Detection and characterization of adnexal masses. *Radiol Clin North Am.* 2002;40(3):591–608.

Qu E, Zhang M, Ju J, et al. Is hysterosalpingo-contrast sonography (HyCoSy) using sulfur hexafluoride microbubbles (SonoVue) sufficient for the assessment of fallopian tube patency? A systematic review and meta-analysis. *J Ultrasound Med.* 2023;42(1):7–15.

Shwayder JM. Normal pelvic anatomy. *Obstet Gynecol Clin North Am.* 2019;46(4): 563–580.

ULTRASOUND OF THE SCROTUM

Indications

1. Suspected testicular tumour
2. Suspected epididymo-orchitis
3. Hydrocoele
4. Acute torsion. In boys or young men in whom this clinical diagnosis has been made and emergency surgical exploration is planned, US should not delay the operation. Although colour Doppler may show an absence of vessels in the ischaemic testis, it is possible that partial untwisting resulting in some blood flow could lead to a false-negative examination result.
5. Suspected varicocele
6. Scrotal trauma

Contraindications

None

Patient preparation

Verbal consent is usually obtained.

Equipment

7.5- to 15-MHz transducer. Linear array for optimum imaging.

Technique

1. Patient supine with the legs together. Some operators support the scrotum on a towel draped beneath it or in a gloved hand.
2. Both sides are examined with longitudinal and transverse scans enabling comparison to be made.
3. Real-time scanning enables the optimal oblique planes to be examined.
4. In comparing the 'normal' with the 'abnormal' side, the machine settings should be optimized for the normal side, especially for colour

Doppler. They should not be changed until both sides have been compared.

5. The patient can also be scanned standing upright, and a Valsalva manoeuvre can be performed if a varicocele is suspected.

6. Testicular size and volume, echogenicity and presence of focal lesions to be noted. Epididymides are seen posterolaterally. The presence of cysts and inflammatory changes needs to be noted. Also look for hydrocele, noted as free fluid outside the testes in the tunica.

Further Reading

Alkhori NA, Barth RA. Pediatric scrotal ultrasound: review and update. *Pediatr Radiol.* 2017;47(9):1125–1133.

Kim W, Rosen MA, Langer JE, et al. US MR imaging correlation in pathologic conditions of the scrotum. *Radiographics.* 2007;27(5):1239–1253.

Pearl MS, Hill MC. Ultrasound of the scrotum. *Semin Ultrasound CT MR.* 2007;28(4): 225–248.

Rebik K, Wagner JM, Middleton W. Scrotal ultrasound. *Radiol Clin North Am.* 2019;57(3):635–648.

COMPUTED TOMOGRAPHY OF THE REPRODUCTIVE SYSTEM

Indications

8

1. Staging of vaginal, ovarian, endometrial and cervical cancers
2. To evaluate causes of raised CA125 levels
3. In postoperative settings such as evaluation for intestinal obstruction or collections

Technique

CT staging is usually performed with IV contrast to evaluate for metastatic disease. Local staging in endometrial and cervical cancers is performed with MRI scan. CT of the thorax, abdomen and pelvis is indicated in endometrial cancers with advanced local disease, aggressive histology and sarcomas. Local staging in cervical cancer is also performed with MRI scan, but CT of the abdomen may be indicated in assessment of extent of nodal disease into the abdomen. CT of the abdomen and pelvis is generally used for staging of ovarian cancer but is of limited value in characterization of ovarian lesions, in which MRI is more useful.

MAGNETIC RESONANCE IMAGING OF THE REPRODUCTIVE SYSTEM

Indications

1. Staging of cervical and endometrial cancers
2. Characterization of complex ovarian mass
3. Suspected Müllerian tract anomalies

4. Investigation of endometriosis
5. Staging of ovarian cancer, although CT is often necessary
6. Assessment of the pelvic floor
7. Scrotal MR can be used, generally after US, to further characterize a mass as intra- or extratesticular and to determine the location of intraabdominal undescended testis
8. Localization and morphology of uterine fibroids before consideration for uterine artery embolization.

Artefacts

Artefact from small-bowel peristalsis and, to a lesser extent, colonic peristalsis can occasionally be a problem in the pelvis, and IV Buscopan 20 mg may be used to minimize this. Respiratory artefact is less of a problem in the pelvis than in the upper and mid abdomen. Movement from anterior abdominal wall fat can be suppressed using a saturation band. Fasting for 3 h before MRI scan can also help to reduce bowel movements.

It is also important that the urinary bladder is not too full because it limits evaluation.

Pulse Sequences

For midline structures (uterus, cervix and vagina) sagittal T2-weighted spin-echo (SE) sequences can be augmented with further high-resolution, small-field-of-view T2 axial and coronal sequences angled to regions of interest are required.

Inclined axial and coronal images perpendicular and parallel to the long axis of the uterus or the long axis of the cervix are helpful for uterine and cervical abnormalities, respectively. This technique is also mandatory for accurate local staging of uterine and cervical cancers.

The ovaries may be assessed with axial T1-weighted and three orthogonal planes T2-weighted SE sequences. T1-weighted fat saturated sequences are used to identify haemorrhage (e.g. within endometriomas) and to help identify fat-containing masses.

Diffusion-weighted imaging (DWI) is now routinely used in pelvic MRI. Restricted diffusion in cancer cells makes pathology bright on sequences with higher b-values (measured in seconds per square millimetre). Usually higher b-values of 800–1000 s mm^{-2} are used in gynaecology imaging. Thus, DWI helps in detection and characterization of tumours and assessment of treatment response to cancer.[1] Apparent diffusion coefficient (ADC) values may make it possible to differentiate between normal and cancerous tissues in the uterine cervix and endometrium.

Perfusion imaging of the uterus can be used to assess the effectiveness of uterine fibroid therapy.

MRI is also used to measure the pelvic outlet in pelvimetry to avoid radiation dose.

Scrotal MR is generally performed with the scrotum supported as in US, using a surface coil. High-resolution axial, sagittal and coronal T2-weighted SE scans are obtained with a T1-weighted scan to identify haemorrhage. Large field-of-view scans should be performed to assess the inguinal canal for the presence of a hernia. Gadolinium IV can be given if necessary to assess perfusion. Scans should include the pelvis and kidneys if an undescended testis is being investigated.

Reference
1. Motoshima S, Irie H, Nakazono T, et al. Diffusion-weighted MR imaging in gynecologic cancers. *J Gynecol Oncol.* 2011;22(4):275–287.

GYNAECOLOGICAL MALIGNANCY

There are two commonly used staging systems for gynaecological cancers, namely Fédération Internationale de Gynécologie et d'Obstétrique (FIGO) and Tumour, Node and Metastases (TNM); the former is recommended for use in current UK practice.

CERVICAL CANCER

The initial diagnosis is made on clinical history, abnormal smear results, direct examination and biopsy. Regular cervical smears are recommended in disease prevention.

Staging

MRI is the technique of first choice for staging cervical cancer. It is of limited use in clinical stage less than 1B1. If the tumour is larger than 4 cm, then it is staged as 1B2 and not suitable for surgery and warrants radiotherapy. If there is spread of tumour outside pelvis, CT scan may be necessary to evaluate distant metastatic disease. PET-CT may be useful if extensive pelvic exenteration surgery is needed.

The FIGO system does not take nodes into consideration for staging; hence, the presence of nodes should be indicated in the final report.

Pulse Sequences

1. Axial T1 weighted: whole pelvis (slice thickness, 5–7 mm)
2. Axial, coronal and sagittal T2 weighted, high resolution (3-mm slices)
3. Axial DWI sequences with high b-values (B0, B800–1000 s/mm^2)

Use of IV hyoscine or the other antiperistalsis agent may be useful to reduce artefacts from bowel movements.

Additional sequences may be necessary and be varied according to local protocol.

When reporting comment on regional nodes: paracervical, parametrial, internal iliac, obturator, common iliac, external iliac, presacral and lateral sacral.

Follow-up

Clinical and imaging follow-up as appropriate and according to local protocol.

8

If recurrence is suspected, local spread is best assessed by MRI. More extensive and distant spread is assessed by CT scan. Treatment decisions are usually made in multidisciplinary meetings.

UTERINE CARCINOMA

Uterine cancer usually presents as postmenopausal bleeding. An initial evaluation is performed with US measuring endometrial thickness. Endometrial thickness greater than 4 mm in postmenopausal women warrants further hysteroscopy and biopsy.

MRI staging should be performed in biopsy positive cases for local staging. However, in more aggressive tumours on histology, a CT scan of the thorax, abdomen and pelvis is necessary to exclude distant metastases.

Pulse Sequences

A surface coil is used for pelvic imaging.
  Suggested sequences are:

1. Axial, coronal and sagittal T2-weighted high-resolution 3-mm slices with a small field of view
2. Axial T2-weighted whole pelvis 5-mm thickness
3. Axial T1-weighted whole pelvis 5- to 7-mm thickness
4. T1-weighted fat-saturated gradient echo sagittal and axial dynamic at 30, 60 and 180 s postgadolinium

DWI may improve the overall staging accuracy.
  IV hyoscine or another antiperistaltic agent may be given to improve image quality.

Follow-up

Clinical and imaging follow-up in accordance with local protocol. The optimal imaging strategy should be determined after discussions in multidisciplinary meetings.

OVARIAN CANCER

US is the initial mode of investigation in evaluation of ovarian mass lesion. Most of the simple cysts may be characterized by transvaginal US.

Indeterminate cysts on US can be characterized by MR scans. Adding a fat-saturated T1-weighted sequence may be useful in characterizing dermoid cysts because of their fat content. Haemorrhagic cysts, which have high T1 signal, do not show suppression on fat-saturated sequences.

Malignant cysts show solid components that show postcontrast enhancement.

DWI sequences also help in identifying malignant components, which appear bright because of restricted diffusion on higher b-values. ADC mapping may also complement analysis.

Highly increased CA125 levels suggest the possibility of metastatic disease and warrant a CT scan.

Typical spread of ovarian cancer is to the omentum, retroperitoneal nodes and surface liver deposits. The diagnosis can be obtained by omental biopsy. It is not recommended to biopsy ovarian masses percutaneously because of the risk of dissemination of disease into the peritoneum.

OMENTAL BIOPSY

Omental biopsy is usually best performed under US or CT guidance. This can be performed as a day case or with overnight hospitalization.

A full blood count and clotting need be performed to exclude coagulopathy. If the patient has ascites, it should be drained. This allows better visualization of the omental mass and makes the biopsy easier.

Written consent should be obtained. The risk of bleeding and injury to bowel should be discussed.

The procedure can be performed under local anaesthesia. The largest and most superficial omental mass is chosen for biopsy. With US, omental masses can be confused with bowel and should be performed by experienced radiologists. Omental tissue is more hypoechoic, shows colour Doppler flow and on compression does not show peristalsis.

If unsure, biopsy should be performed under CT guidance. In small-volume disease, when omental disease is difficult to identify on US, sampling based on prebiopsy CT landmarks can help with diagnostic yields.

The procedure is performed with a 18-gauge Tru-Cut biopsy needle. Usually two or three passes can be made to ensure adequate specimen. Care should be exercised to avoid injury to the small bowel because sometimes the tumour can be fixed to the bowel.

Patients need to be under observation for at least 6 h after the procedure.

Percutaneous omental biopsy has significantly reduced the need for diagnostic laparotomy and laparoscopic biopsies.

8

Further Reading
Brown MA, Martin DR, Semelka R. Future directions in MR imaging of the female pelvis. *Magn Reson Imaging Clin N Am.* 2006;14(4):431–437.
Burn PR, McCall JM, Chinn RJ, et al. Uterine fibroleiomyoma: MR imaging appearances before and after embolization of uterine arteries. *Radiology.* 2000;214(3):729–734.
Coakley FV. Staging ovarian cancer: role of imaging. *Radiol Clin North Am.* 2002;40(3):609–636.
Devine C, Viswanathan C, Faria S, et al. Imaging and staging of cervical cancer. *Semin Ultrasound CT MR.* 2019;40(4):280–286.
Hamm B, Forstner R, Kim ES, et al. MRI and CT of the female pelvis. *J Nucl Med.* 2008;49(5):862.
Hill DK, Schmit GD, Moynagh MR, et al. Percutaneous omental biopsy: efficacy and complications. *Abdom Radiol (NY).* 2017;42(5):1566–1570.

Humphries PD, SimpsonJ C, Creighton SC, et al. MRI in the assessment of congenital vaginal anomalies. *Clin. Radiol.* 2008;63(4):442–448.

Lewin SN. Revised FIGO staging system for endometrial cancer. *Clin Obstet Gynecol.* 2011;54(2):215–218.

Martin DR, Salman K, Wilmot CC. MR imaging evaluation of the pelvic floor for the assessment of vaginal prolapse and urinary incontinence. *Magn Reson Imaging Clin N Am.* 2006;14(4):523–535.

McCluggage G, Hirschowitz L, Ganesan R, et al. Which staging system to use for gynaecological cancers: a survey with recommendations for practice in the UK. *J Clin Pathol.* 2010;63(9):768–770.

Pecorelli S. Revised FIGO staging for carcinoma of the vulva, cervix and endometrium. *Int J Gynecol Obstet.* 2009;105(2):103–104.

Perez AA, Lubner MG, Pickhardt PJ. Ultrasound-guided omental biopsy: diagnostic yield and association with CT features based on a single-Institution 18-year series. *AJR Am J Roentgenol.* 2021;217(4):898–906.

Que Y, Wang X, Liu Y, et al. Ultrasound-guided biopsy of greater omentum: an effective method to trace the origin of unclear ascites. *Eur J Radiol.* 2009;70(2):331–335.

Raithatha A, Papadopoulou I, Stewart V, et al. Cervical cancer staging: a resident's primer: women's imaging. *Radiographics.* 2016;36(3):933–934.

Scheidler J, Heuck AF. Imaging of cancer of the cervix. *Radiol Clin North Am.* 2002;40(3):577–590.

Spencer JA, Swift SE, Wilkinson N, et al. Peritoneal carcinomatosis: image-guided peritoneal core biopsy for tumor type and patient care. *Radiology.* 2001;221:173–177.

Respiratory system

Samavia Raza

METHODS OF IMAGING THE RESPIRATORY SYSTEM

1. Plain films
2. Computed tomography (CT)
3. Radionuclide imaging (ventilation/perfusion (V/Q) scans)
4. Ultrasound (US)—for pleural, chest wall disease and diaphragm
5. Magnetic resonance imaging (MRI)
6. Positron emission tomography (PET)

Further Reading
Hansell DM, Lynch DA, Page H, et al. Technical considerations. In: *Imaging of Diseases of the Chest*. Elsevier; 2009:1–37.

COMPUTED TOMOGRAPHY OF THE THORAX

Indications

1. In the assessment of pulmonary masses, chest wall or pleural disease
2. For the staging and follow-up of malignancy in the chest
3. In the assessment (characterization, quantification and follow-up) of diffuse lung disease
4. Evaluation of known or suspected thoracic vascular assessment (congenital or acquired—pulmonary embolus (PE), aortic dissection, arteriovenous malformation and so on)
5. In the assessment of airways disease, bronchiectasis and large airway stenosis
6. Evaluation for thoracic manifestations of known extrathoracic disease
7. Trauma of the chest
8. Performing CT-guided intervention (e.g. lung, pleura or chest wall mass biopsy, bronchial stent insertion, pleural collection drainage, radiofrequency ablation)

Contraindications

When intravenous (IV) contrast medium is to be administered, the presence of impaired renal function, nephrotoxic drugs and history of previous reaction to IV iodinated contrast media must be evaluated.

Technique

1. **Volume scan**—usually performed with intravenous contrast enhancement at a rate of 3–5 mL s^{-1} with a delay of 25–40 s. Bolus tracking software, however, can be used to trigger the scan more precisely to coincide with optimal contrast enhancement of specific structures such as the mediastinum or the aorta in suspected aortic dissection or pulmonary artery in suspected PE. The combination of bolus tracking timing and saline chaser produces higher contrast density, with smaller volume of contrast needed and can wash out streak artefact from dense contrast in the great veins and right side of the heart. (Delayed imaging at 60–65 s can be useful in cases of large pleural effusion to assess for enhancement of otherwise occult underlying soft tissue pleural thickening.)

2. **High-resolution scan.** Non-contrast scan obtained on full inspiration, either:

   (a) 1-mm (or less) slices at 10- to 20-mm intervals or

   (b) Volume acquisition through the lungs with reconstruction of contiguous 1-mm slices:
   - Spatial resolution should be maximized using the smallest field of view possible.
   - Reconstruct images use a high-resolution (high spatial resolution) 'bone' algorithm.
   - A volume acquisition with reconstruction of contiguous slices has the benefit of postprocessing capabilities, particularly multiplanar reformatting, which can help illustrate the cranio-caudal distribution of lung changes.
   - Additional expiratory images can be performed in suspected air-trapping and airways disease. Interspaced expiratory imaging is sufficient in most cases; however, dynamic airway collapse assessment may warrant spiral expiratory phase volume acquisition.
   - Additional prone images are indicated to differentiate reversible-dependent change from early interstitial fibrosis.

3. **Low-dose CT (LDCT) and ultra-low-dose CT (ULDCT) of the chest.** Technological advancements in scanner design, particularly because of tin filter acquisition, have led to increasing use of low-dose CT of the chest (radiation dose <1.5 mSv) instead of conventional dose "plain CT" for most thoracic indications.

   There is no significant difference in image quality or diagnostic ability of LDCT.
   - Spiral acquisition with 0.6- or 1-mm reconstruction is used with lung and mediastinal window reformats.
   - ULDCT techniques with iterative reconstruction deliver radiation doses less than 0.5 mSv with high quality of anatomical detail and are now increasingly being used in clinical practice.
   - ULDCT with doses near to that of a conventional chest radiograph has been considered as an alternative to plain film; however, cost,

widespread availability and ease of bedside acquisition remain significant advantages for plain film.

- ULDCT is more suitable for follow-up of known nodules rather than as an initial diagnostic test.

Recently introduced lung cancer screening programmes include 2-yearly chest CTs in appropriate asymptomatic populations. In the United Kingdom, this eligible population is defined as age 55–74 years with a current or past history of smoking. LDCT imaging with audited dose metrics is essential for demonstrating clinical and cost effectiveness of pilot programmes as national screening is expanded.

Further Reading
Beigelman-Aubry C, Hill C, Brillet P-Y, et al. MDCT of the airways: technique and normal results. *Radiol Clin N Am.* 2009;47(2):185–201.
Kim Y, Kim YK, Lee BE, et al. Ultra-low-dose CT of the thorax using iterative reconstruction: evaluation of image quality and radiation dose reduction. *AJR Am J Roentgenol.* 2015;204(6):1197–1202.
Macri F, Greffier J, Pereira FR, et al. Ultra-low-dose chest CT with iterative reconstruction does not alter anatomical image quality. *Diagn Interv Imaging.* 2016;97(11):1131–1140.
Paul NS, Sebastian Ley S, Metser U. Optimal imaging protocols for lung cancer staging—CT, PET, MR imaging, and the role of imaging. *Radiol Clin N Am.* 2012;50(5):935–949.
Webb WR, Muller NL, Naidich DP. Technical aspects of high-resolution CT. In: *High-Resolution CT of the Lung*: Lippincott Williams and Wilkins; 2015:2–46.
Weininger M, Barraza JM, Kemper CA, et al. Cardiothoracic CT angiography: current contrast medium delivery strategies. *AJR Am J Roentgenol.* 2011;196(3):W260–W272.

9

COMPUTED TOMOGRAPHY–GUIDED LUNG BIOPSY

Indications

1. Investigation of a new or progressing pulmonary opacity when other diagnostic techniques such as bronchoscopy have failed to make a diagnosis
2. Investigation of a new lung, pleural or chest wall lesion in a patient with known malignancy
3. To obtain histological sample for genetic typing in patient with known malignancy (e.g. identifying epidermal growth factor receptor mutation in patient with known lung adenocarcinoma)
4. To obtain material for culture when other techniques have failed to identify the causative organism in a patient with persistent consolidation

All biopsies should be planned after case discussion at a multidisciplinary meeting with a respiratory physician, radiologist, surgeon and oncologist, in which the balance of benefit versus risk can best be assessed. Central lesions are preferably biopsied transbronchially, either by standard bronchoscopy (when there is endobronchial disease) or, if extrabronchial, by transbronchial needle aspiration via 'blind' or, more usually now, with endoscopic ultrasound guidance.

Contraindications

Contraindications are not absolute but should be carefully evaluated by the relevant multidisciplinary team.

1. **Vascular:** bleeding diatheses (including conditions that affect platelet function such as chronic renal failure), patient on anticoagulants, significant pulmonary arterial or venous hypertension
2. **Respiratory:** contralateral pneumonectomy (unless the lesion is pleural based and lung tissue will not be traversed), presence of significant emphysema (particularly bullous disease) or significantly impaired respiratory function such that pneumothorax would not be tolerated. (A forced expiratory volume in 1 second of <1 L or <35% predicted is often used as lower-limit cut-off for biopsy.) Air travel should not be undertaken within 6 weeks after the procedure.
3. **Suspected hydatid disease**
4. **Uncooperative patient** (including intractable cough)

Equipment

1. Sampling needle:
   (a) Fine-needle aspiration can be performed if there is an on-site cytopathology service. Usually 20- or 22-gauge needles are used. Different needles vary by the profile of the needle tip and include Chiba (with a bevelled tip which allows straightforward cytological sample aspiration) and those with modified tips, which allow 'cutting' to obtain small histological fragments as well as aspiration (suitable for more fibrous lesions, e.g. Franseen (Cook Medical) and Westcott (Becton-Dickinson Medical)).
   (b) Cutting needle biopsy needles are larger gauge (usually 18- or 20-gauge) and obtain a solid core of tissue for histological examination. They usually have adjustable throw of the specimen notch for precise sampling of the lesion. Types include Temno and Quick-Core (Cook Medical). Coaxial needle biopsy systems stabilize the cutting needle, allowing resampling without repuncturing the pleura; aid re-angling of the cutting needle; and allow accurate preplanning of depth of passes. The operator should be aware the outer sheath of the coaxial system is one size larger than the sample core size.
2. Full resuscitation equipment, including equipment for pleural aspiration and chest drain insertion

Staff should be prepared for recognition and treatment of complications of pneumothorax, vasovagal episodes, haemoptysis and (very rarely) and air embolus.

Patient Preparation

1. Sedative premedication should be avoided if possible because the patient must remain cooperative so that a consistent breathing pattern can be maintained during the procedure.
2. The procedure can routinely be performed on a day-case outpatient basis, with observation for 4–6 h after the procedure, but a bed should be available in case of complications. Particularly frail patients, those with frail carers or dependants and those living alone should be admitted overnight after the procedure.
3. Clotting screen (ideally international normalized ratio ≤1.5 and platelets >100 × 10^9 L^{-1}). There is no clear evidence that aspirin should be discontinued prebiopsy, but consensus suggests clopidogrel should be stopped 5 days before the procedure.[1]
4. Pulmonary function tests (spirometry)

Technique

Precise technique will vary between operators, but general considerations include:

(a) Procedures are usually carried out under CT guidance, but if a lesion abuts the peripheral pleural surface, US imaging can be utilized.
(b) The procedure should be clearly explained to patient, particularly with regard to breathing instructions—avoid deep breaths and Valsalva manoeuvres, no sudden movements and to obtain a consistent level of breath-hold whilst the needle traverses the lung and samples are taken.
(c) Position the patient in a stable position on the back, front or side, determined by the position of mass and the most expeditious route from the skin to the lesion to avoid fissures, bony structures, cystic or emphysematous lung tissue and so on.
(d) Standard aseptic technique is used.
(e) Inject local anaesthetic into skin and subcutaneous tissues down to the pleura. Try to instil a bleb of anaesthetic immediately extrapleurally without traversing the parietal pleura itself; the anaesthetic will act over a greater area of pleura, and this reduces the number of times that the pleura is crossed (which may reduce incidence of pneumothorax).
(f) A sampling needle is advanced during suspended expiration with regular imaging to monitor position and alignment. It can be advanced on its own through the chest wall and peripheral lung or using a coaxial system because the latter allows more stable positioning of the biopsy needle and facilitates repeated sampling without repuncturing of the pleura.
(g) After an adequate sample has been obtained, limited CT at the end of the procedure will determine if a pneumothorax or parenchymal bleed is present.

9

Aftercare

1. Close observation is provided after the procedure for at least 1 h in a supervised ward or recovery area, with the patient laying in the puncture-site-down position so the weight of the lung helps seal the pleural puncture site; this should be possible for all but anterior approach interventions. The patient should avoid raising intrathoracic pressure unnecessarily, including avoiding sitting up unaided, coughing and talking for the first hour or so.
2. Departmental posteroanterior chest radiographs are taken approximately 1–4 h after the procedure. If a pneumothorax has developed (or progressed), then the further management will depend on the size of the pneumothorax and clinical condition of the patient. Small pneumothoraces in asymptomatic patients may be observed; larger pneumothoraces in symptomatic patients require aspiration or chest drain insertion.
3. High-risk and frail patients, particularly those with preexisting impairment of respiratory function, are best routinely admitted overnight.

Complications[2-4]

Usually occur early after the procedure:

1. Pneumothorax in about 20% (reported rates range from 8%–50%). Chest drain insertion is necessary, however, in only a small minority (~3%). The incidence of pneumothorax is increased if:
   - The operator is inexperienced.
   - A larger gauge needle is used.
   - There is an increased number of needle passes made.
   - There is a greater pleura to lesion depth.
   - Smaller lesions are biopsied.
   - The needle traverses a fissure.
   - The patient is coughing (precipitated by haemorrhage/ haemoptysis).
2. Local pulmonary haemorrhage (10%)
3. Haemoptysis (2%–5%)
4. Other complications, such as haemothorax, implantation of malignant cells along the needle track, spread of infection and air embolism, are all extremely rare.
5. The current documented death rate is 0.15%.

References
1. Malloy PC, Grassi CJ, Kundu A, et al. Consensus guidelines for periprocedural management of coagulation status and hemostasis risk in percutaneous image-guided interventions. *J Vasc Interv Radiol.* 2009;20(7):240–249.
2. Gohari A, Haramati LB. Complications of CT scan-guided lung biopsy: lesion size and depth matter. *Chest.* 2004;126(3):666–668.
3. Yeow K-M, Su I-H I-Hao, Pan K-T, et al. Risk factors of pneumothorax and bleeding: multivariate analysis of 660 CT-guided coaxial cutting needle lung biopsies. *Chest.* 2004;126(3):748–754.

4. Khankan A, Sirhan S, Aris F. Common complications of nonvascular percutaneous thoracic interventions: diagnosis and management. *Semin Intervent Radiol.* 2015;32(2):174–181.

Further Reading
Anderson JM, Murchison J, Patel D. CT-guided lung biopsy: factors influencing diagnostic yield and complication rate. *Clin Radiol.* 2003;58(10):791–797.
Aviram G, Schwartz DS, Meirsdorf S, et al. Transthoracic needle biopsy of lung masses: a survey of techniques. *Clin Radiol.* 2005;60(3):370–374.
Birchard KR. Transthoracic needle biopsy. *Semin Intervent Radiol.* 2011;28(1):87–97.
Lorenz JM. Updates in percutaneous lung biopsy: new indications, techniques and controversies. *Semin Intervent Radiol.* 2012;29(4):319–324.
Manhire A, Charig M, Clelland C, et al. Guidelines for radiologically guided lung biopsy. *Thorax.* 2003;58:920–936.
Richardson CM, Pointon KS, Manhire AR, et al. Percutaneous lung biopsies: a survey of UK practice based on 5444 biopsies. *Br J Radiol.* 2002;75(897):731–735.
Winokur RS, Pua BB, Sullivan BW, et al. Percutaneous lung biopsy: technique, efficacy, and complications. *Semin Intervent Radiol.* 2013;30(2):121–127.

METHODS OF IMAGING PULMONARY EMBOLISM

1. *Plain film chest radiography.* The initial chest radiograph is often normal. Various signs have been described in association with PE, but overall, the chest radiograph is neither specific nor sensitive. It has, however, an important role in identifying other pathology, producing the clinical picture, including infection, pneumothorax and rib fracture.

2. *V/Q radionuclide scanning.* The technique is described later in this chapter. Interpretation of V/Q images is not straightforward, and there are a number of causes for the typical V/Q mismatch. Interpretive criteria divide results into normal, very low and low probability; intermediate (or indeterminate) probability; and high probability. Specificity and sensitivity are such that PE is virtually excluded in the 'normal' group and is very likely (85%–90%) in the high-probability group. A significant proportion of patients, however, are placed in the indeterminate-/intermediate-risk group in which specificity is poor, and further imaging with computed tomography pulmonary angiography (CTPA) is then usually required. The use of V/Q scanning is diminishing as the first-line use of contrast-enhanced CT increases but may continue to have specific indications for, for example, the use of perfusion imaging alone (rather than CT) to reduce the dose in younger or pregnant or lactating patients.

3. *Multidetector CTPA* to diagnose PE down to a subsegmental level (technique described later). It will also assess for the presence of secondary right heart strain and for the presence of other pathology in the chest. (CT venography sequence performed at the same examination as CTPA to assess for underlying deep vein thrombus is of unproven benefit.[1])

9

Dual-energy CTPA can provide more confidence in diagnosis, especially for peripheral PE, and can help salvage a technically suboptimal scan. Iodine maps generated with dual-energy computed tomography (DECT) can help provide quantitative assessment of perfusion effects.

4. *Pulmonary arteriography* was traditionally the 'gold standard' and detects most PE but has been superseded by multidetector CTPA.

5. *MR angiography* has yet to find a role in the routine investigation of suspected PE but may evolve to be used in patients in whom ionizing radiation exposure or the use of iodinated contrast media is relatively contraindicated.

6. In addition,
    (a) *Echocardiography* can be used to assess right heart function or overload (and therefore prognosis) and in some cases may even identify intracardiac thrombus.
    (b) *Doppler US* of pelvic and leg veins can be undertaken to detect deep vein thrombosis.

RADIONUCLIDE LUNG VENTILATION/PERFUSION IMAGING

Indications

1. Suspected PE
2. Assessment of perfusion and ventilation abnormalities (e.g. in congenital cardiac or pulmonary disease, e.g. cardiac shunts, pulmonary arterial stenosis, arteriovenous malformations)
3. Quantitative assessment of right-to-left shunting (perfusion only)
4. Quantitative assessment of differential perfusion and ventilation before lung cancer, lung transplant or lung volume reduction surgery[1–3]
5. Evaluate causes of pulmonary hypertension (to exclude chronic thromboembolism).

Contraindications (to Perfusion Imaging)

1. Right-to-left shunt because of the risk of cerebral emboli
2. Severe pulmonary hypertension

Neither of these are absolute contraindications (indeed, perfusion imaging can be used for assessment of vascular shunts), and it may be considered acceptable to reduce the number of particles administered in these cases.

Radiopharmaceuticals

Perfusion

^{99m}Tc ($T_{1/2}$ 6 h, photopeak 140 keV) labelled macroaggregated albumin particles (MAA), 100 MBq maximum (1 mSv estimated dose (ED)), 10–40 μm in diameter, which occlude small lung vessels (<0.5% of total capillary bed). The biologic half-life of the MAA in the lungs is 1.5–3 h.

Ventilation

1. ^{81m}Kr (krypton) gas, 6000 MBq maximum (0.2 mSv ED). Ideal generator-produced agent with a short $t_{1/2}$ of 13 s and a γ-energy of 190 keV. Simultaneous dual isotope ventilation and perfusion imaging is possible because of different γ-energy to ^{99m}Tc. Wash-in and wash-out studies are not possible. Expensive and limited availability.

2. ^{99m}Tc-Technegas, 40 MBq maximum (0.6 mSv ED).[3] Ultrafine Tc labelled carbon particles, 5–20 nm in size. No simultaneous ventilation and perfusion imaging. Longer residence time in lungs than aerosols, so single-photon emission computed tomography (SPECT) and respiration-gated studies are possible. Similar diagnostic efficacy to krypton. Expensive dispensing system.

3. ^{99m}Tc-DTPA, aerosol, 80 MBq maximum (0.4 mSv ED). Simultaneous ventilation and perfusion imaging not possible. Cheap and readily available alternative to krypton but less suitable in patients with chronic obstructive airways disease or chronic asthma because clumping of aerosol particles is likely.

4. ^{133}Xe (xenon) gas, 400 MBq maximum (0.4 mSv ED) diluted in 10 L and rebreathed for 5 min. Long $t_{1/2}$ of 5.25 days and a γ-energy of 81 keV. Ventilation must precede perfusion study because low γ-energy would be swamped by scatter from ^{99m}Tc. Wash-in and wash-out studies are possible. Poor-quality images and rarely used.

Equipment

1. Gamma camera, preferably multiheaded for SPECT
2. Low-energy general-purpose collimator
3. Gas dispensing system and breathing circuit for ventilation

Patient Preparation

1. For ventilation, familiarization with breathing equipment
2. A current chest radiograph is required to assist with interpretation.

Technique[4]

Perfusion

1. The injection may be given in the supine, semirecumbent or sitting position (MAA particle uptake is affected by gravity).
2. The syringe is shaken to prevent particles settling.
3. A slow IV injection is given directly into a vein (particles will stick to a plastic cannula) over about 10 s. Avoid drawing blood into the syringe because this can cause clumping.
4. The patient must remain in position for 2–3 min while the particles become fixed in the lungs.
5. Imaging may begin immediately, preferably in the sitting position.

Ventilation

^{81m}Kr gas

This is performed at the same time as the perfusion study, either by dual isotope acquisition or by swapping energy windows at each patient position:

9

1. The patient is positioned to obtain identical views to the perfusion images and asked to breathe normally through the mouthpiece.
2. The air supply attached to the generator is turned on, and imaging is commenced.

^{99m}Tc-DTPA aerosol

This scan is performed before the perfusion study, which may follow immediately unless there is clumping of aerosol particles in the lungs, in which case it is delayed for 1–2 h:

1. A DTPA kit is made up with approximately 600 MBq ^{99m}Tc mL^{-1}.
2. ^{99m}Tc-DTPA is drawn into a 5-mL syringe with 2 mL air and then injected into the nebulizer and flushed through with air.
3. The patient is positioned initially with their back to the camera, sitting if possible.
4. The nose clip is placed on the patient who is asked to breathe normally through the mouthpiece. The air supply is turned on to deliver a rate of 10 l min^{-1}.
5. After reaching a sufficient count rate, the air supply is turned off. The patient should continue to breathe through the mouthpiece for a further 15 s.
6. The nose clip is removed, and the patient is given mouthwash; then imaging is commenced.

Images

Anterior, posterior, left and right posterior obliques

Because perfusion and ventilation images are directly compared, it is important to have identical views for each. Foam wedges between the patient's back and the camera assist accurate oblique positioning.

Additional Techniques

1. SPECT imaging appears to significantly improve the specificity of the technique by reducing the number of intermediate-probability scans.
2. SPECT-CT imaging enables correlation of perfusion defects with parenchymal lung lesions, consolidation and bullae. PE can be discounted as a cause when defects co-register with one of these features.
3. Standardized interpretation of images can improve the clinical effectiveness of V/Q scans, and criteria have been published, which are widely used.[4,5]

Aftercare

None

Complications

Care should be taken when injecting MAA not to induce respiratory failure in patients with severe pulmonary hypertension. In these patients, inject very slowly.

COMPUTED TOMOGRAPHY IN THE DIAGNOSIS OF PULMONARY EMBOLI

Technique

The technique depends on individual CT scanner technology. Individual CT manufacturers recommend specific scanning protocols, including delivery of IV contrast medium. CT not only identifies the presence of thrombus but also allows assessment of secondary right heart strain.[1]

Computed Tomography Pulmonary Angiography— Enhanced Scan of Pulmonary Arterial System[1]

1. Volume of contrast medium—100–150 mL or when a dual-phase injector is used, 60–80 mL of contrast medium followed by saline chase of 30–50 mL
2. Delay:
   (a) Preset delay of approximately 15–25 s, depending on scanner type
   OR preferably:
   (b) Bolus tracking. A region of interest (ROI) is positioned over the pulmonary artery at the level of the carina. After the injection commences, a 'tracker scan' monitors the contrast density within the pulmonary artery, and the scan is then triggered when the density at the ROI reaches a preset value—usually 100–120 HU.
3. Rate of injection—4 mL s^{-1}: contrast delivery aiming optimally for main pulmonary artery enhancement of 350 HU
4. Scan from lowest hemidiaphragm to lung apex. Caudocranial scanning may reduce respiratory motion artefact at the lung bases, though this is less of an issue with faster multislice scanners.
5. Image review and postprocessing[2]—images should be reviewed at three settings:
   (a) Mediastinal window (window width or window level, e.g. 400/40 HU)
   (b) PE-specific window (e.g. 700/100 HU, adjusted to remove contrast 'glare')
   (c) Lung window (e.g. W:1500/L:–500 HU)

9

Multiplanar images reformatted along the longitudinal axis of a vessel can be helpful to overcome difficulties encountered with axial sections of obliquely oriented arteries, aiding confidence in diagnosis or exclusion of thrombus. If there is no evidence of PE, then carefully determine the presence of other potential thoracic causes of the patient's clinical picture.

Dual-Energy Computed Tomography Pulmonary Angiography[3]

With the latest dual-energy scanners, high pitch acquisition allows faster scanning with reduced contrast volume and reduced motion artefact. DECT uses two energy levels to enable two data sets from different x-ray spectra and amplify differences in iodinated contrast uptake. Perfusion maps: Data sets from DECT can generate iodine maps based on distribution of iodine within lung after IV contrast administration. When overlayed on CT images can allow quantitative volume analysis. Perfused blood volume (PBV) images can be generated; however, this needs greater than 300 mg I mL^{-1}.

- Peripheral wedge-shaped perfusion defects are seen in acute PE.
- Peripheral clots are shown to have improved detection with DECT. This was explored in COVID patients in different centres to assess for microthrombi in this patient group.
- Semiautomated and fully automated quantitative assessment of PBV can predict adverse outcomes.
- Virtual monoenergetic images at low energy levels gives higher image contrast and may be particularly beneficial in suboptimal scans
- Virtual non-contrast images can also be derived from the DECT data set. This can help in lesion characterization by providing both contrast and non-contrast images with one acquisition.

PULMONARY ARTERIOGRAPHY

Indications

1. Demonstration of PE and other peripheral abnormalities (e.g. arteriovenous malformations) when less invasive investigations have been non-diagnostic (though now rarely needed with modern multislice CT)
2. Planning and performing therapeutic procedures such as catheter-directed thrombolysis or catheter embolectomy (in patients who cannot receive systemic thrombolysis because of bleeding risk and when surgical embolectomy is contraindicated)
3. Before embolization of pulmonary arteriovenous malformations

Contraindications[1]

These include the general contraindications to any form of arteriography, such as contrast allergy, renal failure and bleeding diatheses. There are more specific relative contraindications to diagnostic pulmonary arteriography:

1. Elevated right ventricular end-diastolic pressure (>20 mmHg) or elevated pulmonary artery pressure (>70 mmHg) when the mortality rate is increased to 2%–3% (compared with a documented mortality rate of 0.2%–0.5% when pressures are not elevated). Selective arteriography is advised if the results of arteriography are essential to patient management.
2. Left bundle branch block—right heart catheterization may induce complete heart block. Insertion of a temporary pacemaker may be indicated before the procedure.

Contrast Medium

Low-osmolar contrast material: 370 mg I mL^{-1}; 0.75 mL kg^{-1} at 20–25 mL s^{-1} (maximum, 40 mL)

Equipment

1. Digital subtraction angiography facilities
2. Pump injector
3. Catheter: pigtail (coiled end, end hole and 12 side holes)

Technique

The Seldinger technique is used via the right femoral vein. The catheter is introduced via an introducer sheath (see Chapter 11 for more details). The catheter tip is sited, under fluoroscopic control, to lie 1–3 cm above the pulmonary valve. Pulmonary pressures should routinely be measured during the procedure; lower injection rates are advised if the pressures are raised.

Additional Techniques

1. If the entire chest cannot be accommodated on one field of view, the examination can be repeated by examining each lung. The catheter is advanced to lie in each main pulmonary artery, in turn. For the right lung, the patient (or the tube) is turned 10 degrees right anterior oblique, and for the left lung, 10 degrees left anterior oblique.
2. Forty-degree caudal-cranial view: This view is optimal for the visualization of the bifurcation of the right and left pulmonary arteries, the pulmonary valve, annulus and trunk. With this manoeuvre, the pulmonary trunk is no longer foreshortened and is not superimposed over its bifurcation.

9

Complications

The rate of minor complications is 1%–3%. These include respiratory distress, major dysrhythmias, contrast reactions and renal failure. The current documented mortality rate is 0.2%–0.5%.

For further details regarding general complications related to catheter techniques, see Chapter 11.

MAGNETIC RESONANCE IMAGING OF PULMONARY EMBOLI

A combination of real-time MR (steady-state free precession sequences), MR perfusion imaging (fat three-dimensional (3D) gradient-echo sequences) and contrast-enhanced MR angiography (CE-MRA) can be used to detect PE.[1] Single-centre studies have shown CE-MRA detecting PE with sensitivities of 77%–100% and specificities of 95%–100%; there are, however, significant variations in results with high levels of technically inadequate scans and sensitivities as low as 45% in some institutions. The place of MRI in diagnosing PE is still evolving, but with the additional benefit of performing lower-limb MR-venography during the same examination, may produce a highly sensitive combined investigation for thromboembolic disease.[2]

References

Methods of Imaging Pulmonary Embolism

1. Krishan S, Panditaratne N, Verma R, et al. Incremental value of CT venography combined with pulmonary CT angiography for the detection of thromboembolic disease: systematic review and meta-analysis. *AJR Am J Roentgenol.* 2011;196(5):1065–1072.

Radionuclide Lung Ventilation/Perfusion Imaging

1. Beckles MA, Spiro S, Colis G, et al. The physiologic evaluation of patients with lung cancer being considered for resectional surgery. *Chest.* 2003;123(suppl): 105S–114S.
2. Wang SC, Fischer KC, Slone RM, et al. Perfusion scintigraphy in the evaluation for lung volume reduction surgery: correlation with clinical outcome. *Radiology.* 1997;205(1):243–248.
3. Win T, Tasker AD, Groves AM, et al. Ventilation-perfusion scintigraphy to predict postoperative pulmonary function in lung cancer patients undergoing pneumonectomy. *AJR Am J Roentgenol.* 2006;187(5):1260–1265.
4. Howarth DM, Lan L, Thomas PA, et al. ^{99m}Tc Technegas ventilation and perfusion lung scintigraphy for the diagnosis of pulmonary embolus. *J Nucl Med.* 1999;40(4):579–584.
5. Freitas JE, Sarosi MG, Nagle CC, et al. Modified PIOPED criteria used in clinical practice. *J Nucl Med.* 1995;36(9):1573–1578.

Computed Tomography Pulmonary Angiography

1. Furlan A, Aghayev A, Chang C-CH, et al. Short-term mortality in acute pulmonary embolism: clot burden and signs of right heart dysfunction at CT pulmonary angiography. *Radiology.* 2012;265(1):283–293.
2. Wittram C. How I do it: CT pulmonary angiography. *AJR Am J Roentgenol.* 2007;188(5):1255–1261.
3. Moore AJE, Wachsmann J, Chamarthy MR, et al. Imaging of acute pulmonary embolism: an update. *Cardiovasc Diagn Ther.* 2018;8(3):225–243.

Complications

1. Gotway MB, Reddy GP, Dawn SK. Pulmonary thromboembolic disease. In: Webb WR, Higgins CB, eds. *Thoracic Imaging: Pulmonary and Cardiovascular Radiology.* Lippincott Williams & Wilkins; 2005:609–629.

Magnetic Resonance of Pulmonary Emboli

1. Kluge A, Luboldt W, Bachmann G. Acute pulmonary embolism to the subsegmental level: diagnostic accuracy of three MRI techniques compared with 16-MDCT. *AJR Am J Roentgenol.* 2006;187(1):W7–W14.
2. Stein PD, Chenevert TL, Fowler SE. Gadolinium-enhanced magnetic resonance angiography for pulmonary embolism: a multicenter prospective study (PIOPED III). *Ann Intern Med.* 2010;152(7):434–443.

Further Reading

Methods of Imaging Pulmonary Embolism

Remy-Jardin M, Pontana F, Faivre J-B, et al. New insights in thromboembolic disease. *Radiol Clin N Am.* 2014;52(1):183–193.

Roy PM, Colombet I, Durieux P, et al. Systematic review and meta-analysis of strategies for the diagnosis of suspected pulmonary embolism. *Br Med J.* 2005;331(7511):259.

Stein PD, Woodard PK, Weg JG, et al. Diagnostic pathways in acute pulmonary embolism: recommendations of the PIOPED II investigators. *Radiology.* 2007;242(1):15–21.

Ventilation/Perfusion Imaging

Parker JA, Coleman RE, Grady E, et al. SNM practice guideline for lung scintigraphy 4.0. *J Nucl Med Technol.* 2012;40(1):57–65.

Sostman HD, Stein PD, Gottschalk A, et al. Acute pulmonary embolism: sensitivity and specificity of ventilation-perfusion scintigraphy in PIOPED II study. *Radiology.* 2008;246(3):941–946.

Computed Tomography Pulmonary Angiography

Chen T, Xiao H, Shannon R. Does dual-energy computed tomography pulmonary angiography (CTPA) have improved image quality over routine single-energy CTPA? *J Med Imaging Radiat Oncol.* 2019;63(2):170–174. Erratum in: *J Med Imaging Radiat Oncol.* 2020;64(4):597.

Moore AJE, Wachsmann J, Chamarthy MR, et al. Imaging of acute pulmonary embolism: an update. *Cardiovasc Diagn Ther.* 2018;8(3):225–243.

Raja AS, Greenberg JO, Qaseem A, et al. Evaluation of patients with suspected acute pulmonary embolism: best practice advice from the Clinical Guidelines Committee of the American College of Physicians. *Ann Intern Med.* 2015;163(9):701–711.

Remy-Jardin M, Pistolesi M, Goodman LR, et al. Management of suspected acute pulmonary embolism in the era of CT angiography: a statement from the Fleischner Society. *Radiology.* 2007;245(2):315–329.

Stein PD, Fowler SE, Goodman LR, et al. Contrast enhanced multidetector spiral CT of the chest and lower extremities in suspected acute pulmonary embolism: results of the Prospective Investigation of Pulmonary Embolism Diagnosis II (PIOPED II). *N Engl J Med.* 2006;354:2317–2327.

Wittram C, Maher MM, Yoo AJ, et al. CT angiography of pulmonary embolism: diagnostic criteria and causes of misdiagnosis. *Radiographics.* 2004;24(5):1219–1238.

Investigating Suspected Pulmonary Embolism in Pregnancy

Leung AN, Bull TM, Jaeschke R, et al. American Thoracic Society Documents: an Official American Thoracic Society/Society of Thoracic Radiology Clinical Practice Guideline: evaluation of suspected pulmonary embolism in pregnancy. *Radiology.* 2012;262(2):635–646.

Tirada N, Dreizin D, Khati NJ, et al. Imaging pregnant and lactating patients. *Radiographics.* 2015;35(6):1751–1765.

9

ULTRASOUND OF THE DIAPHRAGM—THE 'SNIFF TEST'

Functional assessment of hemidiaphragmatic movement can be undertaken in patients with dyspnoea and for investigation of a raised hemidiaphragm on the plain chest radiograph or CT. Assessment of diaphragmatic movement can determine if there is dysfunction—weakness or paralysis—present contributing to a patient's respiratory symptoms. US has superseded the use of fluoroscopy, with the added advantages of avoiding the use of ionizing radiation, and can be undertaken at the bedside if necessary.

Technique

The patient is usually scanned sitting upright. It is useful to image the non-elevated diaphragm first to assess the range of movements on the normal side. With the US probe aligned in the vertical plane to visualize the hemidiaphragmatic excursion, the diaphragmatic movement is observed first in quiet respiration, then with deeper breaths and then with the patient asked to take a sharp 'sniff'. With normal diaphragmatic function, each hemidiaphragm should move downwards on inspiration as the chest wall moves outwards and upwards, with the amplitude of excursion increasing as deeper breaths are taken. Sharp inspiration by sniffing is almost exclusively mediated by a rapid downward 'jerk' of the hemidiaphragm, with little or no contribution from chest wall movement. This brisk caudad movement should be clearly evident on the US image.

Scanning of the contralateral, elevated hemidiaphragm determines whether it has a high anatomical position, but normal movement or whether its high position is secondary to weakness or paralysis. A weak hemidiaphragm usually shows decreased excursion, which persists even as deeper breaths and sniffing are undertaken. A paralyzed hemidiaphragm may show no movement at all on normal breathing and characteristically shows a brisk *paradoxical* upward movement when the patient is asked to sniff.

These appearances can be recorded on real-time US cine capture.

Further Reading

Gerscovich EO, Cronan M, McGahan JP, et al. Ultrasonographic evaluation of diaphragmatic motion. *J Ultrasound Med.* 2001;20(6):597–604.
Nason LK, Walker CM, McNeeley, et al. Imaging of the diaphragm: anatomy and function. *Radiographics.* 2012;32(2):E52–E71.

MAGNETIC RESONANCE IMAGING OF THE RESPIRATORY SYSTEM

MRI currently has a limited role in assessing the respiratory system because of the susceptibility artefact from the large volume of air within the lungs. The mediastinum and chest wall, however, are well assessed by MRI because of the ability to image in the coronal and sagittal plane, and in particular, malignant invasion of the mediastinum, pericardium and chest wall can be usefully evaluated. MRI is particularly useful in the assessment of superior sulcus and neurogenic tumours because it can give information on the nature and extent of brachial plexus or intraspinal extension. Fast sequences and cardiac gating may be used effectively to minimize motion artefacts. Multidetector CT, however, is quicker and more widely available and can now give excellent multiplanar and 3D reconstruction.

MR of the chest whilst the patient breathes hyperpolarized helium-3 (^{3}He) allows visualization of the airspaces within the lungs. The technique can detect abnormal distribution of the gas and may develop a clinical role in the assessment of, and subsequent treatment of, airways and parenchymal disease, particularly in asthma, chronic obstructive pulmonary disease and cystic fibrosis (in the latter, allowing regular imaging follow-up without ionizing radiation burden). MR of the lungs, however, is not yet currently used routinely in clinical practice.

Further Reading

Driehuys B, Martinez-Jimenez S, Cleveland ZI, et al. Chronic obstructive pulmonary disease: safety and tolerability of hyperpolarized 129Xe MR imaging in healthy volunteers and patients. *Radiology*. 2012;262(1):279–289.
Kauczor H-U, Ley-Zaporozhan J, Ley S. Imaging of pulmonary pathologies: focus on magnetic resonance imaging. *Proc Am Thorac Soc*. 2009;6:458–463.

POSITRON EMISSION TOMOGRAPHY AND POSITRON EMISSION TOMOGRAPHY–COMPUTED TOMOGRAPHY OF THE RESPIRATORY SYSTEM

In recent years, fluorodeoxyglucose PET has become an essential part of lung cancer imaging, adding functional information to the morphological information provided by CT. The scan can be performed either on a dedicated PET scanner or, more usually now, on integrated PET-CT scanners. PET imaging plays an important role in loco-regional and distant staging of non–small cell lung cancer and is currently recommended when the lesion is larger than 1 cm in size in all patients in whom curative-intent treatment is contemplated. Patient preparation and the technique are fully described in Chapter 13.

In addition to their current primary use in diagnosis and staging of lung cancer, PET and PET-CT have an emerging role in assessment of early metabolic response to therapy, which may allow influence subsequent treatment planning and may, in the future, predict eventual prognosis.

Further Reading

De Wever W, Stroobants S, Coolen J, et al. Integrated PET/CT in the staging of non-small cell lung cancer: technical aspects and clinical integration. *Eur Respir J*. 2009;33:201–212.
Erasmus JJ, Rohren E, Swisher SG. Prognosis and reevaluation of lung cancer by positron emission tomography imaging. *Proc Am Thorac Soc*. 2009;6:171–179.
Paul NS, Ley S, Metser U. Optimal imaging protocols for lung cancer staging: CT, PET, MR imaging, and the role of imaging. *Radiol Clin N Am*. 2012;50(5): 935–949.
Vansteenkiste JF, Stroobants SS. PET scan in lung cancer: current recommendations and innovation. *J Thorac Oncol*. 2006;1(1):71–73.
Weber WA. Assessing tumor response to therapy. *J Nucl Med*. 2009;50(suppl 5): 1S–10S.

Cardiac
Alim Yucel-Finn

METHODS OF IMAGING THE HEART

1. Chest radiography
2. Fluoroscopy and angiocardiography
3. Echocardiography: transthoracic and transoesophageal techniques
4. Computed tomography (CT)
5. Magnetic resonance imaging (MRI)
6. Radionuclide imaging:
   (a) Ventriculography
   (b) Myocardial perfusion imaging

(Chest radiography and echocardiography are not covered in this chapter.)

ANGIOCARDIOGRAPHY

Diagnostic catheterization has largely been replaced by CT coronary angiography and echocardiography (including transoesophageal echocardiography) and, to a lesser extent, radionuclide ventriculography and MRI. Angiocardiography is usually used as part of an interventional therapeutic procedure and can be performed simultaneously with cardiac catheterization, during which pressures and oximetry are measured in the cardiac chambers and vessels that are under investigation. The right heart, left heart and great vessels are examined together or alone, depending on the clinical problem.

Indications

1. Congenital heart disease and anomalies of the great vessels—mostly in the paediatric population. Either for diagnosis or therapeutic procedures such as transcatheter closure of patent foramen ovale, atrial septal defect (ASD), ventricular septal defect (VSD) and patent ductus arteriosus (PDA).
2. To assess valve disease, myocardial disease and ventricular function. Balloon valvuloplasty and, in selected centres, transcatheter aortic valve implantation (TAVI) can be performed to treat stenotic valvular disease.

Table 10.1   Volumes of Contrast Media in Angiocardiography[a]

	Injection Site		
	Ventricle		Aorta or Pulmonary Artery
Adult	1 mL kg⁻¹ at 18–20 mL s⁻¹		0.75 mL kg⁻¹ at 18–20 mL s⁻¹ (maximum, 40 mL)
Child			
First year	1.5 mL kg⁻¹	Injected over 1–2 s	75% of the ventricular volume
2–4 y	1.2 mL kg⁻¹		
5 y	1.0 mL kg⁻¹		

[a]In general, hypoplastic or obstructed chambers require smaller volumes and flow rates, and large shunts require greater volumes and flow rates of contrast medium.

Contrast Medium

Low-osmolar contrast material (LOCM) 370 mg I mL⁻¹ (Table 10.1)

Equipment

1. Biplane digital fluoroscopy and cine radiography with C-arms to facilitate axial projections
2. Pressure-recording device
3. Electrocardiogram (ECG) monitor
4. Blood oxygen analyser
5. Catheter:
   (a) For pressure measurements and blood sampling: Cournand (Fig. 10.1), 4–7 Fr
   (b) For angiocardiography: National Institutes of Health (NIH) (Fig. 10.2) or pigtail (Fig. 10.3) catheters, 4–8 Fr

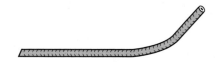

Fig. 10.1 Cournand catheter. End holes, 1; side holes, 0.

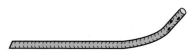

Fig. 10.2 National Institutes of Health catheter. End holes, 0; side holes, 4 or 6.

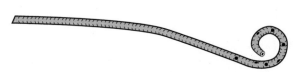

Fig. 10.3 Pigtail catheter. End holes, 1; side holes, 12.

Technique

1. Right-sided cardiac structures and pulmonary arteries are examined by introducing a catheter into a peripheral vein. In babies, the femoral vein may be the only vein large enough to take the catheter. If an ASD is suspected, the femoral vein approach offers the best chance of passing the catheter into the left atrium across the defect. In adults, the right antecubital or basilic vein may be used. The cephalic vein should be avoided because it can be difficult to traverse the catheter past the site where the vein pierces the clavipectoral fascia to join the axillary vein. The catheter, or introducer, is inserted using the Seldinger technique. (The NIH catheter must be introduced via an introducer because there is no end hole for a guidewire.)
2. In children, it is usually possible to examine the left heart and occasionally the aorta by manipulating a venous catheter through a patent foramen ovale. In adults, the aorta and left ventricle are studied via a catheter passed retrogradely from the femoral artery.
3. The catheter is manipulated into the appropriate positions for recording pressures and sampling blood for oxygen saturation. After this, angiography is performed.

Image Acquisition

Using digital angiography at 7.5 frames s^{-1} with alignment to the anatomical axes of the heart (i.e. the x-ray beam is angulated relative to the axial planes of the heart rather than the orthogonal planes of the body). The long axis of the heart is usually oblique to the long axis of the patient's body, and cardiac angiography suites have movable C-arms that allow correct positioning by movement of the equipment alone without disturbing the patient. Supplementary angulations of the x-ray beam from the cardiac axes are used to profile those areas of the heart under examination. Useful views are:

10

1. 40 degrees cranial/40 degrees left anterior oblique (LAO) (hepatoclavicular or four-chamber) view: The beam is perpendicular to the long axis of the heart and aligns the atrial septum and posterior interventricular septum parallel to the beam.
2. Long axial 20 degrees right anterior oblique (RAO) (long axial oblique) view: The lateral tube and image intensifier are angled 25–30 degrees cranially to align with the long axis of the heart and 20 degrees RAO.

CORONARY ARTERIOGRAPHY

Indications

1. Diagnosis of the presence and extent of ischaemic heart disease
2. After revascularization procedures
3. Congenital heart lesions
4. Therapeutic percutaneous coronary intervention: balloon angioplasty and stenting

Diagnostic arteriography can be supplemented by intravascular ultrasound or optical coherence tomography to determine the nature and extent of plaque within the vessel wall and, in some centres, with angioscopy. Pressure wire studies to determine fractional flow reserve (FFR) across stenoses before angioplasty or stenting can be performed; these are particularly useful in assessment of intermediate lesions.

Contrast Medium

LOCM 370 mg I mL^{-1}, 8–10 mL given as a hand injection for each projection

Equipment

1. Digital angiography with C-arm
2. Pressure recording device and ECG monitor
3. Selective coronary artery catheters:
   (a) Judkins (Fig. 10.4) or Amplatz (Fig. 10.5) catheters: The left and right coronary artery catheters are of different shapes. These can be used for both femoral and radial approaches (usually using a smaller Judkins catheter for the left coronary artery).
   (b) Tiger II catheter (Fig. 10.6): Specifically designed for the right radial approach. A single catheter is used for both left and right coronary arteries (reduces procedure time, radiation exposure and less manipulation, leading to less radial artery spasm).
   (c) For assessment of grafts: Judkins, Simmons and others (for both femoral and radial approaches) catheters.

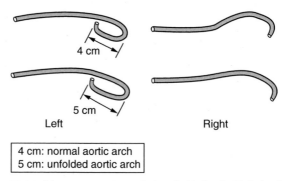

| 4 cm: normal aortic arch |
| 5 cm: unfolded aortic arch |

Left   Right

Fig. 10.4 Judkins coronary artery catheters. End holes, 1; side holes, 0.

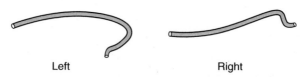

Left   Right

Fig. 10.5 Amplatz coronary artery catheters. End holes, 1; side holes, 0.

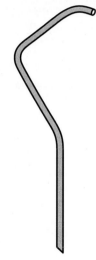

Fig. 10.6 Tiger II coronary artery catheter. End holes, 1; side holes, 0.

Patient Preparation

As for routine arteriography

Preliminary Image

Chest radiography

Technique

The catheter is introduced using the Seldinger technique via the radial (most commonly), brachial or femoral artery and advanced until its tip is seen to engage with the ostium of the coronary artery. Mildly increased radiation doses for the patient and operator have been demonstrated via a radial versus femoral approach, but this is not thought to outweigh the reduction in side effects.

Image Acquisition

Optimum visualization of vessels is obtained with images acquired perpendicular to the vessel under examination, so multiple, compound projections using rotation around the patient axis as well as cranio-caudal angulations of the x-ray beam are used for each coronary vessel.

Angiography (7.5 frames s^{-1}) is performed in the following projections:

1. Right coronary artery
   - RAO 30 degrees
   - LAO 30 degrees
   - LAO 30 degrees, cranial 30 degrees
2. Left coronary artery
   - Posteroanterior
   - LAO 45 degrees, caudad 30 degrees ('spider view')

- RAO 45 degrees, caudad 30 degrees
- RAO 45 degrees, cranial 30 degrees
- LAO 45 degrees, cranial 30 degrees

Each projection provides good visualization of various segments of the other coronary artery.

Complications

In addition to the general complications discussed in Chapter 11, patients undergoing coronary arteriography may be susceptible to:

1. Arrhythmias such as non-sustained atrial fibrillation with right heart catheterization or non-sustained ventricular arrhythmia with left ventriculography
2. Ostial dissection by the catheter
3. Access site complications (more commonly seen with femoral approach), including local haematoma, femoral artery pseudoaneurysm or arteriovenous fistula

Further Reading

Di Mario C, Sutaria N. Coronary angiography in the angioplasty era: projections with a meaning. *Heart*. 2005;91(7):968–976.

Mason PJ, Shah B, Tamis-Holland JE, et al. An Update on Radial Artery Access and Best Practices for Transradial Coronary Angiography and Intervention in Acute Coronary Syndrome: A Scientific Statement from the American Heart Association. *Circ Cardiovasc Interv.* 2018;11(9):e000035.

Tavakol M, Ashraf S, Brener SJ. Risks and complications of coronary angiography: a comprehensive review. *Glob J Health Sci.* 2012;4(1):65–93.

CARDIAC COMPUTED TOMOGRAPHY

The rapid evolution of multidetector CT scanner technology over the past 15 years has resulted in cardiac CT and coronary CT angiography becoming well-established techniques in the investigation and management of cardiovascular disease. Greater temporal resolution (<75 ms), spatial resolution (0.5 mm), sophisticated ECG-gating software and postprocessing algorithms have allowed for the acquisition of 'still' images of the heart and, by extension, the coronaries (see Fig. 10.7). Additionally, when combined with further radiation dose-reducing strategies, cardiac CT can be used widely without a significant dose footprint. CT has a high accuracy in detecting coronary vessel stenoses and a very high negative predictive value in excluding significant disease. It also allows the characterization of plaque morphology. With additional third-party computational analysis, it is possible to establish and model the FFR in a coronary system.

Indications

1. As a screening test in symptomatic patients with typical chest pain but a low clinical probability of significant coronary artery disease

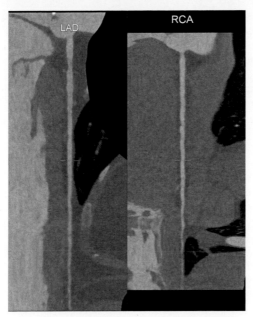

Fig. 10.7 Straightened reformat of two coronary arteries acquired from a dedicated coronary computed tomography angiogram. *LAD,* Left anterior descending artery; *RCA,* right coronary artery.

2. As a screening test in asymptomatic but high-risk patients or patients with atypical chest pain
3. Assessment of aortic stenosis and procedure planning for TAVI
4. Patients with known or suspected chronic coronary artery disease
5. Assessment of suspected anomalous coronary artery anatomy
6. Assessment of coronary artery grafts, including left internal mammary artery (LIMA) grafts, in the acute or chronic setting
7. Assessment of coronary artery dissection
8. Assessment of coronary stent patency
9. As an alternative to diagnostic coronary angiography when planning percutaneous angiographic intervention or as postprocedure follow-up
10. Assessment of left atrium and pulmonary vein anatomy before electrophysiological studies and ablation

Contraindications

1. Standard contraindications to iodinated contrast media administration: previous significant contrast reaction, severe acute renal insufficiency and so on
2. Inability to lie still, breath-hold or cooperate with scan instructions
3. Clinical instability:
   (a) Cardiac failure, acute myocardial infarction (MI), severe hypotension

    (b) Cardiac dysrhythmia, including atrial fibrillation, frequent ventricular extrasystoles and bigeminy
    (c) Elevated heart rate (in the presence of contraindication to beta blockade)

Patient Preparation

1. Avoid caffeine for 24 h. This includes tea, coffee and caffeine-containing soft drinks (including 'decaffeinated' varieties), 'energy' pills and Viagra-type medication.
2. Drugs: Patients should take all their normal cardiac medication as usual on the day of the test.
3. A thorough explanation of the procedure to the patient aids compliance, particularly with regard to breath-hold; suggest patients take a 'three-quarters breath' when instructed, leading them to be less likely to move during scan, and avoid the 'Valsalva' manoeuvre, which affects contrast bolus entering the chest.
4. An 18-gauge cannula in the right antecubital fossa: a siting cannula in the right arm reduces artefact as contrast crosses the mediastinum. For graft studies, this avoids streak artefact from obscuring the origin of LIMA grafts.
5. Assess suitability for administration of beta-blockers and sublingual nitrates (discussed later).

Beta-Blockers

Optimal imaging quality and radiation dose are significantly influenced by heart rate, which ideally should be between 55 and 60 beats/min. With basic precautions and simple monitoring, safe and dose-titratable heart rate reduction can be achieved in the majority of patients using a beta-blocker administered within the radiology department. Metoprolol is commonly used and can be given orally, intravenously or in combination:

- The patient may already be taking oral beta-blockers (either as regular medication or specifically prescribed by the referrer for the purposes of the examination). In most cases, the scan can proceed without further medication.
- If the patient is not taking beta-blockers, requires heart rate reduction to optimize scan and has no contraindication to beta-blocker administration, metoprolol can be given orally or intravenously.

(Contraindications to beta-blockade include heart failure, significant aortic stenosis, heart block, asthma or chronic obstructive pulmonary disease and use of other antiarrhythmic medication, including calcium channel blockers and digoxin.)

- Metoprolol 100 revascularization mg orally 1 h before the scan. Pulse and blood pressure should be monitored regularly until the heart rate reaches the desired level. (If the heart rate does not reach a satisfactory level, additional metoprolol can be given intravenously while the patient is on the scan table.)

- Metoprolol can be given solely in intravenous (IV) form (or to 'top up' an oral dose when an optimal heart rate has not been achieved with oral administration) just before the start of the scan with the patient on the scanner table (5–30 mg IV of metoprolol given in aliquots of 5 mg titrated against the heart rate).

Nitrates

Sublingual glyceryl trinitrate (GTN) 400–800 µg (1–2 tablets) can be given a few minutes before scanning to produce coronary dilation and improve image quality. The temporary effect of hypotension is unlikely to be an issue with the patient lying on the CT table, and transient physiological elevation of heart rate is usually not an issue if the GTN is given 90–120 s before scan acquisition. (Contraindications to nitrates include hypotension, hypovolaemia, severe aortic valve stenosis, hypertrophic cardiomyopathy, recent myocardial infraction, severe anaemia and recent 'Viagra'-type medication.)

Technique

Cardiac CT remains a potentially high-radiation-dose procedure, and careful attention to dose reduction measures while maintaining image quality is essential. The use of 'prospective' rather than 'retrospective' scanning and, when possible, single heartbeat acquisition reduce radiation doses significantly.

Scan technique is determined by the clinical question to be answered and by the patient's heart rate; the exact protocol will be determined by the manufacturer and model of the CT scanner.

Scan Protocol

All scans are ECG gated (Fig. 10.8) to allow for imaging of the heart during fractions of the ECG cycle (considered R–R interval). This is done for the following reasons:

10

1. To allow prospective ECG triggering of the scan whenever possible, with x-ray exposure only during specific parts of the cardiac cycle. Heart motion is minimal during diastole (70%) of the ECG cycle. For patients with elevated heart rates (>80 beats/min), systolic imaging can yield superior results (~30% of the ECG cycle or 250–400 ms after the preceding R wave).
2. For timing of the single heart beat acquisition.
3. If prospective triggering is not possible, to modulate the tube current, by decreasing x-ray exposure during parts of the cardiac cycle when image quality is not so critical (usually systole and early diastole) to reduce overall radiation dose.
4. To allow retrospective reconstruction of images timed to specific points in the cardiac cycle.

Plain computed tomography of the heart

Prospective ECG-triggered non-contrast scan acquired during diastole (usually c. 65%–80% of the R–R interval) over three or four cardiac cycles. Used to detect and quantify coronary artery calcification from

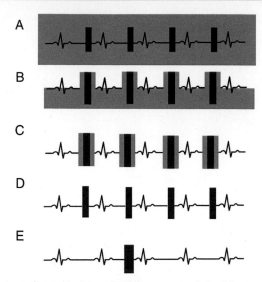

Fig. 10.8 Electrocardiographic gating. *Light brown* represents the tube current levels. *Dark brown* represents the reconstructed acquisition window. **A,** Retrospective, no modulation. **B,** Retrospective, tube modulation. **C,** Prospective, with padding. **D,** Prospective, no padding. **E,** Ultra-high pitch.

which the age- and sex-matched *calcium score* is calculated. Higher scores are associated with increasing risk of significant atheromatous disease, and the technique can be used as a screening tool for subclinical cardiac disease. The absence of coronary artery calcification, however, does not completely exclude atheroma but is associated with a low risk of an adverse coronary event. The aortic valve calcification can also be quantified as a surrogate marker of valve stenosis. The plain scan can then be used to plan the range of the subsequent contrast-enhanced scan.

Contrast-Enhanced Cardiac Scan

Contrast administration

The rapidity of the scan acquisition necessitates very accurate timing of contrast bolus to ensure optimal vessel opacification (but also means that generally smaller volumes of contrast medium can be used). Biphasic injection of contrast followed by a saline 'chaser' or, if desired, diluted contrast improves the geometry of delivery of contrast and 'washes out' the right side of the heart to reduce streak artefact— typically, 90–100 mL LOCM 350 mg I mL^{-1} given at 5–7 mL s^{-1} followed by 40–50 mL saline at 4–7 mL s^{-1}. Graft studies require a higher volume of contrast of 100–120 mL LOCM 350 mg I mL^{-1} at 5–6 mL s^{-1}.

Bolus timing can be achieved using:

1. A 'test bolus': A small initial injection of contrast (e.g. 20- to 30-mL bolus of contrast with a 40-mL saline 'chaser' bolus) is given, the region of interest (ROI) (ascending aorta) is scanned and time to

peak enhancement is derived. The full scan is then performed using this timing delay. (Usually add 3 s to allow for maximal coronary vessel enhancement.) This method is probably the most reliable and accurate.

2. 'Bolus tracking': A selected ROI, usually the ascending aorta, is scanned every second or so after contrast injection, and the full acquisition scan is automatically triggered (after a short delay) when the ROI has enhanced to a preset level (e.g. 120 HU).

3. Empirical delay of c. 25 s: unlikely to yield satisfactory images and not recommended.

Prospective scan

The patient's ECG is monitored allowing the timing of the cycle to be anticipated and predicted. The scanner is triggered at a certain point in the cardiac cycle based on this prediction. For example, for diastolic acquisition, the timing is desired at 70% of the ECG cycle, whereas end-systolic acquisition would be at 30% of the ECG cycle. Based on the ECG, the scanner is triggered at end systole (~45%) with the anticipation that diastole will occur as predicted. This is best achieved with steady heart rates and can be prone to error (e.g. ectopic beats). The acquisition scan can be 'padded' whereby there is additional image acquisition before and after the desired point to help account for beat-beat variations.

In prospective imaging a section of the heart (usually ~3 cm in the z-axis) is imaged during one acquisition window. The patient table moves along the z-axis in between each acquisition, similar to a 'step and shoot' acquisition. These 3-cm segments are combined to form the final image (Fig. 10.9). Dose reduction is up to 90% compared with retrospective acquisition (currently 2–4.5 mSv—comparable to conventional catheter angiogram c. 5 mSv).

Single-beat acquisition

Achieved using the advanced ultra-high-pitch CT technology available on select scanners. This uses dual-source scanners and rapid table movement to cover the entire heart in a single heartbeat. This method is the acquisition of choice for TAVI and graft analysis. This technique needs low and steady heart beats (<60 beats/min ideally). Very low doses are achievable (<1 mSv).

10

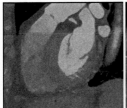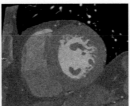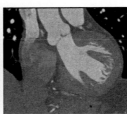

Fig. 10.9 Reconstructed heart images 'stitched together' from three separate prospective acquisitions.

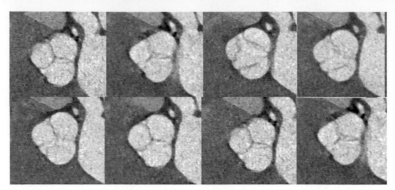

Fig. 10.10 Different phases of a cardiac cycle acquisition reconstructed showing the aortic valve open and closed.

Retrospective scan

Helical acquisition throughout the cardiac cycle, which is high dose, is no longer a routinely used acquisition. Retrospective reconstruction of images from data acquired during diastole (c. 70% of RR) show coronary and cardiac structures and from the entire data set to show functional imaging of entire cardiac cycle. This is a high-radiation-dose procedure (~14 mSv) and was used in patients with higher heart rates (superseded by systolic phase acquisitions) and less stable heart rhythms for graft assessment (superseded by ultra-high-pitch single-beat). It is used in patients in whom functional data from the whole cardiac cycle are required (e.g. opening of the aortic valve (Fig. 10.10), also achievable with systolic imaging) and MRI is not possible. Modulation of tube current in systole and early diastole should be used whenever possible to decrease overall radiation dose (by ≤50%). Image quality is reduced during these less critical parts of the cardiac cycle, but useful functional data are preserved.

Transcatheter aortic valve implantation acquisition

A CT TAVI needs to combine the dataset of an ECG-gated aortic root (including coronaries) with a vascular angiogram (neck to upper thigh). This can be achieved with multiple methods:

1. Single-beat acquisition (timed at midsystole, 250 ms) of the entire volume
2. Separate acquisitions of the ECG-gated aortic root and standard vascular angiogram
3. Combined acquisitions of ECG-gated thorax with switch to non-gated abdomen and thigh

Further Reading

Bastarrika G, Lee YS, Huda W, et al. CT of coronary artery disease. *Radiology.* 2009;253(2):317–338.

Boxt LM. Coronary computed tomography angiography: a practical guide to performance and interpretation. *Semin Roentgenol.* 2012;47(3):204–219.

Kite TA, Ladwiniec A, Arnold JR, et al. Early invasive versus non-invasive assessment in patients with suspected non-ST-elevation acute coronary syndrome. *Heart.* 2022;108:500–506.

Mahesh M, Cody DD. AAPM/RSNA physics tutorial for residents: physics of cardiac imaging with multiple-row detector CT. *Radiographics.* 2007;27:1495–1509.

Pannu HK, Alvarez W, Fishman EK. Review: β-blockers for cardiac CT: a primer for the radiologist. *AJR Am J Roentgenol.* 2006;186(suppl):S341–S345.

Schoepf UJ, Zwerner PL, Savino G, et al. Coronary CT angiography: how I do it. *Radiology.* 2007;244:48–63.

Shriki JE, Shinbane JS, Rashid MA, et al. Identifying, characterizing, and classifying congenital anomalies of the coronary arteries. *Radiographics.* 2012;32(2):453–468.

Sun Z, Ng KH. Prospective versus retrospective ECG-gated multislice CT coronary angiography: a systematic review of radiation dose and diagnostic accuracy. *Euro J Radiol.* 2012;81(2):94–100.

Taylor CM, Blum A, Abbara S. Cardiac CT. Patient preparation and scanning techniques. *Radiol Clin North Am.* 2010;48(4):675–686.

Yucel-Finn A, Nicol E, Leipsic JA, et al. CT in planning transcatheter aortic valve implantation procedures and risk assessment. *Clin Radiol.* 2021;76(1):73.e1–e73.

CARDIAC MAGNETIC RESONANCE IMAGING

Cardiac MRI plays a major role in the assessment of cardiac disease. MRI is well established in the evaluation of cardiac and major vessel anatomy, ventricular volumes and mass; functional imaging to assess ventricular and valve motion; and flow quantification, allowing measurement of blood velocity and volume to assess intracardiac shunts and stenotic and regurgitant, valvular disease. More recently, contrast-enhanced MR has evolved as a powerful tool in assessing myocardial viability and perfusion, both in the evaluation of acute myocardial ischaemia and in the assessment of myocardial viability and potential reversibility before revascularization. Coronary artery MRI can be acquired in very compliant patients but has yet to be developed for routine use and presently has been comprehensively overtaken by recent advances in low-radiation-dose CT coronary imaging.

10

Indications

1. Assessment of chamber dimensions, mass and function
2. Assessment of complex congenital heart disease
3. Diagnosis and evaluation of cardiomyopathies: sarcoid, amyloid, hypertrophic cardiomyopathy, arrhythmogenic right ventricular cardiomyopathy
4. Evaluation of cardiac masses
5. Evaluation of pericardial disease
6. Evaluation of:
   (a) Myocardial viability
   (b) Extent of myocardial necrosis/fibrosis
   (c) Inducible ischaemia to guide revascularization strategies

7. Imaging and quantification of flow:
   (a) To assess valvular disease: stenosis and incompetence
   (b) To assess shunts: ASD, VSD, PDA, partial anomalous pulmonary venous return
   (c) To assess coarctation of the aorta

Contraindications

1. Non–MRI-compatible pacemaker
2. Other active implant or device
3. Claustrophobia

Relative Contraindications

1. Asthma is a relative contraindication in adenosine stress perfusion imaging.
2. Frequent ectopics, bigeminy or rhythms such as atrial fibrillation with fast ventricular response may render functional imaging non-diagnostic.

Patient Preparation

1. Standard MRI safety screening
2. Placement of MRI-compatible ECG electrodes for gating of sequences
3. IV cannulation
4. Patients undergoing adenosine stress imaging must avoid caffeine.

Technique

Technique varies varied depending upon the indication but consists of elements from the following.

Localizer images

Fast/Rapid Gradient echo (fGRE) or steady-state free procession (SSFP)

Thoracic overview, cardiac morphology

Half-Fourier acquisition single-shot turbo spin echo (HASTE) black blood imaging

Functional imaging

Long- and short-axis SSFP multiphase retrospectively gated imaging in the standard cardiac planes viz. echocardiography (fGRE/flash may be used at high field strengths), 6–8 mm with 2- to 4-mm gap (spatial resolution ~1.5 × 1.5 × 8 mm, temporal resolution <50 ms). Postprocessing of these images produces quantification of chamber volumes, myocardial mass and ventricular ejection fraction.

In patients with arrhythmia or an inability to breath-hold, lower resolution untriggered real-time functional imaging can be helpful. Typically temporal resolution is about 40 ms, and spatial resolution is 2–3 mm.

Tissue characterization

1. T2 Turbo spin echo (TSE) or short tau inversion recovery (STIR) imaging of oedema for myocarditis and peri-infarct 'region at risk'

2. T2* mapping for iron load in haemochromatosis in the heart and liver
   T1tse imaging for fatty infiltration, pericardial anatomy and accurate
   two-dimensional (2D) analysis of the endovasculature
3. T1 mapping is a newer technique used to quantitatively characterize
   the myocardium. Native T1 values are acquired before contrast
   administration. Postcontrast T1 mapping calculates the extracellular
   volume. A combination of these two values allows for better
   estimation of myocardial oedema, fibrosis and lipid component.
4. T2 mapping is also used to quantitatively characterize the
   myocardium. T2 predominantly indicates the amount of myocardial
   oedema and is most used in acute inflammation or infarction.

Strain imaging

This process indicates the relative 2D or three-dimensional (3D) motion of the myocardium. Myocardial tagging technique is used to depict foci to reflect myocardial motion. These foci usually manifest as hypointense or black lines in the myocardium, achieved with spatially selective destruction of magnetization. During the normal cardiac cycle, these hypointense foci should deform and reform.

Myocardial perfusion

Distal, mid and basal segment flash/fGRE images every heartbeat during rapid administration of IV gadolinium; this is considered first-pass perfusion. These images are acquired at rest or with the addition of a vasodilator (stress imaging). The vasodilator can be adenosine, dobutamine or regadenoson. Stress images appear the same as rest images in a normal myocardium. In an ischaemic myocardium, there are foci or regions of hypo- or reduced perfusion (they appear dark relative to the bright contrast enhancement).

Low-dose vasodilator doses can be used to assess myocardial viability in very poorly functioning ventricles.

Early gadolinium enhancement

Inversion Recovery fast Gradient Echo (IRfGRE) images immediately following administration of gadolinium chelate to detect or exclude intracardiac thrombus or microvascular obstruction.

Late gadolinium enhancement

Phase sensitive IRfGRE images 10–20 min after administration of gadolinium in the standard cardiac planes. Patterns of enhancement or hyperenhancement are characteristic for MI and for midwall fibrosis and infiltration in various cardiomyopathies.

Flow quantification

Phase contrast imaging with velocity encoding about 120% of expected velocity:

1. For assessment of transvalvular velocities and flow volumes in valve disease
2. For derivation of Qp:Qs ratio in intracardiac shunts
3. For demonstration of shunts, including septal defects and conduits

Magnetic resonance angiography

3D-T1SSFP volumes for coronaries using navigator respiratory gating or 2D breath-hold SSFP

Contrast-enhanced angiography using isovolumetric 3DT1fGRE sequences for demonstration of the aorta, pulmonary artery or pulmonary veins.

Further Reading

Belloni E, De Cobelli F, Esposito A, et al. MRI of cardiomyopathy. *AJR Am J Roentgenol.* 2008;191(6):1702–1710.

Ginat DT, Fong MW, Tuttle DJ, et al. Review: cardiac imaging: part 1, MR pulse sequences, imaging planes, and basic anatomy. *AJR Am J Roentgenol.* 2011;197(4):808–815.

Kramer CM, Barkhausen J, Flamm SD, et al. Standardized cardiovascular magnetic resonance imaging (CMR) protocols, Society for Cardiovascular Magnetic Resonance: Board of Trustees' Task Force on Standardized Protocols. *J Cardiovasc Mag Res.* 2008;10:35.

Moon JC, Messroghli DR, Kellman P, et al. Myocardial T1 mapping and extracellular volume quantification: a Society for Cardiovascular Magnetic Resonance (SCMR) and CMR working group of the European Society of Cardiology consensus statement. *J Cardiovasc Mag Res.* 2013;15:92.

O'Donnell DH, Abbara S, Chaithiraphan V, et al. Cardiac tumours: optimal cardiac MR sequences and spectrum of imaging appearances. *AJR Am J Roentgenol.* 2009;193(2):377–387.

Schwitter J, Arai AE. Assessment of cardiac ischaemia and viability: role of cardiovascular magnetic resonance. *Euro Heart J.* 2011;32:799–809.

RADIONUCLIDE VENTRICULOGRAPHY

Indications

Gated blood-pool study

1. Evaluation of ventricular function, particularly left ventricular ejection fraction (LVEF)
2. Assessment of myocardial reserve in coronary artery disease
3. Cardiomyopathy, including the effects of cardiotoxic drugs

Previous indications of *first-pass radionuclide angiography*—for evaluation of right ventricular ejection fraction and detection and quantification of intracardiac shunts—are now superseded by echocardiography and MR unless for very specialist indications and are not described here.

Contraindications

Significant arrhythmias may make gated blood-pool imaging impossible.

Radiopharmaceuticals

^{99m}Technetium (^{99m}Tc) in vivo–labelled red blood cells, 800 MBq maximum (8 mSv estimated dose (ED))

Before radiolabelling with ^{99m}Tc-pertechnetate, the red blood cells are 'primed' with an injection of stannous pyrophosphate. The stannous ions reduce the pertechnetate and allow it to bind to the pyrophosphate, which adsorbs onto the red blood cells.

Equipment

1. Gamma camera equipped with a low-energy general-purpose collimator
2. Imaging computer: list-mode or multigated acquisition (MUGA)
3. ECG monitor with gating pulse output

Patient Preparation

1. An IV injection of 'cold' stannous pyrophosphate (20 µg kg^{-1}) is given directly into a vein 20–30 min before the pertechnetate injection. (Avoid injection via long plastic Teflon-coated cannula, which may result in a poor label.)
2. Three ECG electrodes are placed in standard positions to give a gating signal.

Technique

1. The patient is supine.
2. The ECG trigger signal is connected.
3. IV injection of ^{99m}Tc pertechnetate is done.
4. One minute is allowed for the bolus to equilibrate before computer acquisition is commenced (see the 'Images' section later in the chapter).

List mode is best, in which individual events are stored as their x,y coordinates along with timing and gating pulses. This allows maximum flexibility for later manipulation and framing of data. About 5 million counts should be acquired. However, MUGA mode is adequate and is still the most commonly used. In this, the start of an acquisition cycle is usually triggered by the R wave of the patient's ECG. A series of 16–32 fast frames is recorded before the next R wave occurs. Each of these has very few counts per individual cycle, so every time the R wave trigger arrives, another set of frames is recorded and summed with the first. The sequence continues until 100–200 kilocounts per frame have been acquired in about 10 min. Some degree of arrhythmia can be tolerated using the technique of 'buffered bad beat rejection', in which cardiac cycles of irregular length are rejected and the data are not included in the images. The length of time to acquire an image set increases as the proportion of rejected beats rises.

Images

A number of views may be recorded, depending on the clinical problem:

1. LAO 35–45 degrees with a 15- to 30-degree caudal tilt, chosen to give best separation between left and right ventricles. The patient is supine. This view is sufficient if only LVEF is required.

2. Anterior, with the patient supine
3. LPO, chosen to give best separation between atria and ventricles. The patient is in the right lateral decubitus position.

Analysis

1. The LVEF is calculated.
2. Systolic, diastolic, phase and amplitude images are generated.
3. The frames can be displayed in cine mode to give good visualization of wall motion.

Additional Techniques

1. Gated blood-pool imaging can be performed during controlled exercise with appropriate precautions to assess ventricular functional reserve. Leg exercise using a bed-mounted bicycle ergometer is the method of choice. Shoulder restraints and hand grips help reduce upper body movement during imaging. For patients who are unable to exercise effectively, stress with dobutamine infusion is used.[2] Under continuous monitoring, the dose is incrementally increased from 5–20 µg kg^{-1} min^{-1}, infusing each dose for 3 min. The infusion is stopped when S-T segment depression greater than 3 mm, any ventricular arrhythmia, systolic blood pressure greater than 220 mmHg, attainment of maximum heart rate or any side effects occur.
2. Gated single-photon emission computed tomography (SPECT) blood-pool acquisition can be used for measurement of left as well as the right ventricular function using special software (Autoquant+) that calculates the left and right ventricular volumes.
3. With gated SPECT using the myocardial perfusion imaging agents ^{99m}Tc-MIBI and ^{99m}Tc-tetrofosmin (see the section Radionuclide myocardial perfusion imaging), it is possible to combine ventriculography and perfusion scans in a single study.[3,4]

When acquiring gated SPECT studies, ventricular parameters are usually measured during the rest study only because of the length of the examination (20 min).

Aftercare

1. Monitor recovery from exercise.
2. Implement normal radiation safety precautions (see Chapter 1).

Complications

Complications are related to the exercise test and include induction of angina, cardiac arrhythmias and cardiac arrest.

References

1. Metcalfe MJ. Radionuclide ventriculography. In: Sharp PF, Gemmell HG, Murray AD, eds. *Practical Nuclear Medicine*. Springer; 2005.
2. Konishi T, Koyama T, Aoki T, et al. Radionuclide assessment of left ventricular function during dobutamine infusion in patients with coronary artery disease: comparison with ergometer exercise. *Clin Cardiol*. 1990;13:183–188.

3. Fukuoka S, Maeno M, Nakagawa S, et al. Feasibility of myocardial dual-isotope perfusion imaging combined with gated single photon emission tomography for assessing coronary artery disease. *Nucl Med Commun.* 2002;23(1):19–29.

4. Anagnostopoulos C, Underwood SR. Simultaneous assessment of myocardial perfusion and function: how and when? *Eur J Nucl Med.* 1998;25:555–558.

RADIONUCLIDE MYOCARDIAL PERFUSION IMAGING

Indications

1. Diagnosis and assessment of extent and severity of myocardial ischaemia or infarction
2. Assessment of myocardial viability
3. Evaluation of prognosis
4. Evaluation of effects of angioplasty and bypass surgery on myocardial perfusion with pre- and postintervention imaging

Contraindications

1. Unstable angina
2. Frequent ventricular arrhythmias at rest
3. Contraindications to pharmacological stress agent
4. Second-degree heart block
5. Severe valvular disease, especially aortic valve stenosis

Radiopharmaceuticals[1,2]

1. ^{99m}Tc-methoxyisobutylisonitrile (MIBI or sestamibi), up to 800 MBq (8 mSv ED) for planar imaging, 800 MBq (8 mSv ED) for SPECT (or 1600 MBq maximum for the total of two injections in single-day rest–exercise protocols). Cationic complex with myocardial uptake in near proportion to coronary blood flow but with minimal redistribution. There are also typically liver uptake and biliary excretion, which can cause inferior wall artifacts on SPECT if care is not taken. Separate injections are required for stress–rest studies, but image timing is flexible because of minimal redistribution.

2. ^{99m}Tc-tetrofosmin (Myoview) (activity and radiation dose as for MIBI). Similar uptake characteristics and diagnostic efficacy to MIBI but with easier preparation.

3. ^{201}Tl-thallous chloride, 80 MBq maximum (18 mSv ED). Thallium is a potassium analogue with initial rapid myocardial uptake in near proportion to coronary blood flow and subsequent washout and redistribution. Hence, unlike the ^{99m}Tc agents, same-day stress–rest redistribution studies can be performed with a single injection. With principal photon energies of 68–72 and 167 keV and $t_{1/2}$ of 73 h, it is not ideal for imaging and gives a higher radiation dose than the newer ^{99m}Tc alternatives. It is increasingly being replaced by ^{99m}Tc agents. However, many still consider ^{201}Tl for assessment of

10

myocardial viability and hibernation, with either reinjection at rest or a separate day rest–redistribution study giving the greatest sensitivity.

4. ^{18}FDG + blood flow positron emission tomography (PET). The radioisotope gold standard for viability assessment but not widely available.[3]

5. Rubidium-82 PET. This study can be used to assess absolute myocardial perfusion. It is not widely available.

Equipment

1. SPECT-capable gamma camera, preferably dual headed
2. Low-energy, high-resolution, general-purpose or specialized cardiac collimators
3. Pharmacological stressing agent (adenosine or dobutamine (dipyridamole now rarely used)) or exercise (bicycle ergometer or treadmill)
4. Nitroglycerin (tablets or sublingual spray) to enhance resting uptake of ischaemic but viable segments
5. ECG monitor
6. Resuscitation facilities including defibrillator
7. Lidocaine to reverse serious arrhythmias caused by dobutamine infusion

Patient Preparation

1. Nil by mouth or light breakfast 4–6 h before test
2. Cessation of cardiac medication on the day of the test if possible. Beta-blockers can be continued and adenosine stress used. Avoid caffeine for 24 h if using dipyridamole or adenosine.

Technique

The principle of the technique is to compare myocardial perfusion under conditions of pharmacological stress or physical exercise with perfusion at rest. Diseased but patent arterial territories show lower perfusion under stress conditions than healthy arteries but show relatively improved perfusion at rest. Infarcted tissue shows no improvement at rest. Hence, prognostic information on the likelihood of adverse cardiac events and the benefits of revascularization can be gained.[4]

Stress regimen

Pharmacological stress has become increasingly widely used instead of physical exercise.[5] The optimal stress technique aims to maximize coronary arterial flow. The preferred pharmacological stressing agent is adenosine infusion (0.14 mg kg^{-1} min^{-1} for 6 min).[6] Adenosine is a potent coronary vasodilator. It reproducibly increases coronary artery flow by more than maximal physical exercise (which often cannot be achieved in this group of patients). It has a short biological half-life of 8–10 s, so most side effects are reversed simply by discontinuing infusion. Stressing with adenosine has now almost completely replaced dipyridamole, which is therefore not discussed here.

There are circumstances when adenosine is contraindicated, such as in patients with asthma, second-degree heart block or systolic blood pressure below 100 mmHg. Dobutamine stress may be used in these circumstances.[7] Dobutamine acts as a β_1 receptor agonist, increasing contractility and heart rate. Under continuous monitoring, the dose is incrementally increased from 5–20 µg kg^{-1} min^{-1}, infusing each dose for 3 min. The infusion is terminated when S-T segment depression of greater than 3 mm, any ventricular arrhythmia, systolic blood pressure greater than 220 mmHg, attainment of maximum heart rate or any side effects occur. Dobutamine is contraindicated in patients with aortic aneurysm. New, more specific targeted agents such as regadenoson (A_{2A} adenosine receptor agonist) are available, which can be used rather than dobutamine in patients with asthma.[8]

^{99m}Tc-MIBI or tetrofosmin rest and stress tests

Because MIBI and tetrofosmin have minimal redistribution, separate injections are needed for stress and rest studies. Two-day protocols are optimal, but it is often more convenient to perform both studies on the same day. A number of groups have shown that this is possible without significantly degrading the results, most effectively when the resting study is performed first.[9]

Two-day protocol (stress and rest)

1. Initiate pharmacological stress or exercise.
2. Up to 800 MBq MIBI or tetrofosmin is administered IV at maximal stress, continuing the stress protocol for 2 min postinjection to allow uptake in the myocardium.
3. At 10–30 min after the injection, a milky drink or similar is given to promote biliary clearance; high fluid intake dilutes bowel contents.
4. Images are acquired 15–30 min after tetrofosmin or 60–120 min after sestamibi injection. If there is excessive liver uptake or activity in small bowel close to the heart, imaging should be delayed by a further 60 min.
5. Depending on the clinical situation, if the stress scan result is completely normal, the patient may not need to return for the rest scan.[10]
6. Preferably 2–7 days later, the patient returns for a resting scan.
7. GTN (two 0.3-mg tablets) or equivalent sublingual spray may be given to improve blood flow to ischaemic but viable segments.[11]
8. Immediately, up to 800 MBq MIBI or tetrofosmin IV is administered; proceed as for stress imaging.

One-day protocol (stress and rest)

1. Initiate pharmacological stress or exercise; up to 400 MBq MIBI or tetrofosmin IV is administered at maximum stress.
2. Image as per the 2-day protocol.
3. A minimum of 2 h after first tetrofosmin injection and minimum of 4 h after sestamibi injection, GTN is administered as noted previously followed by up to 1200 MBq of MIBI or tetrofosmin. (With a longer period between injections, the activity of the second injection may be reduced.)
4. Image as per the 2-day protocol.

10

[201]Tl stress and rest test

Because ^{201}Tl redistributes after injection, stress and rest studies can be performed with a single injection. However, stress image timing is more critical:

1. Initiate pharmacological stress or exercise.
2. Administer 80 MBq ^{201}Tl IV at maximal stress, continuing the stress protocol for 1 min postinjection to allow uptake in the myocardium.
3. Image immediately (<5 min).
4. Image at rest 3–4 h after redistribution period, during which time the patient should not eat.
5. If fixed defects are present in exercise and rest images and assessment of viability and hibernation is required, either:
   (a) Administer a second, smaller dose of 40 MBq ^{201}Tl, giving GTN pre injection, and image 20–30 min later. If defects still persist, image again at 18–24 h *or*
   (b) Perform a separate day rest-redistribution study with 80 MBq ^{201}Tl after GTN and image at 20–30 min and 3–4 h.

Images

Single-photon emission computed tomography

1. Position the patient as comfortably as possible with their arms above their head (or at least the left arm), if possible. SPECT images may be severely degraded by patient movement, so attention should be paid to keeping the patient very still.
2. For the ^{99m}Tc agents, check for activity in bowel loops close to the inferior wall of the heart. This can cause artefacts in the reconstructed images, so if significant activity is seen, delay the imaging to give greater time for clearance.
3. 180-degree orbit from RAO 45 degrees to LPO 45 degrees, elliptical if possible. With modern dual-headed systems, this can be achieved with the heads at 90 degrees to each other to minimize the amount of camera rotation required.
4. Matrix size and zoom to give a pixel size of 6 mm.
5. Sixty projections, with a total imaging time of about 30–40 min for single and 15–25 min for dual-head systems.
6. View the projections as a cine before the patient leaves the department. If available, perform software motion correction. If there is significant movement that cannot be corrected, repeat imaging. Beware of 'diaphragmatic creep', particularly on ^{201}Tl patients breathless after exercise because the average position of the diaphragm changes as they recover.

Analysis[12]

1. Short, vertical long-axis and horizontal long-axis views are reconstructed, taking care to use the same orientation for stress and rest image data sets. (Modern systems have automatic alignment software.)
2. 2D circumferential profile or 'bull's-eye' polar maps may be generated.

Additional Techniques

1. Gated SPECT is now recommended,[13] and special software (e.g. Cedars Sinai QGS package, Emory cardiac tool box) can provide additional information on ventricular wall motion, ejection fraction and chamber volume. It can also improve specificity by reducing artefactual defects caused by regional myocardial motion and wall thickening.

2. Bull's-eye maps can be compared with normal databases and displayed quantitatively in terms of the severity and extent of relative underperfusion.[14]

3. Attenuation and scatter correction using scanning transmission line sources or CT are now available on most modern dual-headed systems. This technique can improve diagnostic specificity by correcting attenuation artefacts and thereby increasing the normalcy rate. However, algorithms are still being improved, so at present, it is wise to view the attenuation-corrected and -uncorrected images together to identify possible introduced artefacts.[15]

4. The combination of rest ^{201}Tl and exercise ^{99m}Tc MIBI or tetrofosmin can be used to assess both ischaemia and viability.[16]

Aftercare

1. Monitoring of patient postexercise
2. Normal radiation safety precautions (see Chapter 1)

Complications

Complications are related to stress and exercise and include induction of angina, cardiac arrhythmias, cardiac arrest and bronchospasm after adenosine.

References

1. Reyes E, Loong CY, Harbinson M, et al. A comparison of Tl-201, Tc-99m sestamibi, and Ic-99m tetrofosmin myocardial perfusion scintigraphy in patients with mild to moderate coronary stenosis. *J Nucl Cardiol.* 2006;13(4):488–494.

2. Kapur A, Latus KA, Davies G, et al. A comparison of three radionuclide myocardial perfusion tracers in clinical practice: the ROBUST study. *Eur J Nucl Med Mol Imaging.* 2002;29(12):1608–1616.

3. Nandalur KR, Dwamena BA, Choudhri AF, et al. Diagnostic performance of positron emission tomography in the detection of coronary artery disease: a meta-analysis. *Acad Radiol.* 2008;15(4):444–451.

4. Travin MI, Bergmann SR. Assessment of myocardial viability. *Semin Nucl Med.* 2005;35(1):2–16.

5. Travin MI, Wexler JP. Pharmacological stress testing. *Semin Nucl Med.* 1999;29:298–318.

6. Takeishi Y, Takahashi N, Fujiwara S, et al. Myocardial tomography with technetium-99m-tetrofosmin during intravenous infusion of adenosine triphosphate. *J Nucl Med.* 1998;39:582–586.

7. Verani MS. Dobutamine myocardial perfusion imaging. *J Nucl Med.* 1994;35:737–739.

8. Iskandrian AE, Bateman TM, Belardinelli L, et al. Adenosine versus regadenoson comparative evaluation in myocardial perfusion imaging:

10

results of the ADVANCE phase 3 multicenter international trial. *J Nucl Cardiol.* 2007;14(5):645–658.

9. Tadehara F, Yamamoto H, Tsujiyama S, et al. Feasibility of a rapid protocol of 1-day single-isotope rest/adenosine stress Tc-99m sestamibi ECG-gated myocardial perfusion imaging. *J Nucl Cardiol.* 2008;15(1):35–41.

10. Lavalaye JM, Shroeder-Tanka JM, Tiel-van Buul MM, et al. Implementation of technetium-99m MIBI SPECT imaging guidelines: optimizing the two-day stress-rest protocol. *Int J Card Imaging.* 1997;13:331–335.

11. Thorley PJ, Sheard KL, Wright DJ, et al. The routine use of sublingual GTN with resting ^{99m}Tc-tetrofosmin myocardial perfusion imaging. *Nucl Med Commun.* 1998;19:937–942.

12. Motwani M, Berman DS, Germano G, et al. Automated quantitative nuclear cardiology methods. *Cardiol Clin.* 2016;34(1):47–57.

13. Travin MI, Heller GV, Johnson LL, et al. The prognostic value of ECG-gated SPECT imaging in patients undergoing stress Tc-99m sestamibi myocardial perfusion imaging. *J Nucl Cardiol.* 2004;11(3):253–262.

14. Schwaiger M, Melin J. Cardiological applications of nuclear medicine. *Lancet.* 1999;354:661–666.

15. Banzo I, Pena FJ, Allende RH, et al. Prospective clinical comparison of non-corrected and attenuation- and scatter-corrected myocardial perfusion SPECT in patients with suspicion of coronary artery disease. *Nucl Med Commun.* 2003;24(9):995–1002.

16. Kim Y, Goto H, Kobayshi K, et al. A new method to evaluate ischemic heart disease: combined use of rest thallium-201 myocardial SPECT and Tc-99m exercise tetrofosmin first pass and myocardial SPECT. *Ann Nucl Med.* 1999;13:147–153.

Arterial system

Christopher Day

NON-INVASIVE IMAGING

Non-invasive methods of imaging are usually preferred before catheter angiography and are usually able to provide sufficient diagnostic information to guide therapeutic procedures.

Methods include the following:

1. Ultrasound (US)
2. Computed tomography (CT)
3. Magnetic resonance imaging (MRI)

VASCULAR ULTRASOUND

US is a reliable, non-invasive, inexpensive test that is well tolerated by patients and widely used for assessment of the arterial system. Intraabdominal or pelvic arteries can be examined with US, but US is best suited to relatively superficial vessels such as those of the neck or lower limb. Chest arteries cannot be assessed by US because the high-frequency sound waves do not adequately penetrate air or bone. The main disadvantages of US are the marked operator-dependent nature of the technique and lengthy examination times for some studies.

The main components of arterial vascular US studies are the following:

1. Grey-scale US: gives anatomical information and detailed assessment of vessel wall, including areas of intimal thickening or calcification.
2. Pulsed-wave Doppler: measures changes in frequency of US waves reflected by moving blood within the vessel (Doppler shift). These data are used to calculate a detailed graph of direction and velocity of flow in the vessel. The normal pattern of flow differs between various arteries, and flow patterns change at sites of disease such as narrowing (i.e. increases in velocity).
3. Colour Doppler: uses the same information as pulsed-wave Doppler but displays flow as colour superimposed within the arterial lumen on grey-scale imaging. Colour encoding represents the direction and velocity of flow with red conventionally indicating

flow towards the US transducer and blue representing flow away from the transducer. Rapid flow is displayed as white or yellow. This is helpful in selection of regions for detailed assessment with pulsed-wave Doppler or detection of arteriovenous fistulae or pseudoaneurysm.

4. Power Doppler: a modification of colour Doppler that is more sensitive to slow flow or flow in small structures. However, it does not give information on direction or velocity of flow.

COMPUTED TOMOGRAPHY ANGIOGRAPHY

Computed tomography angiography (CTA) is performed as a block of very thin axial multidetector computed tomography (MDCT) images obtained during the rapid peripheral intravenous (IV) infusion of iodinated contrast. The acquisition is timed to coincide with the peak density of contrast in arteries, and the images are subsequently reconstructed using postprocessing techniques such as multiplanar reconstruction or maximum-intensity projection.

Although CTA involves administration of iodinated contrast (see Chapter 2) and significant radiation dose, there are many advantages: imaging is very rapid, scanners are readily available, unstable patients can be monitored with standard equipment and diagnostic performance is equivalent to digital subtraction angiography with additional valuable information obtained about the blood vessel wall and surrounding structures (may reveal unsuspected comorbidities). One of the disadvantages of CTA is poor visualization of small vessels with significant vessel wall calcification that is often seen in patients with diabetes or those with significant renal impairment. To try and mitigate this, it may be possible to perform a non-contrast scan, initially allowing the calcification to be subtracted from the contrast enhanced scan.

PERIPHERAL (LOWER LIMB) COMPUTED TOMOGRAPHY ANGIOGRAPHY

Descriptions of other specific CTA methods are found in appropriate chapters.

Indications

1. Lower limb ischaemia
2. Arteriovenous malformation
3. Trauma

Patient Preparation

General precautions for use of ionizing radiation (see Chapter 1) and iodinated contrast (see Chapter 2). The nature and purpose of the examination are explained to the patient.

Technique

For optimum images, an MDCT scanner with at least a 16-slice detector is used:

1. Contrast: 100–150 mL low-osmolar contrast medium 300 mg I mL^{-1} (volume determined by scanner and scan protocol)
2. Contrast injection rate: 4 mL s^{-1} via a peripheral vein
3. Range: lower abdominal aorta to heel or extended as upper abdominal aorta to heel
4. Slice thickness: 3 mm or less
5. Reconstruction increment: 0.6 mm
6. Delay:
   (a) Preset empirical delay using the manufacturer's guidelines for individual scanner. This is not routinely used because of significant variability of blood flow between patients, resulting in suboptimal contrast opacification.
   (b) Bolus tracking technique, choosing a region of interest (ROI) in the aorta just above the upper range of the scan and monitoring contrast density in ROI during injection until it reaches a predetermined value (usually 100–120 Hounsfield units), which triggers the CT acquisition. The technique may be modified to include a second ROI more distally in the popliteal artery. This may be achieved by giving a second bolus of contrast or with the scanner automatically moving to the second ROI after contrast has reached threshold in the first ROI. The time taken for contrast to move between the two ROIs allows more accurate prediction of how long the delay needs to be enabling good contrast opacification of distal vessels.

Aftercare and Complications

For iodinated contrast, see Chapter 2.

MAGNETIC RESONANCE ANGIOGRAPHY

11

Guidelines on MR safety and selection of patients must be followed (see Chapter 1).

Magnetic resonance angiography (MRA) can be contrast-enhanced MRA with IV gadolinium (see Chapter 2) or non-contrast. Gadolinium IV shortens the T1 relaxation time of blood, so blood appears bright when imaged with a very short TR (repetition time), and other structures on the image appear dark. Timing of the contrast injection is critical. Imaging without contrast is used infrequently but may be either a 'bright blood' gradient echo cine technique to demonstrate both anatomical and functional data or 'black blood' imaging, which gives useful morphological information.

Non-contrast techniques have significantly improved with specific sequences developed by different manufacturers. These techniques are particularly useful in patients with impaired renal function. MRA generally provides better detail, particularly in patients with significant vessel wall calcification such as patients with diabetes or renal failure. Time-resolved MRA is able to produce a cine loop from arterial to venous phases, producing an image that appears similar to conventional catheter angiography. This may be useful when looking at vascular malformations.

Further Reading

Cavallo AU, Koktzoglou I, Edelman RR, et al. Noncontrast magnetic resonance angiography for the diagnosis of peripheral vascular disease. *Circ Cardiovasc Imaging*. 2019;12(5):e008844.

Cole DA, Fox BR, Peña CS. The role of imaging in peripheral interventions. *Tech Vasc Interv Radiol*. 2022;25(3):100836.

Cook TS. Computed tomography angiography of the lower extremities. *Radiol Clin North Am*. 2016;54(1):115–130.

Thrush A, Hartshorne T, Deane CR. *Vascular Ultrasound How, Why and When*. 4th ed. Elsevier; 2022.

VASCULAR ACCESS

All invasive arterial procedures begin with arterial access. The same techniques are applicable to all vessels that may be used for access, including veins. Common sites used for arterial access include:

1. Common femoral artery: most frequently used, so this will be described in detail
2. Brachial artery: reserved for patients in whom the common femoral artery is unsuitable
3. Radial artery: more frequently used in cardiology interventions but increasingly used in interventional radiology for visceral and pelvic interventions, mainly limited by the length of available catheters and devices.

Patient Preparation

1. The patient needs admission to hospital. Careful preparation before the procedure and observation afterward are required. Most elective cases may be admitted to a day case unit for discharge the same day, with overnight stays reserved for complex cases and those in which there has been a significant complication requiring extended observation.
2. If the patient is on anticoagulant treatment, blood clotting should be within an acceptable therapeutic 'window'. According to the consensus guidelines issued by the Society of Interventional Radiology (SIR) and Cardiovascular and Interventional Radiological Society of Europe, the international normalized ratio should be less than 1.5, and the activated partial thromboplastin time should be less than 1.5 times the control.
3. The radiologist or a suitably trained person should see the patient, preferably several days before the procedure, in order to:
   (a) Explain the procedure
   (b) Obtain informed consent

(c) Assess the patient, with special reference to renal function, blood pressure and peripheral pulses as a baseline for post-arteriographic problems

Equipment for Vascular Access

Ultrasound

US-guided puncture of the artery is recommended in contemporary practice for all arterial access, particularly with the widespread availability of suitable US machines. It allows the anatomy of the vessel to be delineated, including any anatomical variation that may affect the level of the puncture. Calcification of the vessel wall can be identified and avoided during the puncture. Local anaesthesia is more accurately delivered to the vessel, aiming to produce a 'lake' immediately next to the adventitia to provide the most effective analgesia. US reduces the risk of inadvertent puncture of the vessel during administration. In addition, any change in the vessel compared with previous imaging (e.g. unexpected occlusion) can be identified and an alternative vessel chosen. A non–image-guided technique using palpation of anatomical landmarks is not recommended routinely but is important to understand in the unlikely event that US is not available.

Needle

A bevelled, hollow needle is used to puncture the artery. This allows a guidewire to be advanced through it into the vessel lumen.

Guidewires

Basic guidewires consist of two central cores of straight wire, around which is a tightly wound coiled wire spring (Fig. 11.1). The ends are sealed with solder. One of the central core wires is secured at both ends (a safety feature in case of fracturing). The other is anchored in solder at one end but terminates 5 cm from the other end, leaving a soft flexible tip. Some guidewires have a movable central core, so the tip can be flexible or stiff. Others have a J-shaped tip that is useful for negotiating vessels with irregular walls. The size of the J-curve is denoted by its radius in millimetres. Guidewires are polyethylene coated but may be coated with a thin film of Teflon to reduce friction. Teflon, however, also increases the thrombogenicity, which can be countered by using heparin-bonded Teflon. The most common sizes are 0.035- and 0.038-in diameters as well as smaller diameter wires such as 0.018- and 0.014-in wires, particularly for small arteries such as the infrapopliteal vessels. More recently, hydrophilic guidewires have been developed. These frequently have a metal mandrel as their core. They are very slippery, with excellent torque, and are useful in negotiating narrow tortuous vessels. They require constant lubrication with saline.

Vascular sheaths

These consist of a tube with a haemostatic valve and a 'side arm' consisting of a single tube with a two-way flow switch on the end.

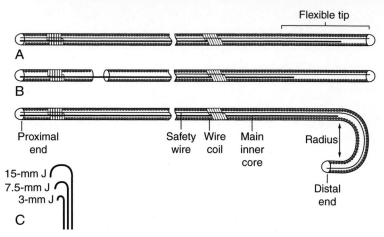

Fig. 11.1 Guidewire construction. **A,** Fixed core, straight. **B,** Movable core, straight. **C,** Fixed core, J-curve.

A dilator is advanced into the sheath through the haemostatic valve to aid insertion through the vessel wall. The sheath provides secure access to the vessel lumen, allowing multiple exchanges of guidewires and catheters without further trauma to the vessel wall or bleeding. The side arm may be used to flush the sheath, inject contrast into the vessel and administer medications during the procedure. Sometimes it may be connected to a pressure monitor, allowing continuous blood pressure monitoring. Sheaths come in various diameters, with 4–7 Fr being the commonest for most procedures.

Catheters

Most catheters are manufactured commercially, complete with end hole, side holes, preformed curves and Luer lock connections. They are made of polyurethane or polyethylene. Details of the specific catheter types are given with the appropriate technique.

Some straight catheters may be shaped by immersion in hot sterile water until they become malleable, forming the desired shape and then fixing the shape by cooling in cold sterile water, but this technique is rarely needed in contemporary practice because of the wide range of available catheter shapes. For the average adult, a 100-cm catheter with a 145-cm guidewire is suitable for reaching the thoracic aortic branches from a femoral puncture. If abdominal aortography or peripheral arteriography of the legs is to be performed, shorter catheters may be used.

Taps and connectors

These should have a large internal diameter that will not increase resistance to flow. Taps should be removed during high-pressure injections.

Relative Contraindications

1. Blood dyscrasias
2. Femoral artery aneurysm or pseudoaneurysm
3. Local soft tissue infection
4. Severe hypertension
5. Ehlers–Danlos syndrome (because the vessel wall is easily torn)

Technique (Fig. 11.2)

1. The patient lies supine on the x-ray table. The target artery is palpated, and the proposed puncture site is chosen, ideally where the vessel passes close to underlying bone (e.g. the femoral head for common femoral artery puncture and distal humerus for brachial artery puncture) to aid postprocedure compression.
2. The appropriate size of sheath is selected and prepared by flushing both the introducer and the sheath (through its sidearm) using heparinized saline. The size of sheath should be large enough to introduce the devices needed to complete the procedure.
3. The guidewire and catheter are selected, and if necessary, their compatibility is checked by passing the guidewire through the catheter and needle. The catheter should be flushed with heparinized saline.
4. US-guided technique: Direct US guidance allows the correct location for puncture to be identified. The US probe is used to identify the proximal and distal ends of the common femoral artery. Proximally, the vessel passes deep to the inguinal ligament, and distally, it divides into superficial femoral and profunda femoris arteries. The puncture point is between these landmarks at a location that avoids calcified atherosclerotic plaque, if possible. The US probe may be held transverse or longitudinal to the artery. Transverse allows the centre of anterior vessel wall to be punctured more accurately but can be more challenging because the probe has to be angled craniocaudally to follow the needle. Longitudinal orientation of the probe allows the needle to be imaged easily from skin to the artery but is more challenging to accurately puncture the centre of the vessel wall. Using aseptic technique, local anaesthetic is infiltrated down to the adventitia of the vessel. US allows accurate infiltration of the local anaesthesia, aiming to form a 'lake' of local anaesthetic adjacent to the artery and then infiltrating the superficial tissues as the needle is withdrawn back to the skin surface. A 2- to 3-mm stab incision is made over the artery, and the needle is advanced under direct vision through the anterior wall of the vessel until the needle tip is in the centre of the vessel lumen and blood flow through the needle is observed (see Fig. 11.2A). Poor flow may be caused by:
   (a) The end of the needle lying in or against the vessel wall or within plaque; this can be checked by direct visualization
   (b) Aorto-iliac stenosis or occlusion, resulting in low femoral artery pressure
   (c) Hypotension due to vasovagal reaction during the puncture

11

5. Non–image-guided technique: not recommended but may be necessary if US is unavailable. The artery is palpated below the inguinal ligament, and fluoroscopy is used to identify the location of the underlying femoral head aiming for the puncture to be performed directly over this bony landmark. Using aseptic technique, local anaesthetic is infiltrated down to the artery, with care taken not to inject it into the artery lumen by aspirating before injection to make sure no blood is seen entering the syringe. A 2- to 3-mm stab incision is made over the artery to reduce binding of soft tissues on the sheath. In thin patients, the artery may be very superficial, and the skin may need to be pinched up or deflected laterally to avoid cutting the artery. The artery is immobilized by placing the index and middle fingers of the left hand on either side of the artery, and the needle is held in the right hand. The needle is advanced through the soft tissues until transmitted pulsations are felt. The needle is advanced through the superficial vessel wall until pulsatile blood flow through the needle is observed (see Fig. 11.2A). Poor flow may be caused by:

   (a) The end of the needle lying in or against the vessel wall or within plaque: Slowly pull back the needle until better flow is observed or try to change the angle of the needle.
   (b) Aortoiliac stenosis or occlusion resulting in low femoral artery pressure
   (c) Hypotension caused by vasovagal reaction during the puncture
   (d) Femoral vein puncture

6. When good flow is obtained, the sheath guidewire is introduced through the needle and advanced gently along the artery (see Fig. 11.2B). Intermittent fluoroscopy may be used if necessary to confirm the guidewire position. Next, the needle is removed, leaving the guidewire in position (see Fig. 11.2C).

7. The vascular sheath with its introducer dilator in place is advanced over the guidewire (see Fig. 11.2D). If this is difficult, it may be necessary to dilate the tract initially with a 4-Fr dilator followed by increasing dilators to the size of the sheath, and it may be necessary to use a stiffer guidewire for more support. When in position, the sheath introducer dilator and guidewire are removed, leaving the sheath in situ (see Fig. 11.2E). The sidearm of the sheath is aspirated then flushed with heparinized saline to confirm its position in the vessel lumen. If the sheath does not aspirate freely, the tip may be against a lesion, and it should be withdrawn until it can be aspirated. Sheath patency can be maintained by continuous flushing from a pressurized bag of heparinized saline (e.g. 2500 units in 500 mL of 0.9% saline) attached through a three-way tap or by intermittent manual flushing throughout the procedure. Continuous flushing is particularly useful when using longer sheaths that are more prone to occlusion and when performing particularly complex procedures in which it is easy to forget to regularly flush the sheath.

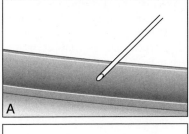

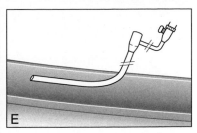

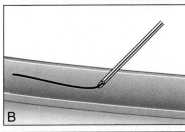

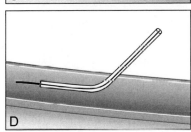

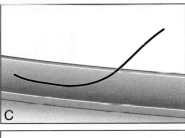

Fig. 11.2 Vascular access technique. **A,** A hollow needle is advanced through the vessel wall. Note that the needle bevel is oriented along the line of the vessel. **B,** A guidewire for the sheath is advanced through the needle into the vessel lumen. The length of wire introduced needs to be enough to allow the tip of the wire to be held whilst the sheath is advanced into position. **C,** The needle is removed with the guidewire left in situ. It may be necessary to apply pressure over the puncture site to reduce haemorrhage at this point. **D,** A vascular sheath with its introducer dilator is advanced over the guidewire into the vessel. Usually the sheath is advanced up to its hub. **E,** The introducer dilator of the sheath and the guidewire are removed with the vascular sheath left in situ.

11

8. At the end of the procedure, the catheter is withdrawn from the sheath. The sheath is flushed through its sidearm with heparinized saline and then withdrawn from the vessel, with manual compression applied to the puncture site. Manual compression is the commonest method used to obtain haemostasis after arterial puncture. It should be directed over the puncture site and the tract from artery to skin surface. Compression should be maintained for 5–10 min (or until haemostasis has been achieved).

9. Closure devices can allow rapid haemostasis at the site of the arterial puncture. They can also speed up mobilization of patients after arterial puncture and may be useful in patients in whom a large sheath or anticoagulants have been used. In addition, they may be useful in patients who are likely to have difficulty complying with

bedrest instructions after manual compression. There are many different closure devices currently on the market, and it is beyond the scope of this text to describe them all in detail (see Further Reading). They may be broadly classified according to their mechanism of action. Plug-based devices introduce material that 'plugs' the hole at the arterial puncture site. Suture-mediated devices introduce a suture into the vessel wall at the site of arterial puncture that is then pulled tight to close the hole. Clip-based devices introduce a clip onto the vessel wall at the site of arterial puncture. In addition, invasive manual compression assist devices are available.

10. Preclosure techniques may be used when introducing large-calibre access sheaths such as during endovascular aneurysm repair that are generally greater than 10 Fr. The technique often involves using two or more suture-mediated closure devices or other devices such as large vascular plugs. As a general rule, one suture is deployed for every 9 Fr of access diameter. For example, two would be used for an 18-Fr sheath and three for a 24-Fr sheath. If two are used, they are deployed at the 11 and 1 o'clock positions on the arterial wall. If three are used, they are positioned at the 10, 12 and 2 o'clock positions. The sutures are deployed but left loose until the end of the procedure when they are tightened sequentially to obtain haemostasis.

Aftercare

1. Bedrest: typically for 4–6 h with the patient lying flat followed by 2 h with the patient in the sitting position but longer at the discretion of the operator. Larger catheters, antiplatelet therapy and anticoagulation require longer observation. Using closure devices can allow more rapid mobilization after the procedure. After the desired period of bedrest has been observed without complication, the patient may be mobilized gently.
2. Careful observation of the puncture site for haemorrhage
3. Pulse and blood pressure observation (e.g. half-hourly for 4 h and then 4 hourly for the remainder of the patient stay)

Further Reading

Patel IJ, Davidson JC, Nikolic B, et al. Consensus guidelines for the periprocedural management of coagulation status and haemostasis risk in percutaneous image-guided interventions. *J Vasc Interv Radiol.* 2012;23:727–736.
Patel R, Muller-Hulsbeck S, Morgan R, et al. Vascular closure devices in radiology practice. *Cardiovasc Intervent Radiol.* 2015;38:781–793.
Rajebi H, Rajebi MR. Optimizing common femoral artery access. *Tech Vasc Interv Radiol.* 2015;18(2):76–81.

GENERAL COMPLICATIONS OF CATHETER TECHNIQUES

Due to the Anaesthetic

See Chapter 21.

Due to the Contrast Medium

See Chapter 2.

Due to the Technique

Diagnostic angiography is an invasive procedure and has associated complications The majority of these are minor (e.g. groin haematoma). Recommended upper limits for complication rates have been produced by the SIR[1]; these rates are included in the following discussion.

Due to Access

The most frequent complications occur at the puncture site. The complication rate is lowest for femoral artery punctures:

1. Haemorrhage or haematoma is the commonest complication. Small haematomas occur in up to 20% of examinations and large haematomas in up to 4%. The SIR threshold for haematomas requiring transfusion, surgery or delayed discharge after diagnostic angiography is 0.5%. Haematoma formation is greater with patients, especially female patients with high systolic blood pressure[1]; larger catheters; more frequent catheter exchanges; and heparin, antiplatelet or thrombolytic agents. Haematoma formation is also greater when the femoral artery is punctured high because of inadequate compression of the artery after catheter removal.
2. Arterial thrombus may be caused by:
   (a) Stripping of thrombus from the catheter wall as it is withdrawn
   (b) Trauma to the vessel wall

   Factors implicated in increased thrombus formation are:
   (a) Large catheters
   (b) Excessive time in the artery
   (c) Multiple catheter changes
   (d) Inexperience of the radiologist
   (e) Polyurethane catheters because of their rough surfaces

   The incidence is decreased by the use of:
   (a) Heparin-bonded catheters
   (b) Heparin-bonded guidewires
   (c) Flushing with heparinized saline
3. Infection at the puncture site
4. Damage to local structures, especially the brachial plexus during axillary artery puncture. Femoral nerve palsy can result from inadvertent infiltration of the nerve with local anaesthetic. It is short-lived but should prompt very cautious subsequent mobilization of the patient in case the leg 'gives way'. More protracted femoral nerve damage can be caused by excessive haematoma or pseudoaneurysm formation in the groin.
5. Pseudoaneurysm. The SIR threshold for diagnostic angiography is 0.2%. It presents as a pulsatile mass at the puncture site any time after arteriography and is caused by communication between the

11

lumen of the artery and a cavity within semisolid or organized haematoma. Arterial puncture below the common femoral artery bifurcation increases the risk of this complication. Some may require surgical or interventional radiological repair.

6. Arteriovenous fistula: rare. SIR threshold is 0.1%. More common with brachial artery puncture because of the two veins that accompany the artery on either side. US-guided puncture reduces the risk.

Reference

1. May O, Schlosser H, Skytte L. A high blood pressure predicts bleeding complications and a longer hospital stay after elective coronary angiography using the femoral approach. *J Interv Cardiol.* 2009;22(2):175–178.

DISTANT

1. Peripheral embolus from stripped catheter thrombus. Emboli to small digital arteries resolve spontaneously; emboli to large arteries may need aspiration thrombectomy through a catheter or surgical embolectomy. The SIR threshold is 0.5%.

2. Atheroembolism: more likely in older patients. J-shaped guidewires are less likely to dislodge atheromatous plaques.

3. Air embolus: may be fatal in coronary or cerebral arteries. It is prevented by:
   (a) Ensuring that all taps and connectors are tight
   (b) Always sucking back when a new syringe is connected
   (c) Ensuring that all bubbles are excluded from the syringe before injecting
   (d) Keeping the syringe vertical, plunger up, when injecting

4. Cotton fibre embolus: occurs when syringes are filled from a bowl containing swabs or when a guidewire is wiped with a dry gauze pad. This is easily avoided:
   (a) Separate bowls of saline for flushing and wet swabs or, preferably,
   (b) A closed system of perfusion

5. Artery dissection: caused by entry of the catheter, guidewire or contrast medium into the subintimal space. It is recognized by resistance to passage of the guidewire or catheter, poor backbleeding from the catheter hub, increased resistance to injection of contrast medium or subintimal contrast medium on fluoroscopy. The risk of serious dissection is reduced by:
   (a) Using floppy J-shaped guidewires
   (b) Using catheters with multiple side holes
   (c) Using a small volume manual test injection before a pump injection
   (d) Careful and gentle manipulation of catheters

6. Catheter knotting: more likely during the investigation of complex congenital heart disease. Non-surgical reduction of catheter knots is discussed by Thomas and Sievers.[1] Withdrawal of the knotted end to the groin followed by surgical removal may be the only solution in some cases.

7. Catheter impaction:
   (a) In a coronary artery produces cardiac ischaemic pain
   (b) In a mesenteric artery produces abdominal pain. There should be rapid wash-out of contrast medium after a selective injection. A sound of sucking air on removing the guidewire and poor backbleeding from the catheter indicate an impacted (wedged) catheter tip.
8. Guidewire breakage—less common with modern guidewires and tended to occur 5 cm from the tip, where a single central core terminates
9. Bacteraemia—rarely of clinical significance

Reference
1. Thomas HA, Sievers RE. Nonsurgical reduction of arterial catheter knots. *AJR Am J Roentgenol.* 1979;132:1018–1019.

Further Reading
Dariushnia S, Gill AE, Martin LG, et al. Quality improvement guidelines for diagnostic arteriography. *J Vasc Interv Radiol.* 2014;25(12):1873–1881.

ANGIOGRAPHY

Indications
1. Arterial ischaemia
2. Trauma
3. Arteriovenous malformations
4. Before endovascular intervention

Equipment
1. Digital fluoroscopy unit with C-arm
2. Pressure injector
3. Guidewires
4. Catheters

Patient Preparation
1. As per introduction to catheter techniques (noted previously)
2. Review all available non-invasive imaging to identify the most appropriate access to image the target vessels

Technique
1. After securing appropriate arterial access, a guidewire is advanced into the target artery over a suitable guidewire. If the angiogram is performed from the aorta, a pigtail catheter is usually used. If a more selective angiogram is being performed, it is performed through the catheter used to access the target artery.
2. Hand injection of contrast may be performed, but use of a pump injector allows for more rapid contrast injection rates and allows the operator to leave the room or at least step away from the patient to reduce their radiation exposure. The rate of contrast injection can be roughly determined by its vessel diameter - 6 mL s^{-1} in a 6-mm vessel, for example.

11

Aftercare

As for the general introduction noted previously

Complications

As for the general complications noted previously

ANGIOPLASTY

Indications

1. Dilation of localized vascular stenoses, mainly of the renal, iliac, lower limb and coronary arteries
2. Recanalization of occluded segments of vessels in selected cases

Equipment

1. Digital fluoroscopy unit with C-arm capable of angiography and preferably with 'roadmapping' facilities
2. Arterial pressure measuring equipment (optional)
3. Catheters may be straight or with a shaped tip to enable better control over the direction of the guidewire. Many different shapes are available, and it is advised that you familiarize yourself with those available in your unit.
4. Guidewires:
   (a) 0.035-in diameter wires, typically 145 cm long; hydrophilic guidewires may be helpful for crossing tight stenosis
   (b) 0.018- and 0.014-in diameter wires may be used for smaller vessels such as the infrapopliteal arteries.
   (c) Weighted-tip guidewires have a specially stiffened tip that exerts a force usually measured in grams. These can be useful for crossing occlusions, particularly in small vessels, and allows the wire to stay within the vessel lumen rather than creating a subintimal dissection.
   (d) 250-cm exchange guidewire, particularly if approaching the lesion from the contralateral side advancing over the aortic bifurcation
5. Angioplasty balloons:
   (a) Plain balloons are used for 'plain old balloon angioplasty' (POBA). Those that can pass over a smaller diameter guidewire are of lower crossing profile and are particularly useful in very tight stenoses.
   (b) Drug-coated balloons are available, in which the drug (paclitaxel) is bonded to the balloon surface by an excipient. When the balloon is inflated, the drug passes into the media of the vessel and eventually into the local tissues. The drug prevents smooth muscle cell proliferation with reportedly improved long-term outcomes compared with POBA.
   (c) High-pressure balloons may be used to treat resistant stenoses and are more often used in the venous system and dialysis arteriovenous fistulas.

(d) Cutting balloon angioplasty involves specially designed balloons that have three or four small blades (endotomes) fixed longitudinally to the balloon that score the atherosclerotic plaque when inflated. This helps control the distribution of dilatation forces during the angioplasty, and it may be helpful in treating resistant stenoses due to the presence of fibrous scar tissue. A similar type of balloon is a scoring balloon with stiff ridges rather than endotomes.

6. Aspiration of thrombus with a suitable aspiration catheter or guide catheter may be used for recently thrombosed vessel, or thrombolytic agent may be infused into recently before angioplasty. If it is clinically appropriate, waiting at least 4 weeks before angioplasty may be considered to allow organization of the thrombus before angioplasty to reduce the risk of distal embolization.

Patient Preparation

1. As per introduction to catheter techniques (noted previously)
2. Review all available non-invasive imaging to identify the most appropriate access to image the target vessels

Technique

1. Heparin 3000–5000 units IV should be administered.
2. The guidewire must be advanced across the lesion to be treated. The wire should stay within the lumen of the vessel if possible, but for an occlusion, the technique of subintimal angioplasty may be required. To perform this, a hydrophilic wire is pushed up to the occlusion and formed into a short loop that is advanced to create and intentional subintimal dissection. The wire usually breaks back into the true lumen distal to the occlusion, and this is confirmed by passing the catheter over the guidewire and gently aspirating blood before injecting contrast.
3. The desired balloon is advanced over the guidewire across the lesion to be treated and inflated using a pressure inflation manometer. The size of balloon should be chosen according to the diameter of the vessel, measured with the preprocedure imaging or from the catheter angiogram. It is important not to oversize the balloon because this may cause vessel rupture. If the patient experiences pain during balloon inflation, it indicates that the balloon diameter may be too large, stretching the vessel adventitia. The balloon should be deflated immediately and angiography performed to make sure the vessel has not been ruptured, and then a smaller diameter balloon should be selected for further angioplasty.
4. Check angiography is performed to ensure that the angioplasty has been successful. A number of complications may be visible immediately after angioplasty:
   (a) Dissection: Inflate the balloon again and leave it inflated for about 1 min and then reimage. If the dissection persists and is flow-limiting, it may be necessary to deploy a stent.

11

(b) Embolus: usually seen at a branch point distal to the angioplasty. An aspiration catheter can be used to aspirate the embolus and restore flow.

(c) Rupture: contrast extravasation from the site of angioplasty. A covered stent deployed at the site of rupture can be used to treat this.

Aftercare

1. The pulses distal to the artery that has been dilated and the colour of the toes should be observed half-hourly for 4 h
2. Best medical therapy
3. Reinforcement of the need to stop smoking

Complications

1. Perforation of artery leading to retroperitoneal haemorrhage
2. Embolization of clot or atheroma distally down either leg. This may be removed by aspiration thromboembolectomy or surgical embolectomy.
3. Occlusion of the main artery
4. Occlusion of the collateral artery
5. Major groin haematoma formation, which may suddenly develop several hours after the procedure is completed
6. False aneurysm formation at the puncture site
7. Cholesterol embolization: Catheter manipulation disrupts atheroma and releases cholesterol crystals into the arterial circulation, causing occlusion at arteriolar level. Pulses may be present and arteries patent angiographically, but patients are restless and develop severe tissue
· ischaemia in the affected vascular territory with skin mottling, limb loss, stroke, bowel infarction and renal failure.

Further Reading
Bukka M, Rednam PJ, Sinha M. Drug-eluting balloon: design, technology and clinical aspects. *Biomed Mater.* 2018;13(3):032001.

Diehm NA, Hoppe H, Do DD. Drug eluting balloons. *Tech Vasc Interv Radiol.* 2010;13(1):59–63.

Loh JP, Barbash IM, Waksman R. The current status of drug-coated balloons in percutaneous coronary and peripheral interventions. *EuroIntervention.* 2013;9(8):979–988.

Tsetis D, Morgan R, Belli AM. Cutting balloons for the treatment of vascular stenoses. *Eur Radiol.* 2006;16:1675–1683.

STENTS

Indications

1. Stenosis resistant to angioplasty
2. Occlusion resistant to angioplasty
3. Vessel dissection
4. Vessel rupture (trauma and iatrogenic)
5. Visceral artery origin stenosis
6. Aneurysms

Equipment

1. Same equipment for angioplasty
2. Stents:
   (a) Self-expanding stents are constrained within a delivery sheath and are deployed by pulling back the sheath so that the stent expands to the diameter of the vessel. After deployment, the stent may need to be postdilated with an appropriate size of balloon. These stents are generally more flexible but have less radial force. They are useful for any vessel but are mostly used for infrainguinal disease.
   (b) Balloon-mounted stents are crimped onto a balloon that is inflated to expand the stent within the vessel lumen. They tend to be less flexible but have greater radial force, and deployment is usually more accurate than with self-expanding stents. They are particularly useful for visceral arterial, common iliac and subclavian lesions, as well as other vessels in which flexibility is not as important. One disadvantage of these stents is that they may be dislodged from the balloon before deployment. To reduce the risk of this happening, the lesion to be treated may be predilated, and the stent should be advanced into position within a long sheath that is then withdrawn before deploying the stent.
   (c) Covered stents may be both balloon-mounted and self-expanding. The stents are covered with a material such as polyester or polytetrafluoroethylene. They are particularly useful for treating vessel ruptures and excluding aneurysms.
   (d) Drug-eluting stents are coated with a drug such as paclitaxel that inhibits smooth muscle proliferation and reduces restenosis.

Patient Preparation

1. As per introduction to catheter techniques (noted previously)
2. Review all available non-invasive imaging to identify the most appropriate access to image the target vessels

11

Technique

1. Heparin 3000–5000 units IV should be administered
2. The guidewire must be advanced across the lesion to be treated
3. Stent is deployed across the lesion to be treated and postdilated, if necessary, with an angioplasty balloon
4. Check the angiogram to ensure that the lesion has been treated adequately

Aftercare

1. The pulses distal to the artery that has been dilated, and the colour of the toes should be observed half-hourly for 4 h
2. Best medical therapy
3. Clopidogrel may help reduce the risk of in-stent restenosis
4. Reinforcement of the need to stop smoking

Complications

1. As for all angiographic procedures
2. Stent deployed in the incorrect position, particularly with self-expanding stents that may migrate proximally or distally during deployment
3. Stent dislodged from the balloon

Further Reading

Lindquist J, Schramm K. Drug-eluting balloons and drug-eluting stents in the treatment of peripheral vascular disease. *Semin Intervent Radiol.* 2018;35(5):443–452.

CATHETER-DIRECTED ARTERIAL THROMBOLYSIS

Indications

Chemical thrombolysis plays a role in the treatment of acute ischaemia of the leg caused by:

1. In situ thrombosis of a stenosed vessel
2. Occluded lower limb arterial bypass graft
3. Thrombosed popliteal aneurysm with no demonstrable distal runoff
4. Infrainguinal embolus (sometimes iatrogenic postangioplasty)

Contraindications

1. Absolute contraindications to thrombolysis include stroke within the preceding 2 months, a recent gastrointestinal (GI) bleed and neurosurgery or head trauma.
2. Relative contraindications are major trauma or surgery, severe hypertension, brain tumour and recent eye surgery.

Patient Preparation

1. Thrombolysis should be undertaken in consultation with a vascular surgeon and should not compromise the leg unnecessarily by delaying surgical treatment. An acute episode less than 24 h old is more likely to respond to thrombolysis. After 14 days, surgery is preferable to thrombolysis.[1]
2. Irreversible limb ischaemia requires amputation to avoid reperfusion syndrome.

Equipment

1. Recombinant tissue plasminogen activator (rt-PA) is the most widely used agent in the United Kingdom. It can be used as local boluses of, for example, 5 mg at 5- to 10-min intervals or as a low-dose infusion at 0.5–2 mg h^{-1}.
2. Specialized catheters may be used to direct the thrombolytic agent into the thrombus. These catheters have multiple side holes over a length (often 10–20 cm) and a method of occluding the distal end of

the catheter, such as a microvalve that shuts when the guidewire is removed (Cragg-McNamara catheter).

Technique

1. Catheter placement for thrombolysis is typically achieved by passing a guidewire alongside or through the thrombus and advancing a catheter into the proximal end. The catheter is firmly fixed to the skin to prevent dislodgement. A bolus of rt-PA followed by infusion is then administered through the catheter, and the patient is returned to a high-dependency ward for observation for signs of haemorrhage. Monitoring of clotting factors such as fibrinogen levels does not predict the likelihood of haemorrhagic complications.
2. Depending on the initial progress and discretion of the operator, the patient returns after several hours for check angiography through the catheter. If necessary, the catheter is advanced, and infusion is continued until satisfactory lysis, or the procedure is discontinued if progress is poor. Successful thrombolysis often reveals underlying stenoses as the cause of the occlusion. These are angioplastied at completion.
3. There are catheters manufactured for delivering fibrinolytics as a high-pressure spray through multiple side holes over several centimetres of occluded vessel. These may be used manually or connected to a dedicated pump that measures and times the 'pulse sprays'. This method has an added mechanical lytic effect and allows faster lysis. Other devices used in thrombolysis include hydrolyzing and mechanical thrombectomy catheters.
4. Bleeding complications are frequent, including haemorrhagic stroke in up to 2%.[2]
5. Thrombolysis is used widely wherever arterial and venous thrombosis occurs in the body.[3] Many applications are not universally accepted and are off-license uses of the thrombolytic agent.

Aftercare

1. When undergoing prolonged thrombolysis, the patient needs to be observed carefully within a higher dependency setting, often with one-to-one nursing.
2. The pulses distal to the artery that has been dilated and the colour of the toes should be observed half-hourly for 4 h.
3. Consider best medical therapy with drugs such as antiplatelets, statins and angiotensin-converting enzyme inhibitors according to local protocols.
4. Reinforcement of the need to stop smoking

Complications

1. Perforation of iliac artery leading to retroperitoneal haemorrhage
2. Embolization of clot or atheroma distally down either leg. This may be removed by aspiration thrombo-embolectomy or surgical embolectomy.
3. Occlusion of the main artery

11

4. Occlusion of the collateral artery
5. Major groin haematoma formation, which may suddenly develop several hours after the procedure is completed
6. False aneurysm formation at the puncture site
7. Cholesterol embolization: Catheter manipulation disrupts atheroma and releases cholesterol crystals into the arterial circulation, causing occlusion at arteriolar level. Pulses may be present and arteries patent angiographically, but patients are restless and develop severe tissue ischaemia in the affected vascular territory with skin mottling, limb loss, stroke, bowel infarction and renal failure.

References
1. Ebben HP, Jongkind V, Wisselink W, et al. Catheter directed thrombolysis protocols for peripheral arterial occlusions: a systematic review. *Eur J Vasc Endovasc Surg.* 2019;57(5):667–675.
2. Ouriel K. Endovascular techniques in the treatment of acute limb ischemia: thrombolytic agents, trials, and percutaneous mechanical thrombectomy techniques. *Semin Vasc Surg.* 2003;16(4):270–279.
3. Working Party on Thrombolysis in the Management of Limb Ischaemia. Thrombolysis in the management of lower limb arterial occlusion—a consensus document. *J Vasc Interv Radiol.* 2003;7(suppl):S337–S349.

VASCULAR EMBOLIZATION

Indications

1. To control bleeding, typically from the GI and genitourinary tracts, from the lungs and after trauma
2. To infarct or reduce the blood supply to tumours or organs
3. To reduce or stop blood flow through arteriovenous malformations, aneurysms, fistulae or varicoceles
4. To reduce the blood flow in high-flow priapism
5. As treatment for uterine fibroids
6. As a treatment for benign prostatic hypertrophy

Equipment

1. Digital fluoroscopy unit with C-arm capable of angiography and preferably with 'roadmapping' facilities
2. Preshaped femorovisceral catheters. These should not have side holes because their presence promotes clumping of particles and fibres at the catheter tip, leading to blockage of the lumen. The size and shape used depend on the particular problem and vascular anatomy. Microcatheters are used to perform more distal embolization in smaller vessels that cannot be reached by conventional catheters. Balloon occlusion catheters and coaxial catheters may also be useful.
3. Embolic materials:
   (a) Liquid: 50% dextrose, alcohol, quick-setting glues and polymers
   (b) Particulate: Gelfoam, polyvinyl alcohol, autologous clot

(c) Solid: metallic embolization coils (these may be detachable to reduce the risk of non-target embolization), vascular plugs and detachable balloon (rarely used now)

The material used depends on the lesion, its site and the duration of the occlusion required. Use of materials other than those listed has been reported.

Patient Preparation

1. As for arteriography
2. Some procedures are painful, and sedoanalgesia may be needed (see Chapter 21).

Technique Principles

1. All therapeutic occlusions are potentially dangerous; the expected gain must justify the risk.
2. Adequate knowledge of the vascular anatomy must be available before commencing. This is usually available from a preprocedure CTA, in which the target vessel can be identified and the route to it planned.
3. The operator must be an experienced angiographer.
4. The lesion must be selectively catheterized. When permanent occlusion is required, the centre of the lesion should be filled with non-absorbable material (e.g. silicone spheres, polyvinyl alcohol, polymer) before the supplying blood vessels are occluded.
5. Reflux of embolic material is likely to occur as the blood flow slows down; injection of emboli should be done slowly with intermittent gentle injections of contrast medium to assess flow and progress.
6. It is safer to come back another day than to continue for too long.

Aftercare

1. Observation of temperature pulse and blood pressure for signs of sepsis or bleeding
2. Observation of the tissues distal to the occluded vessel maintained for 24 h
3. Analgesia as required (patient-controlled administration)

11

Complications

1. Misplacement of embolic material: This may occur without the operator being aware that it has happened.
2. There may be propagation of thrombus, with embolization to the lungs or elsewhere.
3. Postembolization syndrome results from infarcted tissue releasing toxins into the circulation. It comprises pain, fever, malaise, raised white cell count and inflammatory indices and transient impairment of renal function. Infarcted tissue can cause fever for up to 10 days. However, this tissue can also become infected, and antibiotics may be required.

Further Reading

Carnevale FC, Antunes AA. Prostatic artery embolization for enlarged prostates due to benign prostatic hyperplasia. How I do it. *Cardiovasc Intervent Radiol.* 2013;36(6):1452–1463.

Cherian MP, Mehta P, Kalyanpur TM, et al. Arterial interventions in gastrointestinal bleeding. *Semin Intervent Radiol.* 2009;26(3):184–196.

Kim DY, Han KH. Transarterial chemoembolization versus transarterial radioembolization in hepatocellular carcinoma: optimization of selecting treatment modality. *Hepatol Int.* 2016;10(6):883–892.

Lopera JE. Embolization in trauma: principles and techniques. *Semin Intervent Radiol.* 2010;27(1):14–28.

Van Overhagen H, Reekers JA. Uterine fibroid embolization for symptomatic leiomyomata. *Cardiovasc Intervent Radiol.* 2015;38(3):536–542.

THORACIC AND ABDOMINAL AORTIC STENT GRAFTS

Indications

1. Thoracic or abdominal aortic aneurysm
2. Stanford type B aortic dissection
3. Penetrating atherosclerotic ulcer
4. Traumatic aortic injury
5. Iliac aneurysm

Equipment

1. Thoracic stent grafts are made by a number of manufacturers, and readers are advised to familiarize themselves with the grafts available locally. They consist of a tube graft available in a number of different diameters and lengths.
2. Abdominal stent grafts are made by a number of manufacturers, and readers are advised to familiarize themselves with the grafts available locally. They usually consist of a modular design with a main body and iliac limbs.
3. A compliant balloon is used to help fully expand the graft after initial deployment.
4. A stiff guidewire at least 200 cm in length for abdominal aortic stent grafts or 300 cm for thoracic aortic stent grafts.
5. Catheters such as a pigtail for imaging and other shaped catheters, such as a multipurpose catheter, to help advance the guidewire into position.

Preparation

1. CTA to assess suitability, identify important anatomical variants and measure the aorta
2. Considerations for thoracic aortic stent grafts:
   (a) The proximal landing zone should be of sufficient length to provide an adequate seal according to the graft indications for use (IFU).
   (b) The distal landing zone needs to be of sufficient length to provide an adequate seal.

(c) It may be necessary to cover the left subclavian artery, in which case it is important to be aware of a number of anatomical variants that may compromise perfusion of the spinal cord, thus necessitating a bypass graft from the left common carotid artery:
  (i) Dominant left vertebral artery
  (ii) Hypoplastic right vertebral artery
  (iii) Termination of the right vertebral artery as the posterior inferior cerebellar artery in which there is no contribution to the basilar artery

(d) It may be necessary to cover the left common carotid artery, requiring a bypass graft from the right common carotid artery.

(e) Length of graft greater than 20 cm may be at increased risk of spinal cord injury because of the potential compromise of intercostal arteries.

(f) Cerebrospinal fluid drain may be needed if the anatomy is such that it increases the risk of spinal cord injury because of reduced perfusion after deployment of the graft:
  (i) Covering left subclavian artery, particularly with anatomical variants as in (c) above
  (ii) Length of stent graft over 20 cm
  (iii) Previous aortic aneurysm repair
  (iv) Occlusion of the internal iliac arteries

3. Considerations for abdominal aortic stent grafts:
  (a) Proximal landing zone just below the lowest renal artery should be of sufficient length without too much angulation, irregular adherent thrombus or calcification. These differ according to the IFU of each graft.
  (b) Distal landing zone usually at the distal end of the common iliac arteries should be of sufficient length without too much calcification or tortuosity.
  (c) If there is a common iliac aneurysm, it may be necessary to extend the graft into the external iliac artery with two options to manage the internal iliac artery:
    (i) Embolization to prevent endoleak
    (ii) Iliac branch graft to maintain perfusion of the internal iliac artery to reduce the risk of buttock claudication

4. Graft is chosen with 10%–20% oversizing according to the diameter of the landing zones and length sufficient to cover the pathology adequately. This may require more than one stent graft to be used.

Principles

1. Vascular access:
  (a) On the side the stent graft is to be inserted, it may need a surgical cutdown or preclosure technique for percutaneous access, in which sutures are deployed with specially designed devices at the beginning of the procedure to be tightened at the end of the procedure to achieve haemostasis.
  (b) Contralateral vascular sheath to allow a pigtail catheter for imaging. With thoracic stent grafts, a brachial artery approach may be used for this.

11

2. Thoracic stent graft:
   (a) A stiff guidewire is advanced as far as the aortic valve.
   (b) The graft is deployed from the proximal landing zone.
   (c) A compliant balloon is inflated at the landing zones and junction zones (if more than one stent graft is used) to help to fully expand the graft. Balloon inflation when treating a dissection should be done with caution and avoided if possible.
3. Abdominal aortic stent graft:
   (a) A stiff guidewire is advanced as far as the descending thoracic aorta.
   (b) The main body of the graft is deployed from just below the origin of the lowermost renal artery.
   (c) The contralateral limb is catheterized. This is usually undertaken with a hydrophilic guidewire and angled catheter.
   (d) Iliac limbs are deployed to the distal common iliac artery or external iliac artery if excluding a common iliac aneurysm. This may need more than one iliac limb.
   (e) A compliant balloon inflated at the landing zones and junction zones (if more than one stent graft is used) helps fully expand the graft.

Aftercare

1. Patients need lifelong follow-up imaging to look for complications related to the stent graft.
   (a) Plain films to look for graft migration, disconnection of graft components and fracture of stent struts
   (b) Duplex US and contrast US to look for blood flow within the aneurysm sac outside the graft
   (c) CTA
   (d) MRA is less commonly used but may be if the graft materials allow.
2. Protocols vary depending on local expertise.

Complications

1. Endoleaks are a particular complication related to aortic stent grafts:
   Type (a) failure of the primary seal at either the proximal (1a) or distal (1b) landing zones. This needs intervention at the time of stent graft deployment, with further compliant balloon dilation or extension of the graft. Late type 1 endoleaks may occur when there is stent graft migration.
   Type (b) perfusion of the aneurysm sac retrogradely through branches, such as the lumbar or inferior mesenteric arteries in the case of abdominal aortic grafts or intercostal and subclavian arteries in the case of thoracic aortic grafts. These need treatment if there is aneurysm sac expansion and usually involves embolization of the endoleak 'nidus', either through a transarterial approach or direct aneurysm sac puncture.
   Type (c) failure of the graft components such as a hole in the fabric or disconnection of graft components, usually treated by relining the graft

Type (d) porous graft material often seen at the end of the procedure due to heparinization and mostly resolving within 48 hours

Type (e) endotension in which there is continued aneurysm sac expansion without evidence of type 1–4 endoleaks

Further Reading

Bicknell C, Powell JT. Aortic disease: thoracic endovascular aortic repair. *Heart.* 2015;101(8):586–591.

Chung R, Morgan RA. Type 2 endoleaks post EVAR: current evidence for rupture risk, intervention and outcomes of treatment. *Cardiovasc Intervent Radiol.* 2015;38(3):507–522.

Steuer J, Lachat M, Veith FJ, et al. Endovascular grafts for abdominal aortic aneurysm. *Eur Heart J.* 2016;37(2):145–151.

11

Venous system

Christopher Day

METHODS OF IMAGING THE VENOUS SYSTEM

1. Ultrasound (US)
2. Computed tomography (CT)
3. Magnetic resonance imaging (MRI)
4. Contrast venography

Further Reading

Gaitini D. Multimodality imaging of the peripheral venous system. *Int J Biomed Imaging.* 2007;2007:54616.

Katz DS, Hon M. Current DVT imaging. *Tech Vasc Intervent Radiol.* 2004;7(2): 55–62.

Kaufman JA, Lee MJ, eds. *Vascular and Interventional Radiology: The Requisites.* 2nd ed. Elsevier-Mosby; 2013.

Scarvelis D, Wells PS. Diagnosis and treatment of deep-vein thrombosis. *Can Med Assoc J.* 2006;175(9):1087–1092.

ULTRASOUND

US is the most widely used imaging method for the venous system; the advantages are that it is low cost and readily available. It can be used to assess the following:

1. Lower limb veins
2. Upper limb veins
3. Abdominal veins, including renal, hepatic and portal veins as well as the inferior vena cava (IVC)
4. Venous anatomy to assist in central venous line placement (e.g. for the internal jugular or subclavian vein)

US is most commonly used for assessment of patients with suspected venous thrombosis, particularly of the lower limb. It is also useful to assess arteriovenous fistulae, both therapeutic fistulae created for haemodialysis and those occurring as a complication of interventional vascular procedures, and for presurgical planning in patients with varicose veins. Both duplex and colour Doppler techniques are used.

Duplex

Duplex scanning involves a combination of pulsed Doppler and real-time US for direct visualization. Expansion and filling of the normal echo-free lumen can be identified, but slow-moving blood may be misinterpreted as thrombus. Valsalva manoeuvre will cause expansion in the normal vein but is not an entirely reliable sign. Pulsed Doppler assesses flow with demonstration of flow enhancement caused by respiratory excursion or manual calf compression suggests patency. The most reliable sign of patency is compressibility. Direct pressure with the US probe over the vein will cause the normal vein to collapse. If thrombus is present, this will not occur.

Colour Doppler

Colour Doppler examination gives a visual representation of flow over a segment of vein.

LOWER LIMB VENOUS ULTRASOUND

Indications

1. Suspected deep vein thrombosis (DVT)
2. Follow-up of known DVT
3. To guide access for interventional venous procedures

Equipment

5- to 7.5-MHz transducer with colour Doppler

Technique

1. Patient supine with foot-down tilt. The popliteal and calf veins can easily be examined with the patient sitting with the legs dependent or the patient lying on a tilted couch with flexed knees and externally rotated hips. The femoral veins and external iliac veins are examined supine. The popliteal veins may be examined with the patient prone.
2. Longitudinal and transverse scans for external iliac, femoral and popliteal veins. For tibial and peroneal veins, these may be supplemented by oblique coronal scans.
3. Each vein may be identified by real-time scanning and colour Doppler. If in any doubt, it may be confirmed as a vein by the spectral Doppler tracing. A normal patent vein should be completely occluded in real time by directly applied transducer pressure (though this is not always possible for the superficial femoral vein at the adductor canal).
4. The normal venous signal is phasic and in the larger veins varies with respiration. Flow can be stopped by a Valsalva manoeuvre and is transiently augmented by distal compression of the foot or calf. Acute thrombus may be non-echogenic, but the vein should not be completely compressible nor entirely fill with colour Doppler if thrombus is present. Thrombus tends to become echogenic after a few days.

5. Although this technique is less well established for the exclusion of thrombus in the calf vessels, it has been shown to have a sensitivity and specificity close to those of venography. Cannulation of a vein and injection of contrast medium can thus be avoided.

UPPER LIMB VENOUS ULTRASOUND

Indications
As for lower limb US, upper limb US is much less commonly performed.

Equipment
5- to 7.5-MHz transducer with colour Doppler

Technique
1. The patient should be recumbent on a couch wide enough to support the upper limb and trunk comfortably.
2. With the arm in a neutral position at the patient's side, the subclavian vein is assessed either from above or below the clavicle. The image plane is parallel to the long axis of the vein. Diagnostic criteria for upper limb thrombosis are the same as those used for the lower limb, but the Doppler waveform in the upper limb venous system is more pulsatile because of proximity to the heart. The upper limb also has a much more extensive network of potential collateral venous pathways, and care should be taken to avoid confusion of a patent collateral vein with the potentially occluded deep venous structure under examination.
3. The arm is then abducted and the axillary and brachial veins examined. The transducer should be placed high in the axilla to identify the proximal axillary vein and the Doppler characteristics of the axillary and brachial veins followed to assess for spontaneous and phasic flow and appropriate response to augmentation and Valsalva manoeuvre. Both transverse and longitudinal imaging planes should be used, including assessment of response to compression. The examination can be extended to include the cephalic, basilic and forearm veins.

Further Reading
Hamper UM, DeJong MR, Scoutt LM. Ultrasound evaluation of the lower extremity veins. *Radiol Clin North Am.* 2007;45(3):525–547.
Myers K, Clough A. *Making Sense of Vascular Ultrasound: A Hands-on Guide.* Taylor and Francis Group; 2004.
Thrush A, Hartshorne T, Dean CR. *Vascular Ultrasound: How Why and When.* 4th ed. Elsevier; 2021.
Weber TM, Lockhart ME, Robbin ML. Upper extremity venous Doppler ultrasound. *Radiol Clin North Am.* 2007;45(3):513–524.

12

COMPUTED TOMOGRAPHY

Multidetector computed tomography (MDCT) with standard intravenous (IV) contrast and scan delay protocols for the chest or abdomen and pelvis (see Chapter 1) are very effective for the detection of compression or thrombosis of major veins, including the superior vena cava (SVC) and IVC and the iliac and renal veins.

Although it is theoretically possible to perform direct lower limb CT venography after infusion of contrast via a foot vein, this technique has found little application and is not used in clinical practice.

In a group of selected patients with suspected pulmonary embolus (PE), MDCT of the lower limbs from the iliac crest to the popliteal fossa, 2 min after completion of computed tomography pulmonary angiography (CTPA; indirect CT venography), may be used as an alternative to US for detection of lower limb DVT. However, there is a significant associated radiation dose, and it is not recommended as an independent test for suspected DVT, particularly because there is no diagnostic advantage over US.[1] Indirect CT venography should only be used in conjunction with CTPA for suspected PE in patients whom identification of DVT is considered necessary and in those with a high probability of PE, including patients with history of previous venous thromboembolism and possible malignancy.[2,3]

References

1. Goodman LR, Stein PD, Matta F, et al. CT venography and compression sonography are diagnostically equivalent: data from PIOPED II. *AJR Am J Roentgenol.* 2007;189(5):1071–1076.
2. Thomas SM, Goodacre SW, Sampson FC, et al. Diagnostic value of CT for deep vein thrombosis; results of a systematic review and meta-analysis. *Clin Radiol.* 2008;63(3):299–304.
3. Hunsaker AR, Zou KH, Poh AC, et al. Routine pelvic and lower extremity CT venography in patients undergoing pulmonary CT angiography. *AJR Am J Roentgenol.* 2008;190(2):322–326.

MAGNETIC RESONANCE IMAGING

Standard guidance applies on selection of patients suitable for MRI examination (see Chapter 1).

MRI is well suited to imaging the venous system but is infrequently used because of cost and limited availability. Peripheral magnetic resonance venography (MRV)[1] is currently used in selected cases of venous thrombosis in pregnant patients and when fractured limbs are immobilized in casts. It is useful in evaluation of congenital abnormalities of peripheral venous anatomy and venous malformations.

The multiplanar imaging capabilities allow demonstration of complex venous anatomy, and cine sequences, including velocity-encoded phase mapping, can provide functional information regarding direction and velocity of venous blood flow. MRI can be used to 'age' thrombus and differentiate acute from chronic clot. MRV does not involve ionizing radiation, and IV gadolinium has a wider safety profile than iodinated contrast used for CT. Imaging can be performed using slice-by-slice (two-dimensional) or volume (three-dimensional) acquisition. Postprocessing techniques, including maximum-intensity projection images, are used.

MRV sequences can be performed without IV contrast (e.g. time-of-flight imaging or phase contrast imaging sequences). However, these techniques are susceptible to signal loss because of slow flow or turbulence, and IV gadolinium contrast-enhanced MRV studies have been shown to by faster and more accurate. However, new non-contrast MRI sequences are emerging that offer comparable accuracy for patients in whom gadolinium contrast is contraindicated.[2,3] MRV offers unique diagnostic possibilities for abdominal, pelvic and thoracic veins,[4] and development of blood pool contrast agents (see Chapter 2) will further improve clinical usefulness of these procedures.[5]

References

1. Sampson FC, Goodacre SW, Thomas SM, et al. The accuracy of MRI in diagnosis of suspected deep vein thrombosis: systematic review and meta-analysis. *Eur Radiol.* 2007;17(1):175–181.
2. Zhuang G, Tang C, He X, et al. DANTE-SPACE: a new technical tool for DVT on 1.5T MRI. *Int J Cardiovasc Imaging.* 2019;35(12):2231–2237.
3. Treitl KM, Treitl M, Kooijmankurfuerst H, et al. Three-dimensional black-blood t1-weighted turbo spin-echo techniques for the diagnosis of deep vein thrombosis in comparison with contrast-enhanced magnetic resonance imaging: a pilot study. *Invest Radiol.* 2015;50(6):401.
4. Butty S, Hagspiel KD, Leung DA, et al. Body MR venography. *Radiol Clin North Am.* 2002;40(4):899–919.
5. Prince MR, Sostman HD. MR venography: unsung and underutilized. *Radiology.* 2003;226(3):630–632.

PERIPHERAL VENOGRAPHY

IV peripheral venography is an invasive procedure requiring IV injection of contrast medium and the use of ionizing radiation. Marked limb swelling can result in failure to cannulate a vein, which precludes use of the technique. False-negative results do occur. It is still considered the gold standard for diagnosis of DVT but is now only very rarely performed.

LOWER LIMB

12

Method

IV venography

Indications

1. DVT
2. To demonstrate incompetent perforating veins (Doppler US is preferable.)
3. Oedema of unknown cause
4. Congenital abnormality of the venous system

Contraindication

Local sepsis

Contrast Medium

Low-osmolar contrast material (LOCM) 240 mg I mL^{-1}

Equipment

1. Fluoroscopy unit with spot film device
2. Tilting radiography table

Patient Preparation

The leg should be elevated overnight to lessen oedema if leg swelling is severe.

Technique

1. The patient is supine and tilted 40 degrees head up to delay the transit time of the contrast medium.
2. A tourniquet is applied tightly just above the ankle to occlude the superficial venous system. The compression may also occlude the anterior tibial veins, so their absence should not be automatically interpreted as being caused by venous thrombosis.
3. A 19-gauge butterfly needle (smaller if necessary) is inserted into a vein on the dorsum of the foot. If the needle is too near the ankle, the contrast medium may bypass the deep veins and thus give the impression of deep venous occlusion.
4. 40 mL of contrast medium is injected by hand. The first series of spot films is then taken.
5. A further 20-mL bolus is injected quickly whilst the patient performs a Valsalva manoeuvre to delay the transit of contrast medium into the upper thigh and pelvic veins. The patient is tilted quickly into a slightly head-down position, and the Valsalva manoeuvre is relaxed. Alternatively, if the patient is unable to comply, direct manual pressure over the femoral vein whilst the table is being tilted into the head-down position will achieve the same effect. Images are taken 2–3 s after releasing pressure.
6. At the end of the procedure, the needle should be flushed with 0.9% saline to lessen the chance of phlebitis caused by contrast medium.

Images

Collimated to include all veins

1. Anteroposterior (AP) of the calf
2. Both obliques of the calf (foot internally and externally rotated)
3. AP of the popliteal, common femoral and iliac veins

Aftercare

The limb should be exercised.

Complications

Due to the contrast medium

1. As for the general complications of intravascular contrast media (see Chapter 2)

2. Thrombophlebitis
3. Tissue necrosis caused by extravasation of contrast medium. This is rare but may occur in patients with peripheral ischaemia.
4. Cardiac arrhythmia. This is more likely if the patient has pulmonary hypertension

Due to the technique

1. Haematoma
2. PE caused by dislodged clot or injection of excessive air

UPPER LIMB

Method
IV venography

Indications
1. Oedema
2. To demonstrate the site of venous occlusion or stenosis
3. SVC obstruction

Contrast Medium
LOCM 300 mg I mL^{-1}

Equipment
Fluoroscopy unit with spot film device

Patient Preparation
None

Technique
For IV venography:

1. The patient is supine.
2. An 18-gauge butterfly needle is inserted into the median cubital vein at the elbow. The cephalic vein is not used because this bypasses the axillary vein.
3. Spot films are taken of the region of interest during a hand injection of 30 mL of contrast medium. Alternatively, a digital subtraction angiographic run can be performed at 1 frame s^{-1}.

Aftercare
None

Complications

Due to the contrast medium
See Chapter 2.

12

CENTRAL VENOGRAPHY

SUPERIOR VENA CAVOGRAPHY

Indications

1. To demonstrate occlusion or stenosis of the central veins
2. As a preliminary examination in transvenous interventional techniques
3. Congenital abnormality of the venous system (e.g. left-sided SVC)

Contrast Medium

LOCM 370 mg I mL^{-1}, 60 mL

Equipment

A C-arm with digital subtraction angiography

Patient Preparation

None

Technique

1. The patient is supine.
2. 18-gauge butterfly needles are inserted into the median antecubital vein of both arms.
3. Hand injections of contrast medium 30 mL per side are made simultaneously, as rapidly as possible, by two operators. The injection is recorded by rapid serial radiography (see the Images section later in the chapter). The image acquisition is commenced after about two-thirds of the contrast medium has been injected.

If the study is to demonstrate a congenital abnormality, or on the rare occasion that the opacification obtained by this method is subopitmal, a 5-Fr catheter with side holes, introduced by the Seldinger technique, may be used.

Images

Images are obtained at a rate of 1 frame s^{-1} for 10 s.

Aftercare

None unless a catheter is used.

Complications

Due to the contrast medium

See Chapter 2.

INFERIOR VENA CAVOGRAPHY

Indications

1. To demonstrate the site of venous obstruction, displacement or infiltration

2. As a preliminary examination in transvenous interventional techniques (e.g. IVC filter insertion)
3. Congenital abnormality of the venous system

Contrast Medium

LOCM 370 mg I mL^{-1}, 40 mL

Technique

1. With the patient supine, the sheath is placed into the femoral vein using the standard vascular access technique (see Chapter 11). A Valsalva manoeuvre may facilitate venepuncture by distending the vein. Puncture of the femoral vein is preferably carried out under direct US guidance, but if US is not available, blind puncture may be performed aiming for the medial side of the palpable common femoral artery pulse.
2. Any obstruction to the passage of the catheter may indicate thrombus in the iliac veins or that the catheter and wire have entered an ascending lumbar vein. Fluoroscopy and gentle hand injection of contrast will clarify.
3. An injection of 40 mL of contrast medium is made at 20 mL s^{-1} by a pump injector and recorded by rapid serial radiography or as a digital subtraction run at 2 frames s^{-1}.

Aftercare

1. Pressure at venepuncture site
2. Routine observations for 2 h

Complications

Due to the contrast medium

See Chapter 2.

Due to the technique

See Chapter 11—complications of catheter technique.

PORTAL VENOGRAPHY

12

Methods

1. Late-phase superior mesenteric angiography
2. Transsplenic approach (discussed later)
3. Paraumbilical vein catheterization
4. Transjugular transhepatic approach[1]

Indications

1. To demonstrate before surgery the anatomy of the portal system in patients with portal hypertension
2. To check the patency of a portosystemic anastomosis

Contrast Medium

LOCM 370 mg I mL^{-1}, 50 mL

Equipment

1. Digital radiography unit
2. Arterial catheter (superior mesenteric angiography (SMA) approach)
3. 10-cm needle (20 gauge) with stilette and outer plastic sheath (e.g. long-dwell (transsplenic approach))

Patient Preparation

1. Admission to hospital. A surgeon should be informed in case complications of procedure arise (for the transsplenic approach).
2. Clotting factors are checked.
3. Severe ascites is drained.
4. Nil orally for 5 h before the procedure.
5. Premedication, according to local protocols.

Technique

Superior mesenteric angiography

Using standard angiographic technique (see Chapter 11), the splenic, superior mesenteic and portal veins are visualized on the late phases.

For transsplenic approach

1. With the patient supine, the position of the spleen is percussed or identified with US. The access point is as low as possible in the midaxillary line, usually at the level of the 10th or 11th intercostal space.
2. The region is anaesthetized using a sterile procedure.
3. The patient is asked to hold their breath in mid-inspiration, and the needle is then inserted inwards and upwards into the spleen (about three-quarters of the length of the needle is inserted, i.e. 7.5 cm). The needle and stilette are then withdrawn, leaving the plastic cannula in situ. Blood will flow back easily if the cannula is correctly sited. The patient is then asked to breathe as shallowly as possible to avoid trauma to the spleen from excessive movement of the cannula.
4. A test injection of a small volume of contrast medium under screening control can be made to ensure correct siting of the cannula. If it has transfixed the spleen, simple withdrawal into the body of the spleen is not acceptable because any contrast medium subsequently injected would follow the track created by the withdrawal. A new puncture is necessary.
5. When the cannula is in a satisfactory position, the splenic pulp pressure may be measured with a sterile manometer (normally 10–15 cm H_2O).
6. A hand injection of 50 mL of contrast medium is made over 5 s and recorded by rapid serial radiography or digital subtraction angiography. The cannula should be removed as soon as possible after the injection to minimize trauma to the spleen.
7. Occasionally, a patent portal vein will fail to opacify, owing to major portosystemic collaterals causing reversed flow in the portal vein. The

final arbiter of portal vein patency is direct mesenteric venography performed at operation. The maximum width of a normal portal vein is said to be 2 cm.

Images

Rapid serial radiography or digital subtraction runs: 1 image s^{-1} for 10 s

Aftercare

1. Blood pressure and pulse: initially quarter-hourly; subsequently 4 hourly.
2. The patient must remain in hospital overnight.

Complications

Due to the contrast medium

See Chapter 2.

Due to the technique

1. Haemorrhage
2. Subcapsular injection
3. Perforation of adjacent structures (e.g. pleura, colon)
4. Splenic rupture
5. Infection
6. Pain (especially with an extracapsular injection)

Due to the catheter

See Chapter 11.

Reference
1. Rösch J, Antonovic R, Dotter CT. Transjugular approach to the liver, biliary system, and portal circulation. *AJR Am J Roentgenol.* 1975;125(3). 602–608.

Further Reading
Tamura S, Kodama T, Kihara Y, et al. Right anterior caudocranial oblique projection for portal venography; its indications and advantages. *Eur J Radiol.* 1992;15(3):215–219.

12

TRANSHEPATIC PORTAL VENOUS CATHETERIZATION

Indications

To localize pancreatic hormone-secreting tumours before operation.

Contraindications

There are none specific to the technique. Ascites and hepatic cirrhosis make the procedure more difficult.

Contrast Medium

LOCM 370 mg I mL^{-1}, to demonstrate anatomy and position of catheter.

Technique

1. 5-mL samples of blood are taken at points along the splenic vein, superior mesenteric vein and first part of the portal vein. The samples are numbered sequentially, and the site from which each was taken is marked on a sketch map of the portal drainage system. Simultaneous peripheral blood samples should be obtained at the same time as each portal sample to assess changing blood levels.
2. The accuracy of sampling can be improved by selective catheterization of pancreatic veins using varying shapes of catheter.[1]

Reference

1. Reichardt W, Ingemansson S. Selective vein catheterization for hormone assay in endocrine tumours of the pancreas: technique and results. *Acta Radiol Diagn.* 1980;21(suppl 2A):177–187.

VENOUS INTERVENTIONS

Many of the techniques used in the arterial system may also be applied to the venous system. In addition, a number of procedures may be used for the treatment of venous thromboembolic disease and its complications. These include the following:

1. Venous angioplasty and stents
2. Embolization
3. IVC filters
4. Venous thrombolysis
5. PE treatment

VENOUS ANGIOPLASTY AND STENTS

Indications

1. Venous stenosis or chronic occlusion
2. Following thrombolysis
3. May-Thurner syndrome
4. Flow-limiting venous stenosis in arteriovenous dialysis fistulae
5. Symptomatic SVC obstruction

Patient Preparation

1. See general catheter angiography techniques (see Chapter 11).
2. Non-invasive imaging of the venous system to identify the pathology and plan the approach to treatment.

Equipment

1. For vascular access (see Chapter 11).
2. Stents (see the discussion on arterial stents in Chapter 11). Specific venous stents are also available that have higher radial force and also have an obliquely shaped end, allowing deployment at a venous confluence (e.g. near the confluence of the iliac veins with the IVC).
3. Angioplasty balloons (see the discussion on angioplasty in Chapter 11).
4. Intravascular US is particularly useful during these procedures. This involves a specialized catheter and US machine allowing imaging of the vein lumen. This allows accurate localisation of vein confluences (particularly with the IVC) and better visualization of any residual stenosis after the procedure.

Technique

The same techniques described for arterial angioplasty and stent apply to the venous system (see Chapter 11).

Aftercare

Similar aftercare to arterial interventions (see Chapter 11), except that the patient does not need to be kept on bed rest for more than 1–2 h because of the venous puncture (rather than the high-pressure arterial puncture).

Complications

The same as for the arterial system (see Chapter 11).

Further Reading
Hrdman RL. Management of chronic deep vein thrombosis in women. *Semin Intervent Radiol.* 2018;35(1):3–8.
Williams DM. Iliocaval reconstruction in chronic deep vein thrombosis. *Tech Vasc Interv Radiol.* 2014;17(2):109–113.

GONADAL VEIN EMBOLIZATION

12

Indications

1. Testicular varicocele with any of the following:
   (a) Pain
   (b) Cosmesis because of the size of the varicocele
   (c) Infertility
2. Pelvic congestion syndrome (symptomatic ovarian vein insufficiency)

Patient Preparation

1. Admit as a day case procedure.

Equipment

1. For vascular access and angiography (see Chapter 11)
2. Embolic agents:
   (a) Embolization coils
   (b) Liquid embolic agents such as Na-tetradecyl-sulphate (STS) made into a foam by mixing with air

Technique

1. Vascular access is usually through the common femoral vein, but access through the internal jugular or basilic vein may also be considered.
2. The ovarian or testicular vein is catheterized with an angle catheter, and the catheter is advanced over a guidewire into the inferior vein.
3. Venography is performed by hand injection when the patient is performing the Valsalva manoeuvre.
4. Embolization is performed with coils, STS foam or both. STS foam is useful because it scleroses collateral veins that may or may not be visible. Embolization is performed through the whole length of the gonadal vein. Detachable coils may be advantageous near the confluence of the gonadal vein with the left renal vein or IVC, avoiding non-target embolization caused by maldeployment of a coil.
5. Manual compression after the procedure.

Aftercare

1. One to two hours' bedrest flat if common femoral vein puncture
2. No specific bedrest needed if internal jugular or basilic vein puncture

Complications

1. Spasm of gonadal vein preventing embolization
2. Rupture of the gonadal vein
3. Non-target embolization:
   (a) Renal vein from the upper gonadal vein
   (b) Pulmonary arteries from large iliac veins
4. Pain: usually mild to moderate
5. Ureteric injury caused by fibrosis related to blood or foam extravasation

Further Reading

Balabuszek K, Toborek M, Pietura R. Comprehensive overview of the venous disorder known as pelvic congestion syndrome. *Ann Med.* 2022;54(1):22–36.
Iaccarino V, Venetucci P. Interventional radiology of male varicocele: current status. *Cardiovasc Intervent Radiol.* 2012;35(6):1263–1280.

INFERIOR VENA CAVA FILTERS

Indications

1. Thromboembolic disease with one or more of the following:
   (a) Contraindication to anticoagulation
   (b) Complication of anticoagulation

(c) Failure of anticoagulation
(d) Recurrent PE despite anticoagulation
(e) Progression of DVT despite anticoagulation
(f) Massive PE with residual DVT
(g) Iliofemoral or IVC thrombus that is free floating
(h) Perioperative period when anticoagulation needs to be
    temporarily discontinued
2. Prophylaxis against PE:
   (a) Severe trauma without DVT or PE
   (b) Head injury
   (c) Spinal cord injury
   (d) Patients at high risk

PATIENT PREPARATION

1. Review of any previous cross-sectional imaging of the abdomen
   (e.g. CT) is useful to identify the level of the renal veins and any
   anatomical variant of the renal veins, such as circumaortic left renal
   vein and accessory renal veins, that may alter the level at which the
   filter should be placed.
2. General preparation for catheter techniques (see Chapter 11).

Equipment

1. For vascular access and general angiography (see Chapter 11).
2. IVC filters have many different designs by different manufacturers,
   and readers are advised to familiarize themselves with the filters
   available in their department.
3. General equipment for vascular access and angiography.

Technique

1. Vascular access in the internal jugular vein or common femoral
   vein. The same technique as for arterial access is used (see
   Chapter 11).
2. A pigtail catheter is advanced over a guidewire into the IVC, and
   venography is performed with 20–30 mL of iodinated contrast at
   10–15 mL s^{-1}. The presence of any thrombus in the IVC should
   be determined, the level of the renal veins identified and the
   diameter of the IVC measured to ensure that it is not too big
   for the filter (this will vary depending on the exact device to be
   used).
3. After removing the catheter, leaving the guidewire in situ, the filter
   deployment sheath is advanced into position and the filter deployed
   just below the level of the renal veins (so that if the filter causes IVC
   occlusion, the renal veins should remain patent). However, the filter
   can be placed in the suprarenal IVC if necessary (e.g. IVC thrombus).
   The exact mechanism of deployment will depend on the filter being
   used, and readers should familiarize themselves with the device
   available in their department.
4. Haemostasis with manual compression

12

Aftercare

1. Bedrest flat (if common femoral vein puncture) or sitting (if internal jugular vein puncture) for 1–2 h
2. The filter should be removed as soon as possible if it is for temporary insertion. This can present logistical problems, and plans should be made to ensure that this occurs. It may be useful to maintain a database of all filter insertions to ensure reminders are sent to referring clinicians.

Complications

1. General complications of vascular access (see Chapter 11)
2. Occlusion of the IVC caused by thrombosis
3. Penetration through the IVC wall
4. Filter embolization
5. Filter migration or change in orientation
6. Filter fracture with possible embolization
7. Filter thrombosis causing occlusion of the IVC
8. Failure to remove filter at attempted retrieval

Further Reading

Caplin DM, Nikolic B, Kalva SP, et al. Quality improvement guidelines for the performance of inferior vena cava filter placement for the prevention of pulmonary embolism. *J Vasc Interv Radiol.* 2011;22:1499–1506.

Funaki B. Inferior vena cava filter insertion. *Semin Intervent Radiol.* 2006;23(4):357–360.

THROMBOLYSIS

Indications

1. Phlegmasia cerulea dolens
2. Iliofemoral DVT in selected patients:
   (a) Onset of symptoms less than 21 days
   (b) Good functional status
   (c) Good life expectancy
3. Paget-Schroetter syndrome
4. Occlusion venous side of haemodialysis fistula

Patient Preparation

1. Thrombolysis should be undertaken in consultation with a vascular surgeon.
2. If catheter-directed thrombolysis is being used, the patient will need one-to-one nursing care for the duration of treatment.
3. Consider using an IVC filter when treating iliofemoral DVT.

Equipment

1. Recombinant tissue plasminogen activator (rt-PA) is the most widely used agent in the United Kingdom. It can be used as local boluses of, for example, 5 mg at 5- to 10-min intervals or as a low-dose infusion at 0.5–2 mg h^{-1}.

2. Specialized catheters may be used to direct the thrombolytic agent into the thrombus. These catheters have multiple side holes over a length (often 10–20 cm) and a method of occluding the distal end of the catheter such as a microvalve that shuts when the guidewire is removed (Cragg-McNamara catheter).

3. Advanced mechanical thrombectomy catheters are designed to fragment the thrombus using high-velocity saline jets, a high-speed impeller or a combination of mechanical maceration with aspiration of thrombus at the same time.

Technique

1. Catheter-directed thrombolysis:
   (a) Catheter placement for thrombolysis is typically achieved by passing a guidewire alongside or through the thrombus and advancing a catheter into the proximal end. The catheter is firmly fixed to the skin to prevent dislodgement. A bolus of rt-PA followed by infusion is then administered through the catheter, and the patient is returned to a high-dependency ward for observation for signs of haemorrhage. Monitoring of clotting factors such as fibrinogen levels does not predict the likelihood of haemorrhagic complications.
   (b) Depending on the initial progress and discretion of the operator, the patient returns after several hours for check angiography through the catheter. If necessary, the catheter is advanced and infusion continued until satisfactory lysis, or the procedure is discontinued if progress is poor. Successful thrombolysis often reveals underlying stenoses as the cause of the occlusion. These are angioplastied at completion.

2. A mechanical thrombectomy device may be advanced into the main pulmonary arteries or lobar branches and activated to fragment and remove the clot.

3. Aspiration catheters of sufficient size (6–8 Fr) may be used to aspirate thrombus.

4. Bleeding complications are frequent, including haemorrhagic stroke in up to 2%.[2]

5. Treat any underlying stenotic disease with angioplasty or stent.

12

Aftercare

The patient should have follow-up imaging. This may include US, but catheter venography may be preferred because any recurrent lesion may be treated at the same time to reduce the risk of further episodes of DVT.

Complications

1. Access site complications, particularly haematoma formation if using thrombolysis

2. PE: Often patients have an IVC filter to reduce this risk.

References
1. Comerota AJ, Gravett MH. Iliofemoral venous thrombosis. *J Vasc Surg*. 2007;46(5):1065–1076.
2. Liu D, Peterson E, Dooner J, et al. Diagnosis and management of iliofemoral deep vein thrombosis: clinical practice guidelines. *Can Med Assoc J*. 2015;187(17): 1288–1296.

PULMONARY EMBOLISM

Indications

1. Acute massive PE, defined by the American Heart Association as acute PE with sustained hypotension (blood pressure <90 mmHg or reduced by >40 mmHg for >15 min) requiring inotropic support and not due to any other cause
2. Failed systemic thrombolysis
3. Contraindication to systemic thrombolysis

Patient Preparation

1. CTPA to confirm the diagnosis and identify the location of the embolus (see Chapter 9).
2. The decision to treat such patients is usually made with multidisciplinary discussion between the physician, cardiothoracic surgeon and interventional radiologist and often depends on local expertise.
3. The patient requires anaesthetic support.

Equipment

1. General equipment for vascular access
2. Pigtail catheter for angiography, which may also be used to fragment the thrombus
3. Aspiration catheter using suction to remove thrombus
4. Angioplasty balloon to fragment the thrombus
5. Advanced mechanical thrombectomy catheters are designed to fragment the thrombus using high-velocity saline jets, a high-speed impeller or a combination of mechanical maceration with aspiration of thrombus at the same time.
6. Thrombolytic agent such as tissue plasminogen activator (tPA)

Technique

1. Vascular access (see Chapter 11), usually through the common femoral vein with a sheath of sufficient size for the devices to be used
2. A guidewire is advanced through the right atrium and right ventricle into the pulmonary artery (wire passes through both tricuspid and pulmonary valves). This often requires the use of a shaped catheter to help direct the wire.
3. A pigtail catheter is advanced over the wire, and angiography is performed with 50 mL at 25 mL s^{-1} for the main pulmonary artery or 30 mL at 15 mL s^{-1} for left or right pulmonary arteries.

4. A thrombolytic agent such as 5 mg of tPA is injected through the catheter to provide local thrombolysis.
5. The pigtail catheter may be spun to mechanically fragment the clot.
6. Mechanical thrombectomy device may be advanced into the main pulmonary arteries or lobar branches and activated to fragment and remove the clot.
7. Aspiration catheters of sufficient size (8 Fr) may be used to aspirate thrombus.
8. When the patient's haemodynamic status has improved, the procedure is stopped.
9. Manual compression for haemostasis.

Aftercare

Patients are generally transferred to a high-dependency unit for ongoing care.

Complications

1. Of thrombolysis (see Chapter 11)
2. Of vascular access (see Chapter 11)
3. Distal embolization of thrombus
4. Failure to adequately clear the thrombus and death

Further Reading

Jaff MR, McMurtry SM, Archer SL, et al. Management of massive and submassive pulmonary embolism, iliofemoral deep vein thrombosis, and chronic thromboembolic pulmonary hypertension: a statement from the American Heart Association. *Circulation*. 2011;123(16):1788–1830.

Kuo WT. Endovascular therapy for acute pulmonary embolism. *J Vasc Interv Radiol*. 2012;23:167–179.

THORACIC DUCT EMBOLIZATION

Indications

High-output chyle leak (chylothorax, chylopericardium, or chylous ascites) that fail to respond to conservative medical treatment. These arise as a result of direct trauma most commonly after cardiothoracic and upper gastrointestinal surgery or after occlusion of the thoracic duct from malignancy or systemic disease.

12

Contraindications

1. Uncorrectable coagulopathy
2. Pregnancy
3. Allergy to iodinated contrast medium (Lipiodol is an oil-based iodinated contrast medium)

Equipment

1. Digital fluoroscopy unit with C-arm
2. Guidewires
3. Catheters
4. Embolization coils

Patient Preparation

1. If the patient is on anticoagulant treatment, blood clotting should ideally be within an acceptable therapeutic 'window' with international normalized ratio less than 1.5, and the activated partial thromboplastin time less than 1.5 times the control.
2. The radiologist or a suitably trained person should see the patient before the procedure to:
   (a) Explain the procedure.
   (b) Obtain informed consent.
3. Review all available non-invasive imaging to identify a potential site of the chyle leak.
4. Prophylactic IV antibiotics can be administered at the initiation of the procedure.

Technique

Lymphangiography is required to guide thoracic duct embolization and was previously performed via pedal lymphatic cutdown; however, intranodal lymphangiography provides a newer less invasive alternative and is described next.

1. An US examination of both groins is performed to identify the largest inguinal lymph node, which is subsequently punctured using a 21- to 22-gauge needle under US guidance.
2. A maximum of 15–20 mL of Lipiodol is injected by hand at a rate of 0.2–0.4 mL min^{-1}, and the progression of Lipiodol through the lymphatic system is monitored under intermittent fluoroscopy until visualization of the cisterna chyli or thoracic duct.
3. The cisterna chyli or thoracic duct is then directly punctured at the level of L1 to L2 and cannulated with a control wire which is subsequently exchanged for a 2.4- to 2.7-Fr microcatheter system.
4. Contrast is then injected via the microcatheter to confirm position and delineate the site of the chyle leak.
5. A detachable coil is then inserted below the leak followed by a mixture of tissue adhesive glue, which is also injected along the course of the thoracic duct as the microcatheter is pulled out under fluoroscopic guidance.
6. Completion radiographs are subsequently obtained of the chest, abdomen and pelvis for reference of embolic position.

Aftercare

1. Bedrest, typically for 4–6 h
2. Careful observation of the puncture site for evidence of extravasation of Lipiodol or haemorrhage
3. Monitoring of chyle leak output via chest or abdominal drain to assess the success of treatment

Further Reading

Kariya S, Komemushi A, Nakatani M, et al. Intranodal lymphangiogram: technical aspects and findings. *Cardiovasc Intervent Radiol.* 2014;37(6):1606–1610.

Kim SK, Thompson RE, Guevara CJ, et al. Intranodal lymphangiography with thoracic duct embolization for treatment of chyle leak after thoracic outlet decompression surgery. *J Vasc Interv Radiol.* 2020;31(5):795–800.

Nadolski G, Itkin M. Feasibility of ultrasound-guided intranodal lymphangiogram for thoracic duct embolization. *J Vasc Interv Radiol.* 2012;23(5):613–616.

12

Radionuclide imaging in oncology and infection

Greg Chambers and Sriram Vaidyanathan

POSITRON EMISSION TOMOGRAPHY IMAGING

Positron emission tomography (PET) imaging is a modality used to detect and accurately stage malignancy, to differentiate benign and malignant disease and to assess response to treatment. It is also used for imaging infection and inflammation. PET imaging is established in clinical practice and forms part of the standard of care in the imaging work-up of many solid and haematological malignant conditions. PET uses cyclotron-produced radionuclides such as [18]Fluorine (^{18}F), [11]Carbon (^{11}C), [13]Nitrogen and [15]Oxygen, with half-lives of 110, 20, 10 and 2 min, respectively, or generator-produced radionuclides such as [68]Gallium (^{68}Ga) and [82]Rubidium with half-lives of 68 and 1.3 min, respectively. [18]F is the only one of these with a half-life sufficiently long enough to allow it to be produced offsite. This permits 2-[^{18}F]fluoro-2-deoxy-d-glucose (^{18}F-FDG), the most commonly used PET radiopharmaceutical, to be used by sites without their own cyclotron.

The widespread acceptance of PET as a major advance is due to two major factors:

1. There is increased recognition in the literature of the role of the main PET tracer ^{18}F-FDG, a glucose analogue that is taken up in tissue in proportion to cellular glucose metabolism. FDG is phosphorylated by the enzyme hexokinase to a polar intermediate, which does not cross cell membranes well and is therefore trapped in the cell. This is particularly useful for tumour imaging because most tumours have increased glycolysis even in the absence of oxygen and therefore concentrate FDG (the Warburg effect). This is due to multiple factors such as increased glucose transporter molecules (GLUT-1 and -3) at the cancer cell surface and increased hexokinase levels and activity. In addition, the reverse reaction (glucose-6-phosphatase) is slow, and the enzyme is commonly deficient in cancer cells. FDG is a nonspecific biomarker of glycolysis and accumulates through the same mechanisms in cells mediating acute and chronic inflammation and infection. Therefore, ^{18}F-FDG PET-CT cannot reliably differentiate between malignancy and inflammation.

2. All current PET scanners integrate PET and computed tomography (CT) as standard of care. These units have both PET and CT scanners installed in the same gantry. The patient undergoes a conventional CT scan (usually performed with low-exposure factors to reduce radiation dose) immediately followed by a PET scan on the same tabletop. This allows fusion of the anatomical information from CT with the functional data from the PET scan and hence more accurate anatomical localization of metabolically active disease and recognition of normal anatomical and physiological uptake. The density data from the CT scan are also used to correct the PET data for differential attenuation of the emitted photons from different regions within the patient.

Normal physiological uptake of 18-FGD tracer is seen in organs that are major metabolizers of glucose, especially the brain and the heart, or in active or recently active skeletal muscle. Variable uptake is seen in the gut, and there is normal excretion of tracer in the urinary tract. One confounding factor for interpretation may be the presence of normal physiological uptake in brown fat, particularly in the neck and paraspinal regions. It is important to be aware of the physiological sites of FDG uptake and normal variants when interpreting these scans. Differentiation of this normal activity from pathology is greatly aided by the image registration afforded by combined PET-CT scanners.

However, FDG is not specific for cancer cells because any hypermetabolic cell will show increased uptake of FDG such as those in sites of inflammation or infection (and indeed may be utilised specifically for this purpose), so interpretation with reference to the full clinical picture and other imaging is important to avoid false-positive scan results.

FDG is the most widely available and used PET pharmaceutical. Other fluorine-labelled radiopharmaceuticals such as ^{18}F-choline and ^{18}F-PSMA (prostate-specific membrane antigen) are being produced and have a role in imaging of prostate cancer metastases, for example. Radiopharmaceuticals tagged with carbon-11 or other short-lived isotopes are restricted to sites with a dedicated cyclotron. Generator-produced ^{68}G-labelled pharmaceuticals have rapidly evolved in neuroendocrine and prostate tumour imaging.

2-[^{18}F]FLUORO-2-DEOXY-D-GLUCOSE POSITRON EMISSION TOMOGRAPHY SCANNING

Indications (Oncology)

General

1. Establishing the stage of disease (e.g. lung cancer, lymphoma)
2. Establishing whether there is recurrent or residual disease (e.g. lymphoma, teratoma, seminoma)
3. Establishing the site of disease in the face of rising tumour markers (e.g. colorectal, germ cell tumours)

4. Establishing the response to therapy (pre-, during and posttherapy imaging)
5. Help distinguishing benign from malignant disease in conjunction with clinical risk stratification and morphological imaging (e.g. lung nodules, brain lesions)
6. Establishing the grade of cancer (e.g. brain tumours) or tumour de-differentiation (e.g. neuroendocrine cancer)
7. Identifying occult malignancy (e.g. paraneoplastic syndrome or the unknown primary in the setting of proven metastatic disease)

Specific

The following tumours are commonly imaged for staging and follow-up purposes and in cases of diagnostic difficulty:

1. Lung cancer*
2. Lymphoma*
3. Oesophageal cancer*
4. Head and neck cancer*
5. Hepatopancreaticobiliary cancer
6. Melanoma*
7. Breast cancer*
8. Sarcoma
9. Gynaecological cancer
10. Colorectal cancer
11. Anal cancer
12. Myeloma
13. Thyroid cancer
14. Seminoma or teratoma

*Most common cancers staged with PET-CT.
A full list of tumour-specific indications can be found in the 2022 guidance document produced by the Royal Colleges of Physicians and Radiologists, listed under Further Reading.

Relative Contraindications

1. Recent chemotherapy: minimum interval of 2–3 weeks recommended, ideally, more than 6 weeks after end of chemotherapy when possible.
2. Recent radiotherapy: minimum interval of 12 weeks recommended.
3. Recent surgery: minimum of 6–8 weeks.
4. Poorly controlled diabetes (i.e. serum glucose >8.5 mmol L^{-1}) at time of scanning. A blood glucose up to 10–12 mmol L^{-1} can be accepted given the clinical indication. The issue is not the serum glucose but the hyperinsulinaemia that causes altered biodistribution of FDG.

Patient Preparation

1. Fasting for 4–6 h, with plenty of non-sugary fluids. Even a small snack or sweet can alter the biodistribution of FDG.

13

2. Measure blood glucose before injection to ensure it is not elevated. Elevated blood glucose levels result in raised insulin levels, which cause diversion of glucose to muscle.
3. The patient should be informed to refrain from strenuous exercise 24 h before the examination to reduce muscular uptake.
4. Positive oral contrast, although not routinely used, may be administered to aid interpretation of the CT. Previous concerns about attenuation correction artefact on the PET images secondary to the high-density contrast have been shown to be not clinically significant.

Technique

1. 3.5 MBq kg^{-1} body weight ^{18}FDG intravenously (7.6 mSv effective dose (ED)) is administered. Newer generation scanners allow reduced scan times or reduced dose.
2. To reduce muscle uptake of FDG, patients should remain in a relaxed environment such as lying in a darkened room (without talking if the head and neck area are being imaged) between the injection and scan.
3. Image at 1 h after injection.
4. Imaging is preferred with the arms above the head to reduce beam-hardening artefact on the CT.
5. CT:
   (a) Low dose (e.g. exposure factors 120 kV, 80 mAs, ED ~5 mSv)
   (b) Intravenous (IV) contrast medium is not generally used
   (c) Positive or negative oral contrast agents according to local protocol are sometimes used
6. PET:
   (a) From the base of skull to upper thighs (extended to vertex for head and neck cancer, lymphoma and so on; whole body for myeloma, limb cancer and occasionally melanoma)
   (b) 2–4 min for each of five or six bed positions for the PET or equivalent with continuous table movement
7. In some instances, a diagnostic standard-dose CT with IV contrast may be acquired as well, but in routine practice, a diagnostic scan is usually already available. A scan performed with IV contrast may result in attenuation artefacts on the reconstructed PET images if used for attenuation correction, but this is not commonly observed.

Other Applications

Coronary artery disease
Assessment of myocardial viability (see Chapter 10).

Neurology
1. Location of epileptic foci (interictal)
2. Assessment of dementia (see Chapter 16)

Imaging of Infection and Inflammation
See the last section of this chapter.

Further Reading

Cook GJ, Wegner EA, Fogelman I. Pitfalls and artifacts in [18]FDG PET and PET/CT oncologic imaging. *Semin Nucl Med*. 2004;34(2):122–133.

Kapoor V, McCook BM, Torok FS. An introduction to PET CT imaging. *Radiographics*. 2004;24(2):523–543.

Rohren EM, Turkington TG, Coleman RE. Clinical applications of PET in oncology. *Radiology*. 2004;231(2):305–332.

The Royal College of Radiologists, Royal College of Physicians of London. Royal College of Physicians and Surgeons of Glasgow, Royal College of Physicians of Edinburgh, British Nuclear Medicine Society, Administration of Radioactive Substances Advisory Committee. *Evidence Based Indications for the Use of PET-CT in the United Kingdom*. Author; 2022.

von Schulthess GK, Steinert HC, Hany TF. Integrated PET/CT: current applications and future directions. *Radiology*. 2006;238(2):405–422.

OTHER POSITRON EMISSION TOMOGRAPHY RADIOPHARMACEUTICALS

^{18}F-FLUOROETHYLCHOLINE

Choline can be labelled with ^{11}C and ^{18}F, but fluorine is preferred because of the improved logistics of the longer half-life.

Tumours show increased cell membrane turnover and upregulation of choline kinase, leading to incorporation and trapping of choline as phosphatidylcholine (lecithin) in the tumour cell membrane.

Choline is not cancer specific but is a useful agent for imaging of prostate cancer. Non-oncological indications include imaging localization of parathyroid lesions in hyperparathyroidism.

Technique

1. Similar to FDG. Some centres do dynamic and dual time point acquisition.
2. Blood glucose: not relevant
3. 3.5 MBq kg^{-1} body weight ^{18}F-FEC (fluoroethylcholine) intravenously (10 mSv ED) is administered.
4. Image at 1 h after injection. Some authorities use a dynamic early acquisition or a delayed acquisition.

^{18}F-FLUORIDE

This is a useful bone scanning agent with a similar mechanism of uptake to ^{99m}Tc-methylene diphosphonate (^{99m}Tc-MDP) but with greater sensitivity and resolution afforded by PET. It has an evolving role in coronary plaque instability.

[68]GALLIUM-LABELLED PHARMACEUTICALS

This radioisotope is produced by the decay of [68]Germanium ([68]Ge) in a generator that afford greater accessibility and resilience. The parent isotope [68]Ge has a half-life of 271 days and can therefore be used for in-hospital production. The half-life of ^{68}Ga is 68 min.

13

It is widely available outside of the United Kingdom, and one of the fastest growing indications is labelling PSMA, which is overexpressed in metastatic prostate cancer. There are multiple large randomized clinical trials. Preliminary work suggests that it is significantly better than choline PET.

It is used to label peptides (e.g. ^{68}Ga Dotatate (DOTA-DPhe^1, Tyr^3-octreotate) or Dotatoc (DOTA^0-Phe^1-Tyr^3-octreotide) for somatostatin receptor imaging as expressed by neuroendocrine tumours). Gallium PET is significantly more accurate than single-photon emission computed tomography (SPECT) with ^{111}Indium (^{111}In) or ^{99m}Tc-labelled octreotide.

^{67}GALLIUM RADIONUCLIDE TUMOUR IMAGING

In contrast to the PET isotope ^{68}Ga, ^{67}Gallium (^{67}Ga) is a γ-ray rather than a positron emitter. This has almost universally been superseded by cross-sectional techniques and PET scanning. It is not therefore described further in detail. The main disadvantages are the high radiation dose, the extended nature of the investigation, its non-specific nature and difficulties in interpretation in the abdomen because of normal bowel activity. It was used:

1. For Hodgkin's and non-Hodgkin's lymphoma: assessment of residual masses after therapy and early diagnosis of recurrence.
2. With variable success in a variety of other tumours (e.g. hepatoma, bronchial carcinoma, multiple myeloma and sarcoma).
3. In benign conditions such as sarcoidosis and for localization of infection or in suspected orthopaedic infection.

There are some niche applications in which ^{67}Ga citrate may be helpful such as skull base osteomyelitis response assessment.

Further Reading
Afshar-Oromieh A, Avtzi E, Giesel FL, et al. The diagnostic value of PET/CT imaging with the ^{68}Ga-labelled PSMA ligand HBED-CC in the diagnosis of recurrent prostate cancer. *Eur J Nucl Med Imaging*. 2015;42(2):197–209.

Hofman MS, Lau WFE, Hicks RJ. Somatostatin receptor imaging with ^{68}Ga DOTATATE PET/CT: clinical utility, normal patterns, pearls and pitfalls in interpretation. *Radiographics*. 2015;35(2):500–516.

RADIOIODINE (^{123}I OR ^{131}I) METAIODOBENZYLGUANIDINE SCAN

Metaiodobenzylguanidine (mIBG) is a noradrenaline (norepinephrine) analogue. It is taken up actively across cell membranes of sympathetic and adrenal medullary tissue into intracellular storage vesicles. There is no further metabolism, and it remains sequestered and localized in the storage vesicles of catecholamine-secreting tumours and tumours of neuroendocrine origin.[1]

Indications

Localization and staging of the following tumours of neuroendocrine origin:

1. Neuroblastoma
2. Phaeochromocytoma and paraganglioma
3. Neuroendocrine cancer (when the somatostatin receptor imaging result is negative)
4. Medullary thyroid carcinoma

Contraindications

None. A single case report of anaphylaxis after mIBG has been reported. Note, however, that a wide range of medications can interfere with mIBG.

Radiopharmaceuticals

1. ^{123}Iodine (I)-mIBG, 250 MBq typical, 400 MBq maximum (6 mSv ED with thyroid blockade). The 13-h half-life of ^{123}I allows imaging up to 48 h.
2. ^{131}I-labelled mIBG is also available and is still in common use outside Europe, where ^{123}I-mIBG is not made commercially. However, the higher photon energy of the emitted γ-rays renders it an inferior imaging agent and results in a higher radiation dose to the patient. It should only be considered where ^{123}I-mIBG cannot be obtained.

Equipment

1. Gamma camera, preferably with whole-body imaging and SPECT-CT capabilities. Most centres are now using hybrid SPECT-CT cameras for improved anatomical localization and consequently improved specificity.
2. Medium-energy general-purpose collimator for ^{123}I

Patient Preparation

1. When possible, stop medications that interfere with mIBG uptake.[2] There are many medications that can interfere with the scan, including tricyclic antidepressants, antihypertensives, cocaine, sympathomimetics, decongestants containing pseudoephedrine, phenylpropanolamine and phenylephrine (many available over the counter), among others.
2. Thyroid blockade to reduce radiation dose to the thyroid continuing for 24 h after ^{123}I-mIBG injection:
   (a) Adults: either oral potassium perchlorate (400 mg 1 h before mIBG injection; then 200 mg every 6 h) or oral potassium iodate (85 mg twice daily starting 24 h before mIBG injection).
   (b) Children: Lugol's iodine 0.1–0.2 mL diluted with water or milk three times a day starting 48 h before mIBG injection. Potassium iodate is more palatable; the tablets need splitting for paediatric dosage.

13

Technique

1. mIBG is administered slowly IV over 1–2 min (a fast injection may cause adrenergic side effects)
2. Imaging at 24 h (sometimes additionally at 4 or 48 h), emptying the bladder before pelvic views

Images

1. Anterior and posterior abdomen, 10–20 min per view
2. Whole-body imaging for metastases
3. SPECT-CT for anatomical localization and characterization

Additional Techniques

1. If therapy with ^{131}I-mIBG is being considered, dosimetric assessment can be performed using geometric mean and attenuation correction to calculate percentage of administered dose residing in tumour at 24 h.
2. ^{111}In-octreotide, which binds to somatostatin receptors frequently expressed in paraganglioma and medullary thyroid cancer, is an alternative imaging agent to mIBG.
3. PET imaging with radiopharmaceuticals such as ^{18}F fluorodopamine and ^{18}F fluorodopa has limited availability but has been reported to offer additional value over mIBG.[3,4] Conventional ^{18}F FDG PET imaging is also of value in assessing metastatic disease and non–mIBG-avid neuroblastoma (~10%); however, mIBG remains superior to FDG PET in advanced disease, mainly in detecting bone or marrow metastatic disease.[5]

Aftercare

Normal radiation safety precautions (see Chapter 1).

Complications

None

References

1. Ilias I, Divgi C, Pacak K. Current role of metaiodobenzylguanidine in the diagnosis of phaeochromocytoma and medullary thyroid cancer. *Semin Nucl Med.* 2011;41:364–368.
2. Solanki KK, Bomanji J, Moyes J, et al. A pharmacological guide to medicines which interfere with the biodistribution of radiolabelled meta-iodobenzylguanidine (MIBG). *Nucl Med Commun.* 1992;13(7):513–521.
3. Chrisoulidou A, Kaltsas G, Ilias I, et al. The diagnosis and management of malignant phaeochromocytoma and paragangliomas. *Endocrine-Related Cancer.* 2007;14:569–585.
4. Timmers H, Chen C, Jorge A, et al. Comparison of ^{18}F-fluoro-L-DOPA, ^{18}F-fluoro-deoxyglucose, and ^{18}F-fluorodopamine PET and 123I-MIBG scintigraphy in the localization of phaeochromocytoma and paragangliomas. *J Clin Endocrinol Metab.* 2009;94:4757–4767.
5. Sharp SE, Shulkin BL, Gelfand MJ, et al. 123I-MIBG scintigraphy and 18F-FDG PET in neuroblastoma. *J Nucl Med.* 2009;50(8):1237–1243.

SOMATOSTATIN RECEPTOR IMAGING

Somatostatin is a physiological neuropeptide that has biological effects, including inhibition of growth hormone release, and suppression of insulin and glucagon excretion. Octreotide (a long-acting analogue of the human hormone somatostatin) can be used therapeutically to inhibit hormone production by carcinoids, gastrinoma, insulinoma and so on. Several tumours, particularly those of neuroendocrine origin, express somatostatin receptors when they are well-differentiated. Imaging after the administration of radionuclide-labelled somatostatin analogues such as octreotide thus allows their localization.[1]

Indications

Localization and staging of the following tumours of neuroendocrine origin:

1. Neuroendocrine cancer, most commonly midgut carcinoid
2. Gastrinoma
3. Phaeochromocytoma as an alternative to mIBG
4. Medullary cell cancer thyroid as an alternative to mIBG
5. Small cell lung cancer
6. Pituitary

Although sometimes used for the assessment of insulinomas, these latter tumours are more variably perceptible with octreotide (~50%) than carcinoids, gastrinomas and phaeochromocytomas, which are seen in 80%–100% of cases.

Contraindications

None

Radiopharmaceuticals

^{111}In pentetreotide (a DTPA (diethylenetriaminepentaacetic acid) conjugate of octreotide) 220 MBq IV (ED 17 mSv). A new alternative is ^{99m}Tc-EDDA/HYNIC-TOC (Tektrotyd) scintigraphy, which has advantages of the superior imaging resolution and shorter time to scan of ^{99m}Tc.

Equipment

1. Gamma camera, preferably with whole-body imaging and SPECT-CT capabilities
2. Medium energy for ^{111}In, LEHR for ^{99m}Tc

Patient Preparation

1. Some centres use bowel preparation.
2. Oral hydration to help with renal clearance. There is usually high renal uptake.

13

3. In patients with possible insulinoma, IV glucose should be available because of a small risk of inducing hypoglycaemia.
4. Discontinue long-acting somatostatin to avoid competitive inhibition.

Technique

Image at 24 h and if necessary 48 h.

1. Anterior and posterior whole body, 10–20 min per view.
2. Whole-body imaging for comprehensive search for metastases.
3. SPECT-CT will help anatomical localization and improve specificity by differentiating tumour uptake from bowel uptake, for example.

Additional Techniques

mIBG may be positive in octreotide-negative tumours and vice versa.

^{68}Ga DOTA PET is being increasingly used especially outside of the United Kingdom and has superior sensitivity and specificity to octreotide scan because of higher affinity for somatostatin receptor subtype 2 (see previous section on PET).

Aftercare

Normal radiation safety precautions (see Chapter 1).

Complications

None

Reference

1. Krenning EP, Kwekkeboom DJ, Bakker WH, et al. Somatostatin receptor scintigraphy with [^{111}In-DTPA-D-Phe1] and [^{123}I-Tyr3]-octreotide: the Rotterdam experience with more than 1000 patients. *Eur J Nucl Med.* 1993;20(8):716–731.

LYMPH NODE AND LYMPHATIC CHANNEL IMAGING

1. Radiography: not used for this indication anymore
2. Indirect signs such as enlarged lobulated hila on a chest radiograph or eggshell calcification of nodes after lymphoma treatment

ULTRASOUND

Advantages

1. Non-invasive and no ionizing radiation
2. High accuracy in the neck and axilla, especially with morphological characterization and Doppler analysis and ultrasound (US)-guided fine-needle aspiration or core biopsy
3. Endoscopic probes allow access to nodes poorly visualized with percutaneous technique.

Disadvantages

1. Intestinal gas is a major factor in poor visualization of abdominal nodes.
2. Unsuitable for the mediastinum
3. Operator dependent

COMPUTED TOMOGRAPHY

The technique is dealt with in other chapters.

Advantages

1. Can image all nodes
2. Technically easy to perform

Disadvantages

1. Internal nodal structure is not seen
2. Gives no indication of nature, apart from on the basis of size and shape, and possibly on the basis of enhancement characteristics

MAGNETIC RESONANCE IMAGING

The technique is dealt with in other chapters.

Advantages

1. Can image most nodes
2. Multiparametric magnetic resonance imaging (MRI) can assess signal change, haemorrhage, heterogeneity, enhancement and diffusion restriction, among other features.

Disadvantages

1. Internal structure Is not seen.
2. Patient tolerability can be a factor.

RADIOGRAPHIC LYMPHANGIOGRAPHY

This is a technically difficult and invasive examination, requiring limited operative exposure of lymphatic vessels for cannulation, usually in the feet, or direct US-guided lymph node injection most frequently of an inguinal node. It has been superseded by cross-sectional imaging techniques, such as US, CT and MRI, and functional assessment with radionuclide imaging procedures.

13

RADIONUCLIDE LYMPHOSCINTIGRAPHY

Lymphoscintigraphy provides a less invasive alternative to conventional lymphography. High-resolution anatomical detail is not possible (see the discussion on MR lymphangiography under the following section on further techniques).

Indications

1. Localization of the 'sentinel' node in breast carcinoma,[1,2] malignant melanoma[3] penile and vulval malignancies using a handheld probe. In recent years, this has become the major indication for lymphoscintigraphy. The technique in itself does not diagnose nodes affected by malignancy; rather, it identifies the node most likely to be involved and therefore to guide histological sampling. Although still awaiting completion of long-term clinical trials, the early indications are that if the first or 'sentinel' node in the lymphatic drainage chain from the primary site is shown to have negative histology (~60% of cases in breast cancer), then more extensive nodal clearance and associated morbidity can be avoided. SPECT-CT can improve anatomical localization, which aids the surgical exploration.[3] Intraoperative radioguided surgery using a gamma probe or even intraoperative SPECT-CT adds another dimension to the test and improves sampling accuracy and reduces surgical time.
2. Differentiation of lymphoedema from venous oedema
3. Assessment of lymphatic flow in lymphoedema[4]
4. For assessing chyle leaks such as chylous ascites or chylothorax and providing a guide for subsequent thoracic duct embolization

Contraindications

Hypersensitivity to human albumin products

Radiopharmaceuticals

1. [99mTc]-nanocolloidal albumin (particle size <80 nm), 40 MBq maximum (0.4 mSv ED) total for all injections. The colloid is injected intradermally to assess the superficial lymphatic system and is cleared from the interstitial space by lymphatic drainage.
2. A number of other colloids are used around the world for sentinel node imaging, and other radiopharmaceuticals have been used for lymphoscintigraphy such as [99mTc]-Tilmanocept, which targets mannose receptors expressed on the surface of reticuloendothelial cells in lymph nodes.

Equipment

1. Gamma camera
2. Low-energy-high-resolution (LEHR) collimator

Patient Preparation

Clean injection sites.

Technique

1. Sentinel node imaging:
   Example protocols are:
   (a) Breast carcinoma: Inject [99mTc]-colloid in approximately 5-mL volume intradermally for palpable lesions and around the tumour under US guidance for non-palpable lesions.

(b) Melanoma: Inject ^{99m}Tc-colloid intradermally in a ring of locations around the melanoma site, with a volume of about 0.1 mL for each injection.

Static images are taken at intervals until the first node is seen. For breast cancer, take anterior and left or right lateral images with the arm raised as for surgery. Mark the skin over the node in both axes to guide surgical incision and intraoperative location with a gamma-detecting probe.

With effectively no background activity in the body, anatomical localization on the images is needed. A ^{57}Cobalt flood source (usually available for routine camera quality assurance) is placed for a short period under the imaging couch to produce a body outline on the image.

2. Other anatomical sites of investigation or for investigation of lymphatic drainage or lymphoedema:

(a) ^{99m}Tc-colloid in 0.1- to 0.3-mL volume is injected intradermally at sites, depending upon the area to be studied (e.g. for nodes below diaphragm and lower limb drainage). Injections are done in each foot in the first and second web spaces for drainage or over the lateral dorsum of the foot for lymphatics or for axillary nodes and upper limb drainage injections in each hand in the second and third web spaces.

(b) Static images are taken of the injection site(s) immediately followed by the injection site, drainage route and liver images at intervals (e.g. 15, 30, 60 and 180 min), continuing up to 24 h or until the liver is seen. Visualization of the liver indicates patency of at least one lymphatic channel (except early prominent liver activity within 15 min, which implies inadvertent intravascular injection of colloid).

Analysis

If more frequent imaging or a long dynamic study is performed, time–activity curves for regions along the drainage route can be plotted and used to quantify flow impairment.

Aftercare

Normal radiation safety precautions

Complications

Anaphylactic reaction: rare

Other Techniques: Magnetic Resonance Lymphangiography[5]

Although this technique has not yet been widely taken up, this is equivalent to radionuclide lymphoscintigraphy in principle but provides high-resolution anatomical imaging and direct visualization of draining lymph vessels. Instead of radionuclide agents, small volumes of gadolinium-based MR contrast agents are injected intracutaneously into the web spaces of the feet or other relevant anatomical area.

13

T2-weighted imaging is used to demonstrate the lymphoedema, and postcontrast, a three-dimensional spoiled gradient-echo sequence (volumetric interpolated breath-hold examination) at multiple time intervals up to 1 h is used to demonstrate the lymph channels directly.

References

1. Krynyckyi BR, Kim CK, Goyenechea MR, et al. Clinical breast lymphoscintigraphy: optimal techniques for performing studies, image atlas, and analysis of images. *Radiographics.* 2004;24(1):121–145.
2. Husarik DB, Steinert HC. Single-photon emission computed tomography/computed tomography for sentinel node mapping in breast cancer. *Semin Nucl Med.* 2007;37(1):29–33.
3. Intenzo CM, Truluck CA, Kushen MC, et al. Lymphoscintigraphy in cutaneous melanoma: an updated total body atlas of sentinel node mapping. *Radiographics.* 2009;29(4):1125–1135.
4. Witte CL, Witte MH, Unger EC, et al. Advances in imaging of lymph flow disorders. *Radiographics.* 2000;20(6):1697–1719.
5. Lohrmann C, Foeldi E, Speck O, et al. High-resolution MR lymphangiography in patients with primary and secondary lymphoedema. *AJR Am J Roentgenol.* 2006;187(2):556–561.

RADIONUCLIDE IMAGING OF INFECTION AND INFLAMMATION

The round-the-clock availability and sensitivity for collections and inflammation of anatomical imaging techniques such as MRI, CT and US have reduced the demand for radionuclide procedures.

A number of radionuclide techniques exist for complex cases in which standard imaging has not revealed an abnormality or in instances when MRI is contraindicated because of the presence of metalwork or a pacemaker. Traditional scintigraphic techniques have largely been superseded by FDG PET-CT imaging, which benefits from increased sensitivity and specificity thanks to the higher resolution of PET and the greater anatomical localization of CT. A distinct advantage of FDG PET-CT over white cell scintigraphy is the former's ability to image chronic infection and inflammation unlike the latter. The most commonly used scintigraphic technique is radionuclide-labelled leucocyte imaging.[1,2]

Indications

1. Diagnosis and localization of obscure infection and inflammation in soft tissue and bone, particularly sites of chronic disease[3]
2. Assessment of inflammatory activity in disorders such as inflammatory bowel disease, especially when MRI is contraindicated

Contraindications

None

Radiopharmaceuticals

1. ^{111}In-labelled leucocytes, 20 MBq maximum (9 mSv ED): ^{111}In-oxine, tropolonate and acetylacetonate are highly lipophilic complexes that

label leucocytes, erythrocytes and platelets. The leucocytes have to be labelled in vitro and the labelled cell suspension reinjected. ABO/Rh-matched donor leucocytes can be used with neutropenic patients or to reduce infection hazard in human immunodeficiency virus–positive patients.[111]In has a half-life of 67 h and principal gamma emissions at 171 and 245 keV. There is no confounding uptake in the bowel, and this technique may be more suitable for chronic or more low-grade infections because of the longer imaging window (4–48 h).

2. ^{99m}Tc-hexamethylpropyleneamineoxime (HMPAO)-labelled leucocytes, 200 MBq maximum (3 mSv ED): HMPAO is also a highly lipophilic complex, which preferentially labels granulocytes. The cell-labelling technique is similar to that for ^{111}In, but HMPAO has the advantage that kits can be stocked and used at short notice. There is more bowel uptake as a result of biliary excretion than with ^{111}In-labelled leucocytes, so images must be taken earlier than 4 h after injection for diagnosis of abdominal infection. The ^{99m}Tc label delivers a lower radiation dose than ^{111}In-labelled leucocytes and has better imaging resolution, which can, for example, help identify inflammation in the small bowel.

3. [67]Ga citrate, 150 MBq maximum (17 mSv ED): This localizes in inflammatory sites. Formerly the most commonly used agent, it has now largely been replaced by labelled leucocyte imaging. There is significant bowel activity up to 72 h, so delayed imaging may be necessary for suspected abdominal infection, and accuracy in the abdomen is less than appears elsewhere. [67]Ga, with a half-life of 78 h and principal γ-emissions at 93, 185 and 300 keV, delivers a significantly higher radiation dose than ^{99m}Tc-HMPAO and ^{111}In-labelled leucocytes, but it has the advantage of requiring no special preparation.

4. [99m]Tc or ^{111}In-human immunoglobulin (HIG): This is an agent for which a commercial kit is available for ^{99m}Tc labelling. It has the advantage of not requiring a complex preparation procedure, but its place relative to labelled leucocytes is still a matter of debate. There is a risk of allergic reaction.

5. ^{99m}Tc-sulesomab: This is another commercial agent, consisting of a labelled antigranulocyte monoclonal antibody fragment. It also has a simple preparation procedure and is finding a role in the diagnosis of orthopaedic infections. Thirty percent of patients will develop human antimurine antibodies on administration.

Equipment

1. Gamma camera, preferably with a whole-body imaging facility
2. Low-energy, high-resolution collimator for ^{99m}Tc, medium-energy for ^{111}In, medium- or high-energy for [67]Ga

Patient Preparation

None

Technique

1. The radiopharmaceutical is administered intravenously.
2. Image timing depends upon the radiopharmaceutical used and the suspected source of infection. Whole-body imaging may be used for all of the radiopharmaceuticals:
   (a) ^{111}In-labelled white cells: Static images are acquired at 3 and 24 h after injection. Further imaging at 48 h may prove helpful.
   (b) ^{99m}Tc-HMPAO-labelled white cells: For suspected abdominal infections, image at 0.5 and 2 h (i.e. before significant normal bowel activity is seen). For other sites, image at 1, 2 and 4 h. Additional 24-h images may be useful.
   (c) ^{67}Ga-citrate: Images are acquired at 48 and 72 h for regions where normal bowel, urinary and blood-pool activity may obscure abnormal collection sites. Later images may prove helpful in non-urgent cases. The extremities and urgent cases may be imaged from as early as 6 h. If not contraindicated, laxatives given for 48 h after injection help clear bowel activity.
3. SPECT-CT is helpful in many cases.

Additional Techniques

1. The diagnosis of bone infection may be improved by combination with three-phase radioisotope bone scanning or bone marrow imaging.
2. Comparison with a radiocolloid scan may help discriminate between infection in the region of the liver, spleen and bone marrow and normal uptake in these organs.

Aftercare

Normal radiation safety precautions (see Chapter 1).

Complications

None

References

1. Peters AM, Editorial Lavender JP. Imaging inflammation with radiolabelled white cells: ^{99m}Tc-HMPAO or ^{111}. *Nucl Med Commun.* 1991;12:923–925.
2. Love C, Palestro CJ. Radionuclide imaging of infection. *J Nucl Med Technol.* 2004;32(2):47–57.
3. Vaidyanathan S, Patel CN, Scarsbrook AF, et al. FDG PET/CT in infection and inflammation—current and emerging clinical applications. *Clin Radiol.* 2015;70(7):787–800.

Bones and joints
Philip Robinson and James J. Rankine

Imaging Modalities

1. **Plain films:** These are inexpensive, widely available, and valuable screening tools in the preliminary assessment of joint symptoms. Standard views require a minimum of two views perpendicular to each other (e.g. anteroposterior (AP) and lateral projections). Pathological processes producing underlying osteolysis or osteosclerosis (e.g. infection, tumours, articular erosions) are usually well advanced before they become radiographically visible, and radiographs may appear normal despite the presence of significant bone and joint disease. Although there are limitations, plain films are very useful in the characterization and differential diagnosis of disease (e.g. trauma, bone tumours, arthritis). Despite the recent advances in imaging techniques, radiography remains a crucial investigation in the characterization of bone tumours.

2. **Arthrography:** The injection of radiographically positive (iodinated) and negative (air) contrast medium directly into the joint allows radiographic assessment of articular structures in conventional arthrography. The examination can then be supplemented with computed tomography (CT) arthrography, which provides more detailed assessment of intraarticular structures using bone and soft tissue window settings. For optimal evaluation, reformatted CT images in three planes with multidetector computed tomography (MDCT) are obtained. Magnetic resonance (MR) arthrography using a dilute gadolinium-diethylenetriamine pentaacetic acid (DTPA) solution (2 mmoL L^{-1} at 1.5 T) is frequently used in the study of joint disease.

3. **Radionuclide imaging:** This includes conventional imaging such as bone scans, radiolabelled white blood cells and ^{67}gallium citrate and expanding high-resolution modalities such as positron emission tomography (PET)-CT typically using ^{18}fluorine fluorodeoxyglucose (^{18}FDG). Conventional nuclear medicine techniques have high sensitivity but low specificity. The low specificity can be improved to an extent with single-photon emission computed tomography (SPECT)-CT, which harnesses the hybrid aspects of functional and structural imaging and can be useful for identifying pain generators in the limbs and spine after complex surgery. In many areas, conventional nuclear medicine imaging has been superseded

by magnetic resonance imaging (MRI), which demonstrates high sensitivity and increased specificity (e.g. for infection and stress injuries and fractures). FDG PET-CT has high sensitivity and specificity and is recommended as an alternative in scanning spondylodiscitis and limb osteomyelitis when MRI is contraindicated and in the presence of metalwork. Conventional radionuclide imaging continues to be widely used in the detection and follow-up of metastatic disease, painful joint arthroplasties in which infection is suspected. FDG PET-CT is also increasingly used in the systemic staging of bone tumours. However, emerging MRI technologies such as metal reduction techniques, whole-body MRI and PET-MRI are now challenging these indications but are not yet widely available.

4. **Ultrasound (US):** Musculoskeletal US is now commonly used for evaluating disorders in both adult and paediatric age groups. Periarticular structures (capsule, ligaments, and tendons) are optimally imaged. Under US guidance, therapy to soft tissue disease can be accurately targeted, joint fluid aspirated and arthrographic agents instilled into joints.

5. **CT:** This is very useful in complex bone trauma for accurate surgical planning and in many applications, including assessment of bone tumours and infection. CT optimally depicts joint anatomy and pathology in joints that are difficult to image with plain radiography in two perpendicular planes and where there is bone overlap (e.g. shoulder, hip, sternoclavicular, and sacroiliac joints). When used as CT arthrography, the intraarticular status of joints can be optimally assessed to a very high resolution.

6. **MRI:** MRI is the best imaging modality for joint assessment. In many joints, such as the knee, it can be used as the first and only form of imaging required. In other joints, such as the shoulder, MRI alone is used to image the rotator cuff, but MR arthrography is required for optimal imaging of the ligaments, capsule and labrum in posttraumatic instability. MR arthrography can also be used in the hip primarily to image the labrum and in the wrist to assess the interosseous ligaments of the proximal carpal row and the triangular fibrocartilage. However, the optimal technique is constantly evolving because higher-field MRI (3 T) is now increasingly used to assess the hip labrum and wrist ligaments without the need for arthrography. Indirect MR arthrography after intravenous (IV) injection of gadolinium-DTPA, which quickly diffuses into the joint via the synovium, is used in the detection and quantification of active synovitis (e.g. rheumatoid arthritis) and to produce articular cartilage maps. This is particularly valuable in small joints and in the postoperative assessment of large joints. MRI is widely used in the assessment of bone pathology, such as tumour or infection. Metal reduction techniques now allow MRI to be used to evaluate postsurgical implants for most common complications.

MUSCULOSKELETAL MAGNETIC RESONANCE IMAGING: GENERAL POINTS

1. There is a large variety of MR sequences providing an opportunity to tailor the sequences to the tissues that need to be optimally imaged (Table 14.1).
2. IV gadolinium-DTPA is used in musculoskeletal imaging for:
   (a) Infections to differentiate abscess from phlegmon
   (b) Tumours to differentiate viable tumour from necrosis and to differentiate solid from cystic components
   (c) Postoperative spine to differentiate recurrent disc herniation from scar tissue
   (d) Synovial disease (e.g. rheumatoid arthritis) to determine activity and response to treatment
   (e) Avascular necrosis (e.g. Perthes' disease, scaphoid fracture) to show viable tissue
   (f) Indirect MR arthrography to delineate articular cartilage status and meniscal repair
3. MR arthrography: Direct MR arthrography involves joint puncture and the intraarticular injection of a dilute gadolinium solution. (Saline and local anaesthetic can also be used.) The concentration of gadolinium needed to produce contrast by shortening the T1 effect of fluid is very small (2 mmoL L^{-1} at 1.5 T), but a high concentration of gadolinium DTPA results in signal loss of the fluid ('blackout'). The joint is distended and the recesses filled, delineating the intraarticular structures and separating them from adjacent tissues. In the lower

Table 14.1 Optimizing Magnetic Resonance Imaging Sequences for Musculoskeletal Tissues

Tissue Type	Optimal Magnetic Resonance Imaging Sequences		
Bone	T1	STIR	T2 fat saturated
Cartilage	PD fat saturated	T2 fat saturated	PD fat saturated
Labrum	T1 fat saturated (MR arthrogram)	PD fat saturated (MR arthrogram)	PD fat saturated
Meniscus	PD fat saturated	T2 fat saturated	T1
Tendons and ligaments	T2 fat saturated	PD fat saturated	T1
Muscle	T1	T2 fat saturated	STIR
Marrow	T1	STIR	PD fat saturated
Synovium	T1 fat saturated (IV gadolinium)	T1 spin-echo (IV gadolinium)	PD fat saturated

IV, Intravenous; *MR,* magnetic resonance; *PD,* proton density; *STIR,* short tau inversion recovery.

14

limb, it allows accurate visualization of the labrum of the hip, the operated meniscus in the knee, and demonstrates associated osteochondral defects, loose bodies and synovial pathology, although as hardware and sequences evolve, the need for arthrography is now no longer necessary for many conditions (e.g. hip labrum evaluation, many osteochondral defects, ankle impingement). In the upper limb, it is still a valuable technique in unstable shoulders to assess the damaged osteoarticular and ligamentous structures but is rarely needed for the elbow and wrist joints and ligaments. T1 spin-echo and T1 fat-saturated sequences are traditionally used routinely in MR arthrography, along with a T2 sequence in at least one plane to detect cysts, bone, and soft tissue oedema. However, proton density–weighted sequences are now commonly used because they not only show the arthrographic fluid as high signal but also allow better assessment of any intact structure's intrinsic signal (e.g. labrum, cartilage, tendons). Stress views from patient positioning (e.g. abduction and external rotation (ABER) for shoulder anterior labrum or applied traction) improve visualization of certain structures (e.g. long head of biceps origin in the shoulder, articular cartilage in the hip). MR arthrography can avoid the requirement for diagnostic arthroscopy and aids in the therapeutic plan.

Further Reading

Chundru U, Riley GM, Steinbach LS. Magnetic resonance arthrography. *Radiol Clin North Am.* 2009;47(3):471–494.

Morrison WB. Indirect MR arthrography: concepts and controversies. *Semin Musculoskelet Radiol.* 2005;9(2):125–134.

Schmaranzer F, Kheterpal AB, Bredella MA. Best practices: hip femoroacetabular impingement. *AJR Am J Roentgenol.* 2021;216(3):585–598.

Sun G, Zhang Y-X, Liu F, et al. Whole-body magnetic resonance imaging is superior to skeletal scintigraphy for the detection of bone metastatic tumors: a meta-analysis. *Eur Rev Med Pharmacol Sci.* 2020;24(13):7240–7252.

Talbot BS, Weinberg EP. MR imaging with metal-suppression sequences for evaluation of total joint arthroplasty. *Radiographics.* 2016;36(1):209–225.

ARTHROGRAPHY: GENERAL POINTS

1. The conventional radiographs should always be reviewed before the procedure.
2. Aspiration of an effusion should always be performed before contrast medium is injected. The aspirate should be sent, when appropriate, for microscopy, culture (aerobic and anaerobic) and sensitivity, crystal analysis, cytology and biochemistry.
3. Conventional plain film arthrography has largely been replaced by standard MRI. Fluoroscopic arthrography is used for diagnosing and treating shoulder adhesive capsulitis and in demonstrating the exact site of abnormal articular communications (e.g. the wrist) but is mostly undertaken as a prelude to either CT or MR arthrography.
4. When a needle is correctly sited within a joint space, a small-volume test injection of contrast medium will stream away from the needle

tip around the joint. However, if it is incorrectly sited, the contrast medium will remain in a diffuse cloud around the tip of the needle. For this reason, it is important that the fluoroscopy-guided needle approach should aim to visualize the needle tip at all times during its trajectory. In the knee, fluoroscopy in the AP plane is used as the needle is advanced from a lateral approach; fluoroscopy of the ankle in the lateral projection allows needle-tip visualization because it is advanced via an anterior approach.

5. Needle placement may be non–image guided ('blind') or under image guidance (e.g. using fluoroscopy, CT, CT fluoroscopy or US). Measured effective doses given by an experienced radiologist show significant differences (in shoulder arthrography, fluoroscopy (0.0015 mSv), single-slice CT (0.18 mSv) and CT fluoroscopy (0.22 mSv)).[1]

6. The contrast medium is absorbed from the joint and excreted from the body within a few hours. However, intraarticular air may take up to 4 days to be completely absorbed from the joint space. Every effort should be made to eliminate air bubbles at injection for MR arthrography because they create image artefacts.

7. Arthrography is well tolerated by patients, with discomfort rated less severe than general MRI-related patient discomfort.[2]

8. Arthrography is a very safe procedure with low complication rates. In a major study, there were rates of 3.8% for minor complications (vasovagal reaction, pain, synovitis) and 0.02% for major complications (anaphylactic reaction, infection, vascular).[3] This included 13,300 MR arthrograms with only a 0.03% complication rate, all of which were minor.

9. In the scheduling of CT and MR arthrography, it is important to ensure that the examination is carried out within 30–45 min of intraarticular contrast medium instillation. After this, time contrast medium absorption can potentially result in a suboptimal examination with resultant difficulties in interpretation.

ARTHROGRAPHY

Indications

1. **Intraarticular structural abnormalities** (e.g. cartilage, labrum): The exact status of cartilage overlying osteochondritis dissecans (knee, ankle), labral tears (shoulder and hip) and anchor point of the long head of biceps may require CT or MR arthrography for accurate diagnosis.

2. **Capsular, ligamentous and tendon injuries:** Information regarding the presence, type, extent, gap and edges of torn capsular and pericapsular structures (glenohumeral ligaments, rotator cuff tendons, lateral ankle ligaments) may require CT or MR arthrography.

3. **Loose body:** Loose bodies can be solitary or multiple, radiolucent or radiopaque. CT arthrography using dilute contrast medium solution best depicts radiolucent bodies. Double-contrast CT arthrography using only a small amount of positive contrast medium is best to

14

delineate radiopaque loose bodies, determine their true size and assess the articular status of the joint.

4. **Paraarticular cyst:** Synovial cysts and ganglia within paraarticular soft tissues and bones can present with space-occupying lesions, which may migrate some distance away from the joint source of origin (popliteal cysts, iliopsoas bursa). Arthrography can demonstrate the articular communication either immediately or on delayed imaging.

5. **Prosthesis assessment** (e.g. loosening, infection): Arthrography demonstrates abnormal interposition of contrast medium indicating loosening at the cement–bone or metal–bone interface, depending on the type of arthroplasty procedure carried out, but joint irrigation and aspiration fluid specimens are needed to confirm associated infection. Subtraction radiographic techniques are used to facilitate interpretation because the metal prosthesis and the barium-impregnated cement are subtracted out of the final image. However, advanced MRI metal suppression techniques now mean that MRI is initially performed for prosthesis assessment before arthrography is considered.

6. **Pain block** (e.g. ropivacaine ± steroid therapy). For difficult therapeutic decisions, diagnostic tests to confirm the pain source origin are increasingly being used by instilling intraarticular 0.5% ropivacaine. The addition of a steroid preparation can also aid in providing a longer period of pain control. If required, the anaesthetic may be injected with the arthrographic agent for MRI.

7. **Diagnosis and distension therapy in adhesive capsulitis:** Usually used in the shoulder in the treatment of frozen shoulder, the combination of anaesthetic, steroid and saline can be used to distend and rupture the joint after arthrographic confirmation of the diagnosis.

8. **Intraarticular chemical therapy** (e.g. hyaluronic acid, fibrinolysis, radioactive synovectomy): The intraarticular injection of hyaluronic acid in joints with mild to moderate osteoarthritis produces viscosupplementation of joint fluid, reducing pain and increasing the articular cartilage thickness. In fibrin-laden effusions caused by chronic rheumatoid arthritis, injected intraarticular fibrinolytic agents aid in the aspiration of the joint fluid.

Contraindications

1. Local sepsis
2. Allergy to iodine or gadolinium
3. Contraindication to MRI (see Chapter 2); consider CT arthrography

Contrast Medium

Conventional or computed tomography arthrography

Low-osmolar contrast material (LOCM) is used. A higher concentration is needed in larger joints, but for the purposes of CT arthrography, especially in tight joints, a dilute solution (100–150 mg I/100 mL) has distinct advantages. The volume of the contrast medium needed is directly proportional to the capacity of the joint in question (e.g.

15 mL in the shoulder, 6 mL in the elbow and 3 mL in the wrist). Double-contrast examination of the knee for a CT arthrogram to assess the patellofemoral joint requires 4 mL of iodinated contrast medium with 40 mL of air.

Magnetic resonance arthrography

1. The contrast used may be made up to contain both dilute gadolinium-DTPA and iodinated contrast (which is needed to confirm correct needle placement during injection), such as a combination of:
   (a) 0.1 mL gadolinium-DTPA,
   (b) 10 mL sterile saline solution, and
   (c) 2 mL LOCM 200 mg I mL^{-1}.
2. Alternatively, iodinated contrast can be initially injected to confirm position and after exchange of syringes, sterile, premixed gadolinium-DTPA (2 mmoL L^{-1}) solution is subsequently injected.

Equipment

1. Fluoroscopy unit with a spot film device and fine focal spot (0.3 mm^2)
2. Overcouch tube

Patient Preparation

None

Preliminary Images

Routine acquisition and evaluation of joint radiographs is recommended.

Radiographic Views

Further radiographic views are rarely performed because most arthrographic studies are a prelude to MR or CT arthrography, except in the wrist, where spot views in radial and ulnar deviation, and views of the radiocarpal, midcarpal and inferior radioulnar joints are useful to document contrast communication between compartments.

Aftercare

Driving immediately after the procedure is not advisable. The patient is warned that there may be some discomfort in the joint for 1–2 days after the procedure. It is also necessary to refrain from strenuous exercise during this time. The injected air for a double-contrast procedure precludes air travel.

Complications

Due to the contrast medium

1. Allergic reactions
2. Chemical synovitis

Due to the technique

1. Pain
2. Infection

14

3. Capsular rupture or extravasation
4. Trauma to adjacent structures (e.g. neural or vascular structures)
5. Air embolus (rare)

Other

Vasovagal reaction

References

1. Binkert CA, Verdun FR, Zanetti M, et al. CT arthrography of the glenohumeral joint: CT fluoroscopy versus conventional CT and fluoroscopy—comparison of image guidance techniques. *Radiology.* 2003;229:153–158.
2. Binkert CA, Zanetti M, Hodler J. Patient's assessment of discomfort during MR arthrography of the shoulder. *Radiology.* 2001;221:775–778.
3. Hugo PC, Newberg AH, Newman JS, et al. Complications of arthrography. *Semin Musculoskelet Radiol.* 1998;2(4):345–348.

Further Reading

Andreisek G, Duc SR, Froehlich JM, et al. MR arthrography of the shoulder, hip, and wrist: evaluation of contrast dynamics and image quality with increasing injection-to-imaging time. *AJR Am J Roentgenol.* 2007;188(4): 1081–1088.

Schmaranzer F, Kheterpal AB, Bredella MA. Best practices: hip femoroacetabular impingement. *AJR Am J Roentgenol.* 2021;216(3):585–598.

Talbot BS, Weinberg EP. MR imaging with metal-suppression sequences for evaluation of total joint arthroplasty. *Radiographics.* 2016;36(1):209–225.

Tehranzadeh J, Mossop EP, Golshan-Momeni M. Therapeutic arthrography and bursography. *Orthop Clin North Am.* 2006;37(3):393–408.

ARTHROGRAPHY: SITE-SPECIFIC ISSUES

There are various needle approaches using image guidance, and the most commonly used ones are described. All arthrography can now be performed under US guidance, but for brevity, this section focuses on fluoroscopic guidance with limited description of US guidance for the most frequently accessed joints, the knee, hip and shoulder.

KNEE

Fluoroscopic Technique

1. The patient lies supine; either a medial or a lateral approach can be used, and it is important to be familiar with both.
2. Using a sterile technique, the skin and underlying soft tissue are anaesthetized at a point 1–2 cm posterior to the midpoint of the patella.
3. A 21-gauge needle is advanced into the joint space from this point by angling it slightly anterior so the tip comes to lie against the posterior surface of the patella. By virtue of the anatomy, the tip of the needle must be within the joint space (Fig. 14.1). A more horizontal approach may result in the needle's penetrating the infrapatellar fat pad, resulting in an extraarticular injection of contrast.

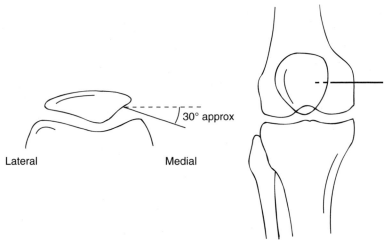

Fig. 14.1 Technique of knee arthrography.

4. Any effusion is aspirated. A test injection of a small volume of contrast medium can be made under fluoroscopic control to ensure the needle is correctly positioned, and if so, the contrast medium should be seen to flow rapidly away from the needle tip. If a satisfactory position is demonstrated, then the full volume of contrast medium (4 mL) and air (40 mL) may be injected for a double-contrast arthrogram.

5. The needle is then removed, and the knee is manipulated to ensure even distribution of contrast medium within the joint; this is easily facilitated by asking the patient to walk around the room several times while bending the knee through as full a movement as possible.

6. The arthrogram is usually followed by CT to assess the patellofemoral articular status and its articular geometric relationship. Patellar tracking in different degrees of knee flexion can be performed if needed. MDCT also assesses the medial and lateral articular and meniscal status optimally.

HIP

Fluoroscopic Technique

1. The patient lies supine on the x-ray table, the leg is extended and internally rotated and the position is maintained with sandbags so that the entire length of the femoral neck is visualized.

2. The position of the femoral vessels may be marked to avoid inadvertent puncture.

3. The skin is prepared in a standard aseptic manner.

4. A metal marker (sterile needle) or a point on the skin is made to show the position of entry (Fig. 14.2), which should correspond to the midpoint of the intertrochanteric line. After local anaesthetic

14

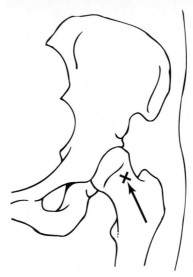

Fig. 14.2 Technique of hip arthrography. *x* indicates the target for the needle tip at the site of entry into the joint.

infiltration, a spinal needle (7.5 cm, 20- or 22-gauge, short bevel) is then advanced vertically with mild forward angulation. The needle tip advances forward toward the femoral neck target under fluoroscopic control, aiming centrally to superolaterally onto the femoral neck immediately below the junction of the femoral head with the neck laterally. The capsule may be thick, and a definite 'give' should be felt when the needle enters the joint.

5. A test injection of contrast medium will demonstrate correct placement of the needle as it freely flows away from the needle tip. Any fluid in the joint should be aspirated at this stage and sent for analysis.

6. Approximately 6–12 mL (1–2 mL in children) of contrast medium is injected until resistance is felt or the patient feels the joint is too tight. The exact amount depends on the capacity of the joint capsule. In MR arthrography, dilute gadolinium solution is used for contrast. Alternatively, in a pain block procedure, 6–8 mL of 0.5% ropivacaine is injected intraarticularly, and this can also act as the contrast medium for a limited MR arthrogram relying on T2 sequences. If examining a prosthetic joint, larger volumes of contrast medium may be required (15–20 mL). By adding a radioactive tracer to the infusate (^{99m}Tc-colloid) and subsequent imaging with a gamma camera, a more accurate assessment of loosening can be made, perhaps because the tracer is less viscous than the contrast medium and extends to a greater extent along the prosthesis.

7. After injection of the contrast medium, the needle is removed, the joint is passively exercised to distribute the contrast medium evenly and the patient is sent to the CT or MR scanning suite accordingly.

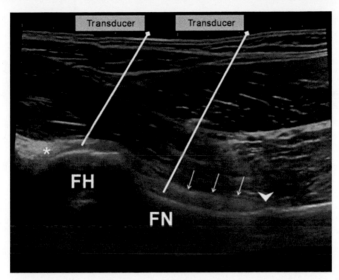

Fig. 14.3 Long-axis ultrasound image of the femoral neck (FN) and head (FH) showing the labrum *(asterisk)*, capsule *(small arrows)* and lower insertion *(arrowhead)*. The two needle positions *(long solid arrows)* for targeting the FH or FN are shown; please see text.

Ultrasound Technique

There are two to three potential approaches to the hip under US guidance. The patient lies supine with the leg extended and internally rotated or in neutral.

1. The hip is visualized in its long axis, and either the femoral head or femoral neck is targeted lateral to the femoral vessels. A point inferior to the long axis of the probe is marked as the entry site for the needle.
2. Using a sterile technique, the skin and soft tissues are anaesthetized immediately adjacent to the marked point. A spinal needle, 21-gauge needle or long 20-gauge needle is inserted and advanced cranially and obliquely down onto the femoral head or neck, depending on the target site chosen (Fig. 14.3). The position of the needle should be confirmed with free flow of contrast on injection, which does not collect around the needle or periarticular soft tissues.
3. Alternatively, the femoral head can be scanned in transverse, and a point lateral to the long axis of the probe is marked as the entry site for the needle. Using a sterile technique, the skin and soft tissues are anaesthetized immediately adjacent to the marked point. A 21-gauge spinal needle or long 20-gauge needle is inserted and advanced medially and obliquely down onto the femoral head.

Radiographic Views in the Paediatric Hip Arthrogram

In children younger than the age of 10 years, the procedure is usually performed under general anaesthesia. A fuller conventional radiographic series is needed to assess the joint dynamics to help in the

14

evaluation of treatment options, particularly in developmental dysplasia of the hip:

1. AP hip
2. Frog lateral
3. Abduction and internal rotation
4. Maximum abduction
5. Maximum adduction
6. Push–pull views to demonstrate instability

SHOULDER

Technique

There are various approaches to needle placement such as anterior (superior or inferior), modified anterior and posterior to the glenohumeral joint.

Anterior (fluoroscopic guided)

1. In the commonly used anterior approach, the patient lies supine, with the arm of the side under investigation close to the body and in external rotation. This is to rotate the long head of the biceps out of the path of the needle. The articular surface of the glenoid faces slightly forward, which is important because it allows a vertically placed needle to enter the joint space without damaging the glenoid labrum.
2. The coracoid process is an important landmark. Using a sterile technique, the skin and soft tissues are anaesthetized at a point 1 cm inferior and 1 cm lateral to the coracoid process. The position of the needle entry point is optimized by fluoroscopy, which also helps ensure that the chosen needle trajectory is not impeded by an elongated coracoid process.
3. A 21-gauge spinal needle is inserted vertically down into the joint space (Fig. 14.4). The vertical direction should intersect the junction of the middle and lower thirds of the craniocaudal plane of the glenohumeral joint. This also allows precise control of the mediolateral course of the needle. The position of the needle should

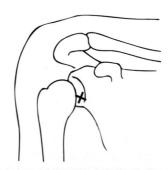

Fig. 14.4 Technique of shoulder arthrography. x indicates the site of entry into the joint.

be checked by intermittent screening. When it meets the resistance of the articular surface of the humeral head, it is withdrawn by 1–2 mm to free the tip. In the modified anterior approach, in which the needle traverses the rotator cuff interval, the needle is aimed towards the upper medial quadrant of the humeral head close to the articular joint line.

4. The intraarticular position of the needle is then confirmed by the injection of a small amount of the contrast medium under fluoroscopic control.

5. Then either the remainder of the iodinated contrast medium (15 mL in total) is injected for a single-contrast examination or sufficient air to distend the synovial sac (12 mL) is injected for a double-contrast examination. CT arthrography can be done after either type. In MR arthrography, a dilute solution of gadolinium needs to be injected into the joint until resistance is felt (usually 6–15 mL). Sterile premixed gadolinium-DTPA solutions are available for use in MR arthrography. Patients with an adhesive capsulitis may experience pain after much smaller amounts. If this is severe, then injection should be stopped. Resistance to injection is common, unlike injection into the knee, and more force is often required.

6. The needle is removed, and the joint is gently manipulated to distribute the contrast medium.

7. CT arthrography examination is performed with the patient supine and positioned slightly eccentrically within the scanner to ensure that the shoulder is as close to the centre of the scanner as possible. The contralateral arm can be elevated above the head to minimize image artefacts. Scanning should be undertaken during arrested respiration to minimize motion artefact.

8. The area of interest in both CT arthrography and MR arthrography should include the acromion to the axillary recess. MDCT provides high-quality reformatted images in the three planes, and MR images should also examine the joint in three planes. In addition when the arm is placed in the ABER position, there are tensioning of the inferior capsule–labral complex and relaxation of supraspinatus to optimally scan these structures for defects.

Posterior (fluoroscopic guided)

1. This approach is increasingly used because fewer soft tissues are traversed in accessing the joint, and many patients prefer not to look at the needle. The patient lies prone, with the side to be injected raised and the arm of the side under investigation close to the body, rotated midway between supination and pronation to relax the posterior capsule.

2. Using a sterile technique, the skin and soft tissues are anaesthetized at a point overlying the inferomedial quadrant of the humeral head within the boundary of the anatomical neck. The position of needle entry point is optimized by fluoroscopy.

3. A 21-gauge spinal needle is inserted vertically down onto the humeral head (Fig. 14.5). The vertical direction should aim for the inferomedial

14

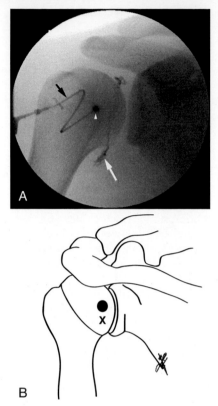

Fig. 14.5 Posterior fluoroscopic-guided approach for shoulder arthrography. The needle *(white arrow head shows the needle entry point)* is inserted vertically over the inferomedial quadrant of humeral head *(black arrow shows the connector to the needle and the white arrow shows the contrast within the joint)* **A,** Fluoroscopic image of the left shoulder. **B,** Diagram of the left shoulder. *x* indicates the site of entry into the joint.

quadrant of the humeral head within the boundary of the anatomical neck. The position of the needle should be checked by intermittent screening. When it meets the resistance of the articular surface of the humeral head, it is withdrawn by 1–2 mm to free the tip.

4. The intraarticular position of the needle is then confirmed by the injection of a small amount of the contrast medium under fluoroscopic control.

Posterior (ultrasound guided)

1. The patient can lie prone, in the same position as for fluoroscopy, or can also lie on their side with the affected side uppermost and the arm in neutral.

2. The posterior shoulder is scanned in transverse, visualizing the posterior joint capsule, labrum and overlying tendons. A point lateral to the long axis of the probe is marked as the entry site for the needle.

3. Using a sterile technique, the skin and soft tissues are anaesthetized immediately adjacent to the marked point. A 21-gauge spinal needle

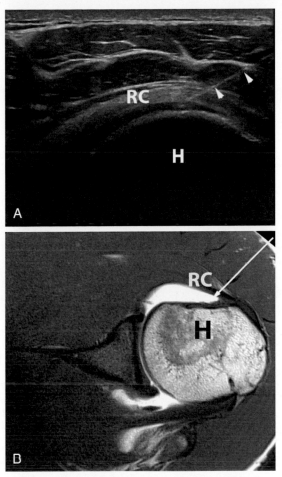

Fig. 14.6 Ultrasound-guided posterior shoulder approach. **A,** Posterior rotator cuff (RC) visualized with the needle *(arrowheads)* seen approaching from a lateral to the transducer onto the humeral head (H). **B,** Magnetic resonance arthrogram image demonstrating the anatomy seen in A with the *arrow* showing the path of the needle.

or long 20-gauge needle is inserted and advanced medially and obliquely down onto the humeral head (Fig. 14.6). The position of the needle should be confirmed with free flow of contrast on injection, which does not collect around the needle or periarticular soft tissues.

ELBOW

Technique

Single contrast

1. The patient sits next to the table with the elbow flexed and resting on the table, the lateral aspect uppermost. Alternatively, the patient lies prone on the table with the shoulder abducted above the head and elbow flexed (the 'superman' position).

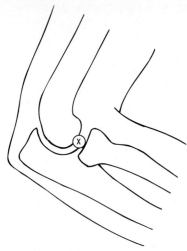

Fig. 14.7 Technique of elbow arthrography. *x* indicates the site of entry into the joint.

2. The radial head is located by palpation during gentle pronation and supination of the forearm. Using sterile technique, the skin and soft tissues are anaesthetized at a point just proximal to the radial head.
3. A 23-gauge needle is then inserted vertically down into the joint space between the radial head and the capitellum (Fig. 14.7).
4. An injection of a small volume of local anaesthetic will flow easily if the needle is correctly sited. This can be confirmed by the injection of a few drops of contrast medium under fluoroscopic control.
5. The remainder of the contrast medium (4–6 mL) is injected (iodinated for CT arthrography or dilute gadolinium for MR arthrography) until resistance is felt, and the joint is gently manipulated to distribute it evenly.

Double contrast

1. Position the patient as for single contrast technique and follow steps 1–4, given previously.
2. Inject 0.5 mL of contrast medium followed by 4–6 mL of air until the olecranon fossa is distended.

WRIST

Technique

Fluoroscopic guidance is usually performed, despite the availability of US for guidance because the iodinated contrast can give vital information on structural defects, which helps interpret the subsequent CT arthrography or MR arthrography.

Radiocarpal joint

1. The patient is seated next to the screening table with the forearm resting in a neutral prone position. Alternatively, the

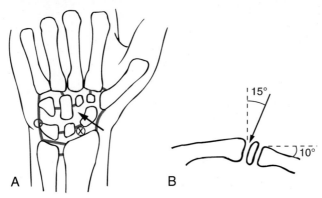

Fig. 14.8 Technique of wrist arthrography. **A,** Anteroposterior view. *x* indicates the point of entry to the radiocarpal joint. The *arrow* indicates the point of entry to the midcarpal joint. **B,** Lateral view. The *arrow* indicates the cranial angulation required for the needle with a dorsal approach to the radiocarpal joint.

patient can lie prone with the arm in the superman position (see the previous discussion of the elbow). The wrist should be supported over a wedge with about 10–15 degrees of flexion. Using a sterile technique, the skin and soft tissues are anaesthetized at a point over the midpoint of the scaphocapitate joint (Fig. 14.8).

2. A 23-gauge needle is inserted into the joint by advancing it downward, at an angle of about 15 degrees proximally toward the scaphoid.

3. Contrast medium (2–4 mL) is injected under fluoroscopic control; if any leakage occurs into the midcarpal joint or distal radioulnar joints, then spot views should be taken. If this is not done, it is possible to miss small tears that later become obscured by the anterior and posterior extensions of the radiocarpal joint. Unlike other joints, the wrist should not be maximally distended because the artefact from extravasation can markedly inhibit accurate assessment of intrinsic ligaments at the subsequent CT arthrography or MR arthrography.

Midcarpal joint

1. The wrist is positioned as for radiocarpal injection but with ulnar deviation because this widens the joint space.

2. The skin and soft tissues are anaesthetized at a point over the midpoint of the scaphocapitate joint (see Fig. 14.8).

3. A 23-gauge needle is inserted vertically into the joint space under fluoroscopic control.

4. Contrast medium (2 mL) is injected under fluoroscopic control, ideally with video-recording facility, until the joint space is full. Without continuous monitoring, it may not be possible to tell which of the ligaments separating the midcarpal from the radiocarpal joint are torn, allowing interarticular communication.

14

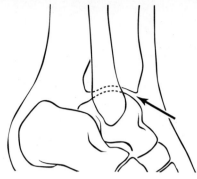

Fig. 14.9 Technique of ankle arthrography. The *arrow* shows the site of entry into the joint.

ANKLE

Technique

Fluoroscopic guided:

1. The patient lies in the lateral decubitus position with the ankle plantarflexed. An anterior approach is used with fluoroscopic guidance of the needle and the ankle in the true lateral projection (Fig. 14.9).
2. Using a sterile technique, the skin is anaesthetized at a point midway to the bimalleolar distance, which places the needle lateral to the dorsalis pedis artery.
3. A 21-gauge needle is inserted and advanced into the anterior joint space, and contrast medium is injected to confirm correct needle position and then to distend the joint (4–6 mL).

Further Reading

Knee

De Filippo M, Bertellini A, Pogliacomi F, et al. Multidetector CT arthrography of the knee: diagnostic accuracy and indications. *Eur J Radiol.* 2008;70(2): 342–351.

Kalke RJ, Di Primio GA, Schweitzer ME. MR and CT arthrography of the knee. *Semin Musculoskelet Radiol.* 2012;16(1):57–68.

Mutschler C, Vande Berg BC, Lecouvet FE, et al. Postoperative meniscus: assessment at dual detector row spiral CT arthrography of the knee. *Radiology.* 2003;228(3):635–641.

Radiographic Views in the Paediatric Hip Arthrogram

Aliabadi P, Baker ND, Jaramillo D. Hip arthrography, aspiration, block, and bursography. *Radiol Clin North Am.* 1998;36(4):673–690.

Devalia KL, Wright D, Sathyamurthy P, et al. Role of preoperative arthrography in early Perthes disease as a decision-making tool. Is it really necessary? *J Pediatr Orthop B.* 2007;16:196–200.

Grissom L, Harcke HT, Thacker M. Imaging in the surgical management of developmental dislocation of the hip. *Clin Orthop Relat Res.* 2008;466: 791–801.

Llopis E, Cerezal L. Direct MR arthrography of the hip with leg traction: feasibility for assessing articular cartilage. *AJR Am J Roentgenol.* 2008;190(4): 1124–1128.

Schmaranzer F, Kheterpal AB, Bredella MA. Best practices: hip femoroacetabular impingement. *AJR Am J Roentgenol.* 2021;216(3):585–598.

Talbot BS, Weinberg EP. MR imaging with metal-suppression sequences for evaluation of total joint arthroplasty. *Radiographics.* 2016;36(1):209–225.

Temmerman OP, Raijmakers PG, Deville WL, et al. The use of plain radiography, subtraction arthrography, nuclear arthrography, and bone scintigraphy in the diagnosis of a loose acetabular component of a total hip prosthesis: a systematic review. *J Arthroplasty.* 2007;22:818–827.

Shoulder

Chung CB, Dwek JR, Feng S, et al. MR arthrography of the glenohumeral joint: a tailored approach. *AJR Am J Roentgenol.* 2001;177(1):217–219.

Dépelteau H, Bureau NJ, Cardinal E, et al. Arthrography of the shoulder: a simple fluoroscopically guided approach for targeting the rotator cuff interval. *AJR Am J Roentgenol.* 2004;182(2):329–332.

Farmer KD, Hughes PM. MR arthrography of the shoulder: fluoroscopically guided technique using a posterior approach. *AJR Am J Roentgenol.* 2002;178(2):433–434.

Fritz J, Fishman EK, Fayad LM. MDCT arthrography of the shoulder. *Semin Musculoskelet Radiol.* 2014;18(4):343–351.

Gokalp G, Dusak A, Yazici Z. Efficacy of ultrasonography-guided shoulder MR arthrography using a posterior approach. *Skeletal Radiol.* 2010;39(6): 575–579.

Llopis E, Montesinos P, Guedez MT, et al. Normal shoulder MRI and MR arthrography: anatomy and technique. *Semin Musculoskelet Radiol.* 2015;19(3):212–230.

Sebro R, Oliveira A, Palmer WE. MR arthrography of the shoulder: technical update and clinical applications. *Semin Musculoskelet Radiol.* 2014;18(4): 352–364.

Elbow

Delport AG, Zoga AC. MR and CT arthrography of the elbow. *Semin Musculoskelet Radiol.* 2012;16(1):15–26.

Dubberley JH, Faber KJ, Patterson SD, et al. The detection of loose bodies in the elbow: the value of MRI and CT arthrography. *J Bone Joint Surg Br.* 2005;87:684–686.

LiMarzi GM, O'Dell MC, Scherer K, et al. Magnetic resonance arthrography of the wrist and elbow. *Magn Reson Imaging Clin N Am.* 2015;23(3):441–455.

Steinbach LS, Schwartz M. Elbow arthrography. *Radiol Clin North Am.* 1998;36(4):635–649.

Waldt S, Bruegel M. Comparison of multislice CT arthrography and MR arthrography for the detection of articular cartilage lesions of the elbow. *Eur Radiol.* 2005;15:784–791.

Wrist

Ali AH, Qenawy OK, Saleh WR, et al. Radio-carpal wrist MR arthrography: comparison of ultrasound with fluoroscopy and palpation-guided injections. *Skeletal Radiology.* 2022;51:765–775.

Cerezal L, de Dios Berna-Mestre J, Canga A, et al. MR and CT arthrography of the wrist. *Semin Musculoskelet Radiol.* 2012;16(1):27–41.

Joshy S, Ghosh S, Lee K, et al. Accuracy of direct MR arthrography in the diagnosis of triangular fibrocartilage complex tears of the wrist. *Int Orthop.* 2008;32:251–253.

14

Moser T, Dosch JC, Moussaoui A, et al. Wrist ligament tears: evaluation with MRI and combined MDCT and MR arthrography. *AJR Am J Roentgenol.* 2007;188:1278–1286.

Ankle

Cerezal L, Abascal F, García-Valtuille R, et al. Ankle MR arthrography: how, why and when? *Radiol Clin North Am.* 2005;43:693–707.

Schmid MR, Pfirrmann CW, Hodler J, et al. Cartilage lesions in the ankle joint: comparison of MR arthrography and CT arthrography. *Skeletal Radiol.* 2003;32:259–265.

TENDON IMAGING

Methods of Imaging Tendons

1. Tenography
2. US
3. CT
4. MRI

GENERAL POINTS

With the advent of CT, US and MRI, the indications for tenography (direct injection of contrast into the tendon sheath) are exceptionally rare. Although CT does show tendons and their relationship to joints and periarticular structures, US and MRI both show the intrinsic tendon structure and differentiate fluid within the sheath from the tendon. The higher resolution of US enables better depiction of internal architecture of superficial tendons. In addition, dynamic assessment to exclude subluxing tendons can be performed sonographically.

ULTRASOUND OF THE PAEDIATRIC HIP

See also Chapter 3.

Indications

1. Developmental dysplasia of the hip
2. Hip effusion
3. Slipped femoral capital epiphysis

Technique

Developmental dysplasia of the hip

With US, the unossified elements of the hip (femoral head, greater trochanter, labrum, triradiate cartilage), as well as the bony acetabular roof can be identified in the first 6 months of life.[1] After 9–12 months, the degree of ossification precludes adequate imaging by US, and plain film radiography becomes superior. There are two main methods, static and dynamic, both of which may be used during one examination.

Static (Graf) method

This assesses the morphology and geometry of the acetabulum. Although independent of the position of the infant, it is recommended that the infant be placed in the decubitus position. A single longitudinal image is obtained with the transducer placed over the greater trochanter and held at right angles to all the anatomical planes. The following landmarks are identified in the following sequence: chondro-osseous boundary between femoral shaft and head, joint capsule, labrum, cartilaginous roof and superior bony rim of the acetabulum. Although most images can be subjectively evaluated, angles can be measured from the image and form the basis for the Graf classification.

Dynamic method

This assesses the stability of the hip when stressed. The hip is studied in the coronal and axial planes with the infant supine. With the hip flexed and adducted, the femur is pushed and pulled with a piston-like action.[2]

Hip-joint effusion

Approximately 50% of children with acute hip pain have intraarticular fluid, and the sensitivity of US for detecting effusion approaches 100%.[3] With the child supine, the hip is scanned anteriorly with the transducer parallel to the femoral neck. Bulging of the anterior portion of the joint capsule can be readily identified.[4] The normal distance between the bony femoral neck and the joint capsule is always less than 3 mm, and the difference between the affected and unaffected sides should not be greater than 2 mm.

Slipped femoral capital epiphysis

Although plain radiographs constitute the usual means of diagnosis, a mild posterior slip can be identified in the acute situation by longitudinal scanning along the femoral neck.

References
1. Yousefzadeh DK, Ramilo JL. Normal hip in children: correlation of US with anatomic and cryomicrotome sections. *Radiology.* 1987;165:647–655.
2. Clarke NM, Harcke HT, McHugh P, et al. Real time ultrasound in the diagnosis of congenital dislocation and dysplasia of the hip. *J Bone Joint Surg Br.* 1985;67:406–412.
3. Dörr U, Zieger M, Hauke H. Ultrasonography of the painful hip. Prospective studies in 204 patients. *Pediatr Radiol.* 1988;19:36–40.
4. Miralles M, Gonzalez G, Pulpeiro JR, et al. Sonography of the painful hip in children: 500 consecutive cases. *AJR Am J Roentgenol.* 1989;152:579–582.

THERMOABLATION OF MUSCULOSKELETAL TUMOURS

14

Introduction

Image-guided interventional techniques are increasingly being used in treating patients with bone and soft tissue musculoskeletal tumours. Radiofrequency (RF) ablation is now the preferred treatment for osteoid osteomas, which are small painful benign tumours that can be difficult to locate at surgery. RF ablation also has a limited role in malignant disease for painful bone tumours[1] as an alternative to radiotherapy because it is more targeted and causes less injury to surrounding tissues. It is most commonly used for metastatic disease in the spine but also has a role elsewhere when surgical intervention is a limited option, with the pelvis being the next most common site. When RF ablation is used for malignant disease, it is usually combined with cementoplasty, which is the injection of cement into the area of bone ablation in the hope that this will provide some structural support.

In this brief section, RF treatment is primarily focused on the treatment of osteoid osteomas, but the basic principles apply to the treatment of malignant disease, although, depending on the size of the malignant tumour, multiple RF ablation needles may be required, and fluoroscopy is needed when the procedure is combined with cementoplasty.

Thermocoagulation

In RF thermal ablation, an alternating current of high-frequency radio waves (>10 KHz) is emitted from an electrode tip, and this dissipates its energy as heat within the surrounding tissues. The tissue around the electrode therefore generate the primary source of heat and not the electrode itself. In response to the RF stimulus, ions within local biological tissues vibrate, leading to ionic agitation. As a direct result of the ions' attempt to change direction with the alternating electrical current, friction is created around the electrode tip, creating heat, which desiccates the soft tissues—'thermal ablation'.[2] The amount of biological tissue that can be ablated is referred to as the 'treatment zone'. The size of the electrode tip will determine the treatment zone, with most commercially available systems offering a range of needles to cover ablation from 1.0–2.0 cm. Effective ablation in living bone is achieved with a temperature of 90°C at the active tip for 4–6 min.[3]

Indications

1. Osteoid osteoma
2. Osteoblastoma
3. Chondroblastoma
4. Metastasis

Rationale

Using CT guidance, the target is accurately localized, and its dimensions are determined. Using a coaxial needle system and drill, a biopsy can be taken and the tip of a thermoablation probe optimally placed in the centre of the lesion. The heat generated causes tumour necrosis over the diameter determined by the size of the electrode tip. Multiple RF probe placements via multiple skin entry points may be needed for large lesions.

Contraindications

1. Cardiac pacemakers are an absolute contraindication because they can be affected by the RF current.
2. Relative contraindications include lesions that are less than 1 cm to neighbouring peripheral nerves, spinal nerves and the spinal cord. Lesions in the hands and feet also have an additional increased risk of skin damage if they lack an adequate soft tissue cover.

Equipment

1. A coaxial bone penetration system that consists of an outer cannula, an inner stylet, a coaxial drill and a coaxial biopsy needle is used. The drill can be manually hand operated or electric.
2. An RF generator is the source of the electric current that passes to the electrode tip into the patient.
3. A single electrode tip is often used for osteoid osteomas. Selection of the correct sized electrode tip to cover the area of the lesion is an important part of the planning of the procedure.

Procedure

After the lesion has been localized by CT, radiopaque markers are placed on the skin. In planning the percutaneous needle route, the most direct path to the lesion with the needle angled perpendicular to the cortex is chosen, avoiding regional neurovascular structures. If this is not possible, a safer but longer route is chosen via the opposite normal cortex.

Because the procedure is painful, it is carried out under a general anaesthetic.

Using CT guidance, the cannula with its inner stylet is guided through the soft tissues to the cortical bone surface. The inner stylet is then replaced by the drill, and this is advanced sequentially through the cortex, ensuring an optimal intraosseous trajectory that is followed by CT spot images, until the tip of the drill reaches the cortical edge of the tumour.[4] The cannula is then advanced over the drill to maintain the position of the drilled intraosseous path, and the drill is removed.

Biopsy

The imaging characteristics of osteoid osteoma, osteoblastoma and chondroblastoma are characteristic, and a biopsy of the nidus is not usually required. Brodie's abscess, intracortical chondroma and stress fracture can mimic the radiological features of osteoid osteoma, and if there is any doubt about the diagnosis, then a biopsy is performed.

The biopsy needle is placed in the cannula and slowly advanced through the lesion, taking a biopsy after confirming that it has negotiated the tumour tissue by CT images.

14

Thermoablation

The RF electrode is passed into the cannula, and its tip is placed in the centre of the lesion. It is essential to partially withdraw the cannula (so that it lies more than 1 cm from the electrode tip) over the electrode to avoid the risk of heating adjacent tissue through contact with the metal cannula. These parameters are double checked by further CT spot images.

Thermal ablation is applied through the RF electrode, typically for a period of 4 minutes, with most modern RF ablation systems automatically adjusting the temperature and ablation time to ensure tissue necrosis occurs.

Post–Radiofrequency Ablation Care

1. Introduce local anaesthetic via the cannula after ablation
2. Sterile dressing
3. Oral analgesia
4. Discharge, usually the same day
5. Avoid strenuous activities if the lesion is in the lower limb for 3 months.
6. No imaging is required in follow-up unless symptoms recur.

Complications

1. Failed treatment can be caused by residual or recurrent tumour. The clinical success rate is greater than 90%[5] and is defined as the absence of pain for 2 years. A second RF ablation can be carried out if necessary.
2. Neural damage
3. Soft tissue necrosis
4. Osteonecrosis
5. Skin burns
6. Infection

References

1. Levy J, Hopkins T, Morris J, et al. Radiofrequency ablation for the palliative treatment of bone metastases: outcomes from the multicenter OsteoCool Tumor Ablation Post-Market Study (OPuS One Study) in 100 patients. *J Vasc Interv Radiol.* 2020;31(11):1745–1752.
2. Organ LW. Electrophysiologic principles of radiofrequency lesion making. *Appl Neurophysiol.* 1976;39(2):69–76.
3. Tillotson CL, Rosenberg AE, Rosenthal DI. Controlled thermal injury of bone: report of a percutaneous technique using radiofrequency electrode and generator. *Invest Radiol.* 1989;24(11):888–892.
4. Pinto CH, Taminiau AH, Vanderschueren GM, et al. Technical considerations in CT guided radiofrequency thermal ablation of osteoid osteoma: tricks of the trade. *AJR Am J Roentgenol.* 2002;179(6):1633–1642.
5. Rimondi E, Mavrogenis AF, Rossi G, et al. Radiofrequency ablation for non-spinal osteoid osteomas in 557 patients. *Eur Radiol.* 2012;22(1):181–188.

RADIONUCLIDE BONE SCAN

Indications

1. Staging of and response to therapy in osteoblastic cancers, especially breast and prostate*
2. Assessment and staging of primary bone tumours*
3. Painful orthopaedic prostheses to detect loosening*

4. Trauma not obvious on radiography such as stress fractures*
5. Assessment of extent multifocal disorders such as Paget's disease and fibrous dysplasia*
6. Bone or joint infection*
7. Detection and grading of cardiac amyloidosis*
8. Persistent bone pain with normal radiographs
9. Avascular necrosis and bone infarction
10. Assessment of non-accidental injury in children
11. Metabolic bone disease for complications such as fractures
12. Arthropathies such as rheumatoid
13. Reflex sympathetic dystrophy

*Common indications.

Contraindications
None

Radiopharmaceuticals
$99m$Tc-labelled diphosphonates such as methyl diphosphonate (MDP) or hydroxyethylidene disphosphonate (HDP) for bone pathology or 3,3-diphosphono-1,2-propanodicarboxylic acid (DPD) for cardiac amyloidosis, 500 MBq typical, 600 MBq maximum (3 mSv effective doses (EDs)). For SPECT, 800 MBq (4 mSv ED). Doses must be appropriately scaled down in paediatric patients based on weight by using resources such as the European Association of Nuclear Medicine (EANM) dosage card.

These compounds are phosphate analogues that bind with a high affinity to hydroxyapatite on native and new bone through chemical adsorption. They are rapidly excreted by the kidneys, providing a good contrast between bone and soft tissue. Bone uptake depends on perfusion, surface area and bone turnover.

Equipment
1. Gamma camera, usually with whole-body imaging with or without SPECT-CT
2. Low-energy high-resolution collimator

Patient Preparation
The patient must be well hydrated.

Technique
1. $99m$Tc-diphosphonate is injected IV. A three-phase study is then performed with arterial, blood-pool and delayed static imaging, although it is increasingly common to perform two phases only (blood pool and delayed). When infection is suspected or blood flow to bone or primary bone tumour is to be assessed, a bolus injection can be given with the patient in position on the camera.
2. The patient should be encouraged to drink plenty and empty the bladder frequently to minimize the radiation dose.

14

3. The bladder is emptied immediately before imaging to prevent obscuring the sacrum and bony pelvis.
4. Delayed static imaging is performed 2 hours or more after injection— up to 4 hours for imaging of extremities and up to 6 hours for patients on dialysis or in renal failure.

Images

Standard

High-resolution images are acquired with a pixel size of 1–2 mm:

1. The whole skeleton: The number of views depends upon the camera specifications, including field of view and whether a whole-body imaging facility is available. Whole-body images have lower resolution than spot views over parts of the skeleton where the camera is some distance from the patient because resolution falls off with distance, but this is less of an issue because almost all modern gamma camera systems have automatic body-contour tracking. Overlapping spot views can be obtained if patients cannot lie still for the duration of the whole-body imaging. Newer gamma cameras have improved detector efficiency, iterative reconstruction and resolution recovery software to reduce scan times, improve image quality and reduce noise.

    Additional non-standard views can be helpful in characterizing unusual foci of activity or when there are overlapping structures (e.g. anterior oblique views of the thorax to separate sternum and spine uptake, arms raised to move the scapula away from the ribs and lateral view to assess sacrum). More commonly, SPECT or SPECT-CT is being used instead of additional planar views to aid with anatomical localization, improve specificity by reducing false-positive results, increase resolution and improve diagnostic confidence.[1,2] In particular, SPECT-CT exploits the hybrid synergy of functional and structural imaging similar to PET-CT. An area of evolving use of SPECT-CT is in assessment of postoperative metalwork complications.[1,2]
2. For imaging small bones and joints, magnified views with pinhole collimation can be useful, but again, SPECT-CT is increasingly used to identify pain generators.

Three phases (most institutions now skip the arterial phase)

1. Arterial phase 1- to 2-s frames of the area of interest for 1 min after injection
2. Blood-pool phase 3-min image of the same area 5 min after injection
3. Delayed phase views 2 hours or more after injection, as for standard imaging

Analysis

1. For the arterial phase, time–activity curves can be created for regions of interest symmetrical about the midline.

2. For SPECT-CT, reconstruction is done of transaxial, coronal, sagittal and possibly oblique slices to demonstrate the lesion.

Additional Techniques

SPECT or SPECT-CT as detailed earlier.[1,2]

Aftercare

Normal radiation safety precautions (see Chapter 1).

Complications

None

Competing Modalities

^{18}F-FDG PET-CT (see Chapter 13) and whole-body MRI (e.g. with diffusion-weighted techniques) are increasingly competitive for oncological purposes and rheumatological conditions.[3] MRI is often preferred for localized orthopaedic applications, and recent advances in MRI techniques now allow excellent assessment of prosthesis.[4] Please see Chapter 13 for other scintigraphic modalities for the musculoskeletal system.

References

1. Waller M, Chowdhury FU. The basic science of nuclear medicine. *Orthop Trauma.* 2021;30(3):201–222.
2. Utsunomiya D, Shiraishi S, Imuta M, et al. Added value of SPECT/CT fusion in assessing suspected bone metastasis: comparison with scintigraphy alone and nonfused scintigraphy and CT. *Radiology.* 2006;238:264–271.
3. Sun G, Zhang Y-X, Liu F, et al. Whole-body magnetic resonance imaging is superior to skeletal scintigraphy for the detection of bone metastatic tumors: a meta-analysis. *Eur Rev Med Pharmacol Sci.* 2020;24(13):7240–7252.
4. Talbot BS, Weinberg EP. MR Imaging with metal-suppression sequences for evaluation of total joint arthroplasty. *Radiographics.* 2016;36(1):209–225.

Further Reading

Brooks M. The skeletal system. In: Sharp PF, Gemmell HG, Murray AD, eds. *Practical Nuclear Medicine.* 3rd ed. Springer-Verlag; 2005:143–161.
Lazzeri E, Bozzao A, Cataldo MA, et al. Joint EANM/ESNR and ESCMID-endorsed consensus document for the diagnosis of spine infection (spondylodiscitis) in adults. *Eur J Nucl Med Mol Imaging.* 2019;12:2464–2487.
Love C, Din AS, Tomas MB, et al. Radionuclide bone imaging: an illustrative review. *Radiographics.* 2003;23:341–358.
Waller M, Chowdhury FU. The basic science of nuclear medicine. *Orthop Trauma.* 2021;30(3):201–222.

14

Spine

James J. Rankine

Methods of Imaging the Spine

Many of the earlier imaging methods (e.g. conventional tomography, epidurography, epidural venography, discography) are now only of historical interest.

1. **Plain films:** These are widely available but with low sensitivity. They are of questionable value in chronic back pain because of the prevalence of degenerative changes in both symptomatic and asymptomatic individuals of all ages beyond the second decade. They are, however, useful in suspected spinal injury, spinal deformity and postoperative assessment.
2. **Myelography:** This is used when magnetic resonance imaging (MRI) is contraindicated or unacceptable to the patient. It is usually followed by computed tomography (CT) for detailed assessment of abnormalities (CT myelography (CTM)).
3. **Facet joint arthrography:** Pain of facet joint origin can be confirmed if it is abolished after diagnostic injection of local anaesthetic and treated by steroid instillation. The radiological appearances of the arthrogram are not helpful for the most part except in showing a communication with a synovial cyst. Vertical and contralateral facet joint communications can arise in the presence of pars interarticularis defects.
4. **Arteriography:** This is used for further study of vascular malformations shown by other methods, usually MRI, and for assessment for potential embolotherapy. It is not appropriate for the primary diagnosis of spinal vascular malformations. It may be used for preoperative embolization of vascular vertebral tumours (e.g. renal metastasis).
5. **Radionuclide imaging:** This is largely performed for suspected vertebral metastases and to exclude an occult painful bone lesion (e.g. osteoid osteoma) using a technetium scintigraphic agent, for which it is a sensitive and cost-effective technique.
6. **CT:** CT provides optimal detail of vertebral structures and is particularly useful in spinal trauma, spondylolysis, vertebral tumours, spinal deformity and postoperative states for the assessment of spinal fusion.

7. **MRI:** This is the preferred technique for virtually all spinal pathology. It is the only technique that directly images the spinal cord and nerve roots. MRI with intravenous gadolinium-DTPA (diethylenetriamine pentaacetic acid) may aid diagnosis in spinal infection, tumours and postoperative assessment.
8. **Ultrasound (US):** This is of use as an intraoperative method and has uses in the infant spine.

IMAGING APPROACH TO BACK PAIN AND SCIATICA

There are a variety of ways to image the spine, many of which are expensive. The role of the radiologist is to ensure that appropriate diagnostic algorithms are selected that promote diagnostic accuracy, clinical relevance and cost-effectiveness. Each diagnostic imaging procedure has a different degree of sensitivity and specificity when applied to a particular clinical problem. A combination of imaging techniques can be used in a complementary way to enhance diagnostic accuracy. The appropriate use of the available methods of investigating the spine is essential, requiring a sensible sequence and timing of the procedures to ensure cost-effectiveness, maximal diagnostic accuracy and clinical effectiveness with minimum discomfort to the patient.

The philosophy underlying the management of low back pain and sciatica encompasses the following fundamental points:

1. Radiological investigation is essential if surgery is proposed.
2. Radiological findings should be compatible with the clinical picture before surgery can be advised.
3. It is vital for the surgeon and radiologist to identify patients who will and who will not benefit from surgery.
4. In patients judged to be in need of surgical intervention, success is very dependent on precise identification of the site and the nature and extent of disease by the radiologist.
5. The demonstration of degenerative disease of the spine cannot be assumed to be the cause of the patient's symptoms because similar changes are often seen in asymptomatic individuals.

The need for radiological investigation of the lumbosacral spine is based on the findings of a thorough clinical examination. A useful and basic preliminary step, which will avoid unnecessary investigations, is to determine whether the predominant symptom is back pain or leg pain. Leg pain extending to the foot is suggestive of nerve root compression, and imaging needs to be directed toward the demonstration of a compressive lesion, typically disc prolapse. This is most commonly seen at the L4–L5 or L5–S1 levels (90%–95%), and MRI should be used as the primary mode of imaging. If the predominant symptom is back pain, imaging is not likely to be helpful because the presence of degenerative disc and facet disease demonstrated by plain films, CT or MRI has no direct correlation with the incidence of clinical symptomatology.

15

CONVENTIONAL RADIOGRAPHY

Radiographs are of most use in older adults for the detection of osteoporotic fractures, which can occur without any history of trauma. Progressive vertebral collapse and even vertebral body avascular necrosis can occur, leading to spinal deformity. The detection of a fracture with a minimal history of trauma should be an indication for performing bone densitometry.

A number of drug therapies are now available for treating patients with osteoporosis, so it is important to make the diagnosis.

In most other circumstances, routine radiographic evaluation at the initial assessment of a patient with acute low back pain does not usually provide clinically useful information. Eighty-five percent of such patients will return to work within 2 months, having received only conservative therapy, indicating the potential for non-contributory imaging. Despite the known limitations of radiographs, it is often helpful to obtain routine radiographs of the lumbar spine before another investigation is requested, and in these circumstances, the role of conventional radiographs can be summarized in the following points:

1. They assist in the diagnosis of conditions that can mimic mechanical or discogenic pain (e.g. infection, spondylolysis, ankylosing spondylitis and bone tumours), though in most circumstances, ^{99m}Tc scintigraphy, CT and MRI are more sensitive.
2. They serve as a technical aid to survey the vertebral column and spinal canal before myelography, CT or MRI, particularly in the sense of providing basic anatomical data regarding segmentation. Failure to do this may lead to errors in correctly interpreting the vertebral level of abnormalities before surgery.
3. Correlation of CT or MRI data with radiographic appearances is often helpful in interpretation, particularly in spinal deformity such as lumbar degenerative scoliosis, which can be difficult to appreciate on MRI sequences obtained in the sagittal plane.

COMPUTED TOMOGRAPHY AND MAGNETIC RESONANCE IMAGING OF THE SPINE

CT and MRI have replaced myelography as the primary method for investigating suspected disc prolapse. High-quality axial imaging by CT is an accurate means of demonstrating disc herniation, but in practice, many studies are less than optimal because of obesity, scoliosis and beam-hardening effects from dense bone sclerosis. For these reasons and because of better contrast resolution, MRI is the preferred technique, and CT is only used when MRI cannot be used. MRI alone has the capacity to show the morphology of the intervertebral disc and can show ageing changes, typically dehydration, in the nucleus pulposus. It provides sagittal sections, which have major advantages for the demonstration of the spinal cord and cauda equina, vertebral alignment and stenosis of the spinal canal and for showing the neural foramina. Far lateral disc herniation cannot be shown by myelography but is readily demonstrated by CT or MRI. CT may be preferred to MRI, when there is a suspected spinal injury, in the assessment of primary spinal tumours of bony origin and in the study of spondylolysis and Paget's disease. MRI in spinal stenosis provides all the required information, showing all the relevant levels on a single image, the degree of narrowing at each level and the secondary effects such as the distension of the vertebral venous plexus. The relative contributions of bone, osteophyte, ligament or disc, although better evaluated by CT, are usually unimportant in the management decisions with the exception of the cervical spine, where ossification of the posterior longitudinal may require a corpectomy surgical procedure (removal of a vertebral body) rather than an anterior cervical discectomy and fusion, which is frequently performed for cervical disc degeneration.

MRI can show conditions that may mimic spinal stenosis such as prolapsed thoracic disc, ependymoma of the conus medullaris and dural arteriovenous fistula.

In addition to the diagnosis of prolapsed intervertebral disc, CT and MRI differentiate the contained disc, in which the herniated portion remains in continuity with the main body of the disc, from the sequestrated disc, in which there is a free migratory disc fragment. This distinction can be crucial in the choice of conservative or surgical therapy and decision of percutaneous rather than open surgical techniques. MRI studies have shown that even massive extruded disc lesions can resolve naturally with time without intervention. Despite the presence of nerve root compression, a disc prolapse can be entirely asymptomatic, and careful clinical correlation is always required. Finally, in the decision as to whether to choose CT or MRI, it should be remembered that lumbar spine CT delivers a substantial radiation dose, which is important, particularly in younger patients.

The main remaining uses of myelography are in patients with claustrophobia or who have contraindications to MRI.

The problems of the 'postlaminectomy' patient or 'failed back surgery syndrome' are well known. Accurate preoperative assessment should limit the number of cases resulting from inappropriate surgery and surgery at the wrong level. The investigation of the postoperative lumbar spine is difficult, and reoperation has a poor outcome in many cases. Although the investigation of the postoperative lumbar spine is difficult, it is vital to make the distinction between residual or recurrent disc prolapse at the operated level and epidural fibrosis to minimize the risk of a negative reexploration. The best available technique is gadolinium-enhanced MRI.

Arachnoiditis is a cause of postoperative symptoms, and its features are shown on myelography, CTM and MRI. In the past, many cases were caused by the use of myodil (Pantopaque) as a myelographic contrast medium. It is likely that the use of myodil as an intrathecal contrast agent caused arachnoiditis in most cases, but only a minority of these became symptomatic. The potentiating effects of blood in the cerebrospinal fluid (CSF), particularly as a result of surgery, have been evident in many cases. New cases of arachnoiditis are now rarely seen, but there is still residue of chronic disease presenting from time to time.

Conclusions

MRI has revolutionized the imaging of spinal disease. Advantages include non-invasiveness, multiple imaging planes and a lack of radiation exposure. Its superior soft tissue contrast enables the distinction of nucleus pulposus from annulus fibrosus of the healthy disc and enables the early diagnosis of degenerative changes. However, up to 35% of asymptomatic individuals younger than 40 years of age have significant intervertebral disc disease at one or more levels on MR images. Therefore, correlation with the clinical evidence is essential before any relevance is attached to their presence and surgery is undertaken.

Further Reading

Boden SD, Davis DO, Dina TS, et al. Abnormal magnetic resonance scans of the lumbar spine in asymptomatic subjects. *J Bone Joint Surg Am.* 1990;72(3):403–408.

Butt WP. Radiology for back pain. *Clin Radiol.* 1989;40(1):6–10.

Cribb GL, Jaffray DC, Cassar-Pullicino VN. Observations on the natural history of massive lumbar disc herniation. *J Bone Joint Surg Br.* 2007;89(6):782–784.

du Boulay GH, Hawkes S, Lee CC, et al. Comparing the cost of spinal MR with conventional myelography and radiculography. *Neuroradiology.* 1990;32(2):124–136.

Horton WC, Daftari TK. Which disc as visualized by magnetic resonance imaging is actually a source of pain? A correlation between magnetic resonance imaging and discography. *Spine (Phila PA 1976).* 1992;17(suppl 6):S164–S171.

Hueftle MG, Modic MT, Ross JS, et al. Lumbar spine: post-operative MR imaging with gadolinium-DTPA. *Radiology.* 1988;167(3):817–824.

MYELOGRAPHY

CONTRAST MEDIA

Modern water-soluble non-ionic iodine contrast agents are very safe in the thecal sac and have not been implicated as a cause of arachnoiditis in the way that early oil-based media were. As with the use of iodine contrast in vascular studies, a history of allergy to iodine may be a contraindication to their use.

CERVICAL MYELOGRAPHY

This is usually performed by introduction of contrast medium into the thecal sac by lumbar puncture and then run up to the cervical spine. Very rarely, a direct cervical puncture at C1–C2 is required.

Indications

Suspected spinal cord pathology or root compression in patients unable or unwilling to undergo MRI.

Lateral Cervical C1–C2 Puncture versus Lumbar Injection

Historically, cervical puncture was frequently performed as a reliable method of getting a sufficient density of contrast into the cervical region to allow diagnostic-quality radiographs, which were performed on the fluoroscopy table. Currently, myelography is always followed by CT, which allows a diagnosis to be made with reduced density of contrast. The dilution of contrast with the patient's CSF, rather than proving a problem for obtaining diagnostic-quality images, is an advantage because it allows imaging of the entire spine to be performed. Cervical myelography is therefore most easily and safely performed as a lumbar injection at the level of the cauda equina and then running the contrast up into the cervical region.

Cervical puncture is indicated when there is severe lumbar disease, which may restrict the flow of contrast medium and may make lumbar puncture difficult, and when there is thoracic spinal canal stenosis. It may also be required for the demonstration of the upper end of a spinal block. It is a relatively safe procedure but is contraindicated in patients with suspected high cervical or craniocervical pathology and where the normal bony anatomy and landmarks are distorted or lost by anomalous development or rheumatoid disease. Complications are rare but include vertebral artery damage and inadvertent cord puncture.

Contrast Medium

Non-ionic contrast medium is used with a total dose not exceeding 3 g of iodine (i.e. 10 mL of contrast medium with a concentration of 300 mg mL^{-1}).

Equipment

Tilting x-ray table with a C-arm fluoroscopic facility for screening and radiography in multiple planes.

Patient Preparation

Mild sedation with oral diazepam is appropriate in anxious patients but is not essential. The skin puncture point is outside the hair line, and no hair removal is generally needed, though the hair should be gathered into a paper cap.

Technique

1. The patient lies prone with arms at the sides and chin resting on a soft pad so that the neck is in a neutral position or in slight extension. Marked hyperextension is undesirable because it accentuates patient discomfort, particularly in those with spondylosis, who are the majority of patients referred for this procedure. In such cases it will further compromise a narrowed canal and may produce symptoms of cord compression. The patient must be comfortable and able to breathe easily.

2. Using lateral fluoroscopy, the C1–C2 space is identified. The beam should be centred at this level to minimize errors caused by parallax. Head and neck adjustments may be needed to ensure a true lateral position. The aim is to puncture the subarachnoid space between the laminae of C1 and C2 at the junction of the middle and posterior thirds of the spinal canal (i.e. posterior to the spinal cord). A 22-gauge spinal needle is used. The needle is inserted in the midline, with periodic screening in both planes to monitor the correct approach. As with single passes of thin-gauge needles elsewhere in interventional procedures, the injection of lignocaine into the subcutaneous tissues is not indicated because the pressure effect of the injected fluid causes more discomfort than the single passage of a needle. Anaesthetizing the tract of the needle approach is only ever indicated if the approach is to be followed by the passage of a wide-gauge needle, such as a biopsy needle.

3. The sensation of the needle penetrating the dura is similar to that experienced during a lumbar puncture, and the patient may experience slight discomfort at this stage. A feature that indicates that the needle tip is close to the dura is the appearance of venous blood at the needle hub as the epidural space is traversed. Severe acute neck or radicular pain indicates that the needle has been directed too far anteriorly and has come into contact with an exiting nerve root. Clumsy technique is known to have caused cord puncture, but permanent neurological damage as a result is unlikely.

4. After removal of the stilette, CSF will drip from the end of the needle, and a sample may be collected if clinically required.

5. Under fluoroscopy, a small amount of contrast medium is injected to verify correct needle-tip placement. This will flow away from the needle tip and gravitate anteriorly to layer behind the vertebral bodies. Transient visualization of the dentate ligaments is obtained.

6. Injection is continued slowly until the required amount has been delivered. The cervical canal should be opacified anteriorly from the foramen magnum to C7–T1. If contrast tends to flow into the head before filling the lower cervical canal, tilt the table feet down slightly and vice versa if contrast is flowing into the thoracic region without filling the upper cervical canal.

Radiographic Views

After needle withdrawal, two anteroposterior (AP) radiographs are obtained, with the tube angulated cranially and caudally in turn along with both oblique views once again with cranial and caudal tube tilt. Soft and penetrated lateral views are needed to ensure full assessment of the cervicothoracic junction. Last, a further lateral view of the craniocervical junction is taken with mild neck flexion because the extended neck position may prevent full visualization of the upper cervical cord up to the foramen magnum. CT is then performed with sagittal and cranial reformats, which provides cross-sectional information equivalent to an MRI examination.

Aftercare

Although many centres request the patient to remain sitting or semi-recumbent for about 6 h, allowing the patient to remain ambulant does not increase the incidence of side effects. A high fluid intake is generally encouraged, although evidence for its efficacy is lacking.

LUMBAR MYELOGRAPHY

This may be performed by injection of contrast medium into the lumbar thecal sac. If for any reason lumbar puncture is not possible (e.g. because of lumbar spine deformity or arachnoiditis), it is possible to introduce the contrast medium from above by cervical injection.

Indications

Suspected lumbar root or cauda equina compression, spinal stenosis and conus medullaris lesions in patients who are unable or unwilling to undergo MRI.

Contraindications

Lumbar puncture is potentially hazardous in the presence of raised intracranial pressure. It may be difficult to achieve satisfactory intra-thecal injection in patients who have had a recent lumbar puncture because subdural CSF accumulates temporarily, and this space may be entered rather than the subarachnoid space. Accordingly, an interval of 1 week or so is advisable.

Contrast Medium

The contrast medium is the same as that used for cervical myelography. The maximum dose is again the equivalent of 3 g of iodine and may be given as 10 mL of contrast medium of 300 mg mL^{-1} concentration, or 12.5 mL of 240 mg mL^{-1}.

Equipment

Tilting fluoroscopic table

Patient Preparation

As for cervical myelography

Preliminary Images

AP and lateral projections of the region under study are taken. Preliminary examination of radiographs is helpful to assess the anatomy of the spine, facilitate the lumbar puncture and assist in interpretation of the images. It is important to draw the surgeon's attention to any question of ambiguous segmentation, either lumbarization or sacralization. There is a potential danger of operating at the wrong level if this is not made explicitly clear in the report. A clear description of any anomaly is required, together with a statement of how the vertebrae have been numbered in the report.

Technique

1. The lumbar thecal sac is punctured at L2–L3, L3–L4 or L4–L5. The higher levels tend to be away from the most common sites of disc herniation and stenosis; therefore, puncture may be easier. In the presence of previous laminectomy decompression, there is a temptation to pass the needle directly into the dura through the laminectomy site because there is no bone to impede the passage of the needle. This temptation should be resisted for a number of reasons. There is likely to be considerable scar tissue, which can deflect the needle's path. The position of the dura is not predictable, possibly lying more posterior than expected if it has prolapsed through the laminectomy site, or it may be reduced in size and distorted by epidural fibrosis. The normal feeling of a 'give' that the operator experiences as the needle passes through the ligamentum flavum into the epidural space is lost, so there is no way of knowing that the needle is about to enter the dura. For all these reasons, it is always advisable to introduce the needle into the spine away from the site of previous surgery.

2. Lumbar puncture can technically be performed in the lateral decubitus position, in the sitting position or in the prone position. In the prone position, the needle is guided under fluoroscopy, usually at the L2–L3 interspinous space with the patient lying on a folded pillow. This is important because in the prone position, the spinous processes are approximated because of lordosis, rendering puncture more difficult. In addition, spinal extension produces a relatively narrow thecal sac. The sitting position is not advisable because it renders the patient prone to fainting. Lumbar puncture is most easily performed in the lateral decubitus position because the interspinous space can be maximally widened with as much spinal flexion as possible within the confines of a narrow fluoroscopy table. The disadvantage of this position is that gravity acts on the needle, tending to drift it off from the midline. The needle is no longer deflected by gravity when it is well into the interspinous ligament, but by then, it is already on a path that the operator has a very limited ability to alter. It is at the point when the needle has just been passed through the skin into the subcutaneous tissue when it is most mobile and the correct path of approach needs to be taken, which coincides with the point when the needle will maximally deflect to the floor if not held in position. The needle should be held with long sterile forceps, which allows the position of the needle to be altered under real-time fluoroscopy without

irradiating the operator's hand. Screening the patient AP will help ensure the needle does not drift off the midline, whilst lateral screening ensures a clear path between the spinous processes, a position that usually requires a slight degree of cranial angulation. When the needle is well embedded in the interspinous ligament, only the position of the bevel will influence its direction. The bevel should point either cranially or caudally to prevent deflection of the needle from the midline. If the needle is drifting too far cranially with risk of hitting the superior lamina, the bevel should be directed cranially, which will deflect the needle away from the bone and vice versa if the needle is drifting caudally.

3. There is a characteristic sudden loss of resistance as the needle passes through the ligamentum flavum into the epidural space. Too cautious advancement of the needle from this point can result in the dura tenting over the needle and injection into the epidural space, in a position where the dural space would usually be expected. It is best at this point to make a brisk advancement of the needle with one push of a centimetre or so; grasping the needle at the required distance from the skin surface will prevent it being pushed in farther than intended. The position aimed for is within the centre of the spinal canal.

4. The central stylet is withdrawn, and dripping of CSF from the needle confirms an intradural position. If the needle has been inserted at a level of spinal stenosis, crowding of nerve roots around the needle tip may prevent the flow of CSF, and gently rotating the needle may result in CSF flow. In any event, if the position of the tip appears satisfactory, cautious injection of contrast under fluoroscopy is performed via a flexible connector, which reduces the chance of disturbing the position of the needle and gets the injecting hand away from the fluoroscopy beam. Flow of contrast away from the needle tip confirms an intradural injection.

5. After the contrast medium has been injected, the patient turns to lie prone, and a series of films is obtained. Before taking films, ensure that the relevant segment of the spinal canal is adequately filled with the contrast medium. This usually requires some degree of feet-down tilt of the table, and a footrest should be in place to support the patient.

Radiographic Views

1. AP and oblique views are obtained. (About 25 degrees of obliquity is typical, but this should be tailored in the individual case to profile the exit sleeves of the nerve roots of the cauda equina.)

2. A lateral view with a horizontal beam is useful, but further laterals in the erect or semierect position on flexion and extension add a dynamic dimension to the study.

Additional Technique

As with all myelography, the examination is followed immediately by thoracic CTM.

THORACIC MYELOGRAPHY

If the thoracic spine is the primary region of interest, the lumbar puncture injection is made with the patient lying on one side, with the head of the table lowered and the patient's head supported on a bolster or pad to prevent contrast medium from running up into the head. If an obstruction to flow is anticipated, about half the volume of contrast medium may be injected and observed as it flows upward. If an obstruction is encountered, the contrast medium is allowed to accumulate against it, and the remainder of the contrast medium is then injected slowly. (This may cause some discomfort or pain, and patience must be used.) This manoeuvre will, in some cases, cause a little of the contrast medium to flow past the obstructing lesion and demonstrate its superior extent. If there is no obstruction, the full volume is injected. When the injection is complete, lateral radiographs may be taken, and the patient is then turned to lie supine. Further AP views are then taken.

CERVICAL MYELOGRAPHY BY LUMBAR INJECTION

The technique proceeds as for thoracic myelography, but the patient remains in the lateral decubitus position until the contrast medium has entered the neck. With the head raised on a pad or bolster, contrast will not flow past the foramen magnum. When all the contrast has reached the neck, the patient is turned to lie prone, and the study is then completed as for a cervical injection study.

COMPUTED TOMOGRAPHY MYELOGRAPHY

In the early days of CT, CTM had to be delayed for up to 4 h after injection to allow dilution of the contrast medium because beam-hardening artefacts occurred because of the density of the contrast. This is not a problem with the current generation of CT scanners, and the CT scan takes place immediately after the injection, provided the patient is rotated a few times to ensure an even distribution and reduce layering effects. The normal lumbar lordosis can present difficulties if the CT scan is performed in the supine position because the contrast layers in the sacrum and thoracic spine away from the lumbar region. This can be prevented by performing the lumbar CT in the prone position. The need for the prone position should be evident to the radiologist at the time of the myelogram by observing the position of the contrast column with the patient lying supine on the fluoroscopy table.

If there is a complete block to the contrast column, then delayed imaging should be performed because the contrast will often pass across through the block and show the full extent of the obstruction. If the block is distal, patients can sit upright for a few hours, and if the block is proximal, they can lie head down on a tilting trolley. Delayed CT is needed in suspected syringomyelia.

PAEDIATRIC MYELOGRAPHY

A few points need to be considered when carrying out myelography in the paediatric age group:

1. General anaesthetic is essential for all children aged 6 years or younger and for many children up to the age of 12 years.
2. Lumbar puncture in cases of spinal dysraphism carries the risk of damaging a low-lying cord because of tethering. The thecal sac is usually wide in these conditions, and the needle should be placed laterally in the thecal sac. In addition, as low a puncture as possible will minimize the risk, though in practice, spinal cord injury is very uncommon or masked by the neurologic deficit already present.
3. In dysraphism, the frequent association of cerebellar tonsillar herniation precludes lateral C1–C2 puncture.

Aftercare

Most patients may be discharged home after being allowed to rest for a few hours following the study. The practice of automatic hospitalization for myelography can no longer be justified in light of improved contrast media with very low rates of serious morbidity. The patient may remain ambulant. A good fluid intake is generally advised, though its value is unproven.

Complications

1. Headache occurs in about 25% of cases and is slightly more frequent in female patients.
2. Nausea and vomiting occur in about 5%.
3. Subdural injection of contrast medium occurs when only part of the needle bevel is within the subarachnoid space. Contrast medium initially remains loculated near the end of the needle but can track freely in the subdural space to simulate intrathecal flow. When in doubt, the injection should be stopped and AP and lateral views obtained with the needle in situ. The temptation to interpret such an examination should be resisted and the patient rebooked.
4. Extradural injection of contrast medium outlines the nerve roots well beyond the exit foramina.
5. Intramedullary injection of contrast medium is a complication of lateral cervical puncture or in a low-lying spinal cord and is recognized as a slitlike collection of contrast medium in the spinal canal. Small collections are without clinical significance.
6. Infection with meningitis is a very rare complication occurring 2–3 days after the procedure. It is an important complication to ensure the patient is aware of during consent for the procedure because symptoms would present well after the patient has left the hospital.

FACET JOINT AND MEDIAL BRANCH BLOCKS

15

Indications

Facet joint and medial branch blocks are both procedures used as a treatment for back pain originating from degenerative facet joints. A facet joint injection is an injection directly into the joint, whereas a medial branch block involves injecting the pericapsular soft tissues, which is the site of the nerve that supplies the joint. There is no evidence to support one procedure over the other, and both can only give temporary relief of symptoms. An injection can also be performed to treat neural compression caused by a facet joint cyst. In this situation, the needle needs to be placed intraarticularly.

Equipment

1. As for myelography
2. A 22-gauge spinal needle

Technique

1. The patient is placed in the prone position on the fluoroscopy table. The C-arm is rotated approximately 20 degrees to the side of the joint to be injected to visualize the joint in profile.
2. The spinal needle is inserted in the plane of the C-arm so that the fluoroscopy looks 'down the eye of the needle'. In the majority of cases, a noticeable 'give' indicates that the capsule is penetrated.
3. Contrast medium injection confirms correct intraarticular placement, but because there is no evidence for an increased effect for intraarticular injection over pericapsular injection, this is not required routinely. Contrast is only required to confirm intraarticular placement if the injection is being performed to treat a facet joint cyst.
4. The facet joint is injected with a long-acting steroid, such as triamcinolone 40 mg, and 0.5 mL of lignocaine 1%.

Further Reading

Fairbank JC, Park WM, McCall IW, et al. Apophyseal injection of local anaesthetic as a diagnostic aid in primary low back syndromes. *Spine (Phila PA 1976)*. 1981;6:598–605.

Maldague B, Mathurin P, Malghem J. Facet joint arthrography in lumbar spondylolysis. *Radiology*. 1981;140(1):29–36.

McCall IW, Park WM, O'Brien JP. Induced pain referral from posterior lumbar elements in normal subjects. *Spine (Phila PA 1976)*. 1979;4(5):441–446.

Mooney V, Robertson J. The facet syndrome. *Clin Orthop Relat Res*. 1976;115:149–156.

PERCUTANEOUS VERTEBRAL BIOPSY

The percutaneous approach to obtaining a representative sample of tissue for diagnosis before therapy is both easy and safe, avoiding the morbidity associated with open surgery. It has a success rate of around 90%. Accurate lesion localization before and during the procedure is required. Vertebral body lesions may be biopsied under either CT or fluoroscopic control. Small lesions, especially those located in the posterior neural arch, are best biopsied under CT control. A preliminary CT scan is helpful, whatever method is finally chosen to control the procedure.

Indications

Suspected vertebral or disc infection and vertebral neoplasia. Note that the presence of a more accessible lesion in the appendicular skeleton should be sought by radionuclide bone scanning or assessment of the bones on a staging CT before vertebral biopsy is undertaken.

Contraindications

Biopsy should not be attempted under any circumstances in the presence of abnormal and uncorrected bleeding or clotting time or if there is a low platelet count.

Equipment

Numerous types of biopsy needle are available, all with the same basic design of a hollow needle with a serrated cutting edge that has a coned tip to aid retrieval of the sample.

Patient Preparation

The procedure can usually be carried out as a day case.

Analgesia and, when necessary, sedation or general anaesthesia are required, preferably administered and monitored by an anaesthetist.

Technique

1. The patient is placed prone for the fluoroscopy- and CT-guided procedures. The skin entry point distances from the midline are about 8 cm for the lumbar region and 5 cm in the thoracic region.
2. If the lesion to be biopsied is in the vertebral body, this can be approached via a direct posterolateral approach through the paravertebral soft tissues. In the thoracic spine, it is safer to go down the pedicle because there is only a very narrow soft tissue plane paravertebrally because of the lungs.
3. Some bone biopsy needles, such as the Bonopty system, have an introducer with a drill that allows an outer guide to be advanced through normal bone and placed adjacent to the lesion. This allows the biopsy to be taken directly from the lesion and prevents a situation in which normal bone can become impacted in the needle, impairing sampling of a lesion more distally, which may be of considerably softer density than normal bone.
4. The biopsy needle is advanced through the lesion using a clockwise rotation, having first withdrawn the central stylet. The needle is then withdrawn while simultaneous suction is applied by a syringe attached to the hub.

5. To remove the specimen, the plunger is inserted at the sharp end of the needle, and the tissue is pushed out. Any blood clot should be included as part of the specimen.

6. In suspected infection, the end plate rather than the disc should be biopsied because all cases of discitis start as osteomyelitis within the end plate. If there is a paravertebral abscess, aspiration and culture of its contents is preferable to vertebral biopsy.

15

Aftercare

The patient can usually be discharged after a few hours of monitoring vital signs and inspection of the skin site.

Complications

These are rare, but there are potential risks to nearby structures in poorly controlled procedures, including the lung and pleura, aorta, nerve roots and spinal cord. Local bleeding is an occasional problem.

Further Reading

Babu NV, Titus VT, Chittaranjan S, et al. Computed tomographically guided biopsy of the spine. *Spine (Phila PA 1976)*. 1994;19(21):2436–2442.

Rankine JJ, Barron DA, Robinson P, et al. The therapeutic impact of percutaneous spinal biopsy in spinal infection. *Postgrad Med J*. 2004;80:607–609.

Shaltot A, Michell PA, Betts JA, et al. Jamshidi needle biopsy of bone lesions. *Clin Radiol*. 1982;33:193–196.

Stoker DJ, Kissin CM. Percutaneous vertebral biopsy: a review of 135 cases. *Clin Radiol*. 1985;36:569–577.

Tehranzadeh J, Tao C, Browning CA. Percutaneous needle biopsy of the spine. *Acta Radiol*. 2007;48(8):860–868.

BONE AUGMENTATION TECHNIQUES

The vertebral bodies can collapse in osteoporosis and metastatic disease. The injection of small amounts of bone cement directly into the vertebral body (vertebroplasty) strengthens the vertebral body and is successful in the control of spinal pain. Preprocedure radiographs and an MRI scan are obtained, while a spinal surgeon is on standby in case any complications require surgical intervention. Multiple levels can be treated in this manner, with placement of the needle in the vertebral body using either a transpedicular approach or a posterolateral approach. The approach and needle insertion technique are as described for vertebral body bone biopsy. Careful aseptic technique and fluoroscopic or CT guidance during cement injection are essential to avoid cement migration into the canal or veins. In addition, an allied technique (kyphoplasty) partially restores vertebral body height in osteoporotic vertebral fractures.

Further Reading

Burton AW, Rhines LD, Mendel E. Vertebroplasty and kyphoplasty: a comprehensive review. *Neurosurg Focus*. 2005;18(3):e1.

Hide IG, Gangi A. Percutaneous vertebroplasty: history, technique and current perspectives. *Clin Radiol*. 2004;59(6):461–467.

NERVE ROOT BLOCKS

LUMBAR SPINE

This is undertaken in difficult diagnostic cases, usually in the presence of multilevel pathology, especially in postoperative situations. If local anaesthetic injected in the associated perineural space abolishes the patient's symptoms, it is concluded that pain is originating from the injected nerve root. Therapeutic instillation of local anaesthetic with steroids (e.g. triamcinolone, betamethasone (Celestone Soluspan)) has proved successful as a means of treating sciatica in patients with disc prolapse, especially in a foraminal location. It is crucial that the MR images are reviewed immediately before the procedure, to confirm that the correct level and side are in accordance with the patient's symptoms. The objective is to place the needle *outside* the nerve root sleeve, so that the injected substances diffuse between the disc prolapse and the compressed nerve. Reduction of the inflammatory response induced by the herniated disc can be slow, and improvement of symptoms can take up to 8–12 weeks.

The accurate placement of the tip of a spinal needle is confirmed by the injection of a small amount of contrast medium. This is important to avoid injection in one of the lumbar vessels because, rarely, paraplegia presumed to be caused by inadvertent intraarterial injection has been reported. This risk needs to be communicated in the informed consent with the patient before the procedure.

The needle is advanced using fluoroscopic or CT guidance to a point inferior and lateral to the ipsilateral pedicle. The extraforaminal nerve roots are outlined by contrast medium and injected with 0.5 mL of 1% lignocaine and steroid.

CERVICAL SPINE

Perineural root sleeve therapy can also be used in cervical radiculopathy. Correct needle placement confirmation using CT and fluoroscopy contrast medium injection is very important before the therapeutic injection of lignocaine and steroids. There is a real risk of inadvertent vascular injection, particularly into the vertebral artery. CT fluoroscopic guidance at the required foraminal level is used to ensure the needle traverses in a horizontal or slightly downward course, posterior to the carotid and jugular vessels. The needle tip is aimed toward the outer rim of the posterior bone outline of the foramen so as to avoid the vertebral vessels and the nerve root.

Further Reading
Blankenbaker DG, De Smet AA, Stanczak JD, et al. Lumbar radiculopathy: treatment with selective lumbar nerve blocks. Comparison of effectiveness of triamcinolone and betamethasone injectable suspensions. *Radiology.* 2005;237(2):738–741.

Herron LD. Selective nerve root block in patient selection for lumbar surgery: surgical results. *J Spinal Disord.* 1989;2(2):75–79.

Schellhas KP, Pollei SR, Johnson BA, et al. Selective cervical nerve root blockade: experience with a safe and reliable technique using an anterolateral approach for needle placement. *AJNR Am J Neuroradiol.* 2007;28(10):1909–1914.

Wagner AL. CT fluoroscopic-guided cervical nerve root blocks. *AJNR Am J Neuroradiol.* 2005;26(1):43–44.

Wagner AL. Selective lumbar nerve root blocks with CT fluoroscopic guidance: technique, results, procedure time, and radiation dose. *AJNR Am J Neuroradiol.* 2004;25(9):1592–1594.

Weiner BK, Fraser RD. Foraminal injection for lateral lumbar disc herniation. *J Bone Joint Surg Br.* 1997;79(5):804–807.

Brain/Neuro

Amit Herwadkar

Methods of Imaging the Brain

Imaging the brain's structure and examining its physiology, both in the acute and elective settings, are now the domain of multiplanar, computer-assisted imaging. The imaging modalities in use today include the following:

1. **Computed tomography (CT):** This is the technique of choice for the investigation of serious head injury for suspected intracranial haemorrhage (ICH), stroke, infection and other acute neurological emergencies. CT is quick, efficient and safer to use in the emergency situation than magnetic resonance imaging (MRI).

2. **MRI:** This is the best and most versatile imaging modality for the brain, constrained only by availability, patient acceptability and the logistics and safety of patient handling in emergency situations. New protocols and higher-field-strength magnets have raised the sensitivity of MRI in epilepsy imaging, acute stroke, aneurysm detection and follow-up posttreatment of neoplastic and vascular disorders. It is the only effective way of diagnosing multiple sclerosis.

3. **Angiography:** This is very important in ICH, especially subarachnoid haemorrhage (SAH), and is essential in intraarterial management of ischaemic stroke. However with the widespread availability of multidetector CT (MDCT) scanners, CT angiography (CTA) is now preferentially used in ischaemic stroke, SAH and ICH. Catheter angiography is still requested for preoperative assessment of tumours and vascular malformations, and angiographic expertise is vital for the performance of many neurointerventional procedures.

4. **Radionuclide imaging:** There are two principal methods. The first is regional cerebral blood flow scanning, which is now regularly used, especially in the investigation of dementia and movement disorders such as Parkinsonism; the second is positron emission tomography (PET). PET can assess focal hypermetabolism using ^{18}F fluorodeoxyglucose ([18]FDG), for example, in epilepsy, and cell turnover may also be shown using ^{11}C-methionine, for example, in tumour studies.

5. **Ultrasound (US):** This is particularly helpful in neonates and during the first year of life to image haemorrhagic and ischaemic syndromes, developmental malformations and hydrocephalus

using the fontanelles as acoustic windows. In adults, transcranial Doppler may be used for intracerebral arterial velocity studies to assess the severity of vasospasm.

6. **Plain films of the skull.** These are of little value except in reviewing shunt settings in patients with intracranial shunts.

COMPUTED TOMOGRAPHY OF THE BRAIN

Indications

CT is the imaging modality that is most commonly used in triaging acute neurological disease. For non-emergency indications, CT is inferior to MR, which has superior tissue contrast and is only used when MR is unavailable or contraindicated. The indications include the following:

1. After major head injury (if the patient has lost consciousness, has impaired consciousness or has a neurological deficit). The presence of a skull fracture also justifies the use of CT. National Institute for Health and Care Excellence (NICE) guidance has been issued on the use of imaging for head injuries for adults and children, specifically CT, listing the criteria for assessment based on best relevant data and consensus recommendations.
2. People who attend an emergency department with head injury if they are taking anticoagulants but have no other risk factors for brain injury.
3. In suspected intracranial infection (the use of contrast enhancement is recommended).
4. For suspected ICH and cases of ischaemic and haemorrhagic stroke. These can be combined with vascular imaging. In patients with SAH, the source of bleed can be identified for treatment planning. In patients with ischaemic stroke, the site of intracranial arterial occlusion and a proximal source can be identified. This information is vital before patient selection for intraarterial thrombectomy. In cases with suspected venous ischaemia or haemorrhage, a CT venogram can confirm venous sinus thrombosis.
5. In suspected raised intracranial pressure and as a precaution before lumbar puncture after certain criteria are fulfilled. These include reduced consciousness (a Glasgow Coma Scale score of <15), definite papilloedema, focal neurological deficit, immune suppression and bleeding dyscrasias.
6. In other situations, such as epilepsy, migraine, suspected tumour, demyelination, dementia and psychosis, CT is a poorer-quality tool. If imaging can be justified, MRI is greatly preferable and is recommended by NICE in these situations except for the first episode of psychosis.

Technique

1. Most clinical indications are adequately covered with thin slices that are 1 mm or less from the skull base to the vertex. In all trauma cases, window width and level should be adjusted to examine

bone and any haemorrhagic, space-occupying lesions. Review of all trauma studies should be done on brain windows, bone and 'blood windows' (i.e. W175 L75). Narrow CT window settings should be used in suspected cases of early cerebral ischaemia (i.e. W8 L32).

2. In suspected infection, tumours, vascular malformations and subacute infarctions, the sections should be repeated following intravenous (IV) contrast enhancement if MR is not available. Standard precautions with regard to possible adverse reactions to contrast medium should be taken.

3. Dynamic studies using iodinated contrast are increasingly being used as a routine in high-velocity head trauma, the assessment of intracerebral bleeding in young patients, aneurysmal SAH, ruptured arteriovenous shunts and dural venous sinus thrombosis. CTA on a typical 64- to 128-slice multidetector scanner is performed using 70–100 mL of contrast and a 50-ml saline chaser injected at 4 mL s^{-1} with a delay of 15 s or triggered by bolus tracking with the region of interest in the aortic arch. Overlapping slices of 0.5–1.0 mm are reconstructed. CT venography involves injecting 90–100 mL of contrast with a delay of 40 s. Images are usually reviewed as both three-dimensional (3D) rendered data and multiplanar reformats.

Further Reading
Yates D, Aktar R, Hill J. Assessment, investigation, and early management of head injury: summary of NICE guidance. *Br Med J.* 2007;335:719–720.

MAGNETIC RESONANCE IMAGING OF THE BRAIN

Indications

MRI is indicated in all cases of suspected intracranial pathology. Techniques in use change with the development of new sequences and higher-field-strength magnets. Therefore, the techniques described as follows are only basic indications as to sequences in use. The greatest advantages in the use of MRI are the improved contrast resolution between the grey and white matter, brain and cerebrospinal fluid (CSF); the removal of artefact caused by bone close to the skull base and in the posterior fossa; and in obtaining multiplanar images for lesion localization.

Technique

1. **Long TR sequences:** The whole brain can be examined with 4-mm sections, with 1-mm interspaces using T2-weighted- turbo spin-echo imaging. Proton density sequences, long TR and short TE, can be used for the assessment of demyelination and intraarticular disc changes in the temporomandibular joints.

2. **Short TR sequences:** T1-weighted sequences are used for the demonstration of detailed anatomy, but gadolinium chelate contrast agents are required to view pathology. Common practice is to obtain a sagittal or coronal T1-weighted sequence as part of a standard

brain study. Volumetric sequences pre- and postcontrast are used for image guidance software interfaces for epilepsy imaging, insertion of deep brain stimulators for movement disorders and the removal of intra- and extraaxial tumours.

3. **Gradient-echo (GE) T2-weighted sequences and susceptibility-weighted imaging (SWI):** Although suffering from various artefacts, the sensitivity of these sequences to susceptibility effects makes them very sensitive to the presence of blood products, as in cases of previous head injury, SAH and cavernomas. Haemosiderin produces marked focal loss of signal in such cases, and all patients with a history of head injury or other causes of haemorrhage should be imaged with this sequence. These sequences identify abnormal mineral deposition and can be used in deposition disorders. SWI sequences have also been used in cerebrovascular disorders, including ischaemic stroke and venous sinus occlusions.

4. **FLAIR sequences (fluid attenuated inversion recovery)** provide very good contrast resolution in the detection of demyelinating plaques and infarcts. These sequences have the advantage that juxtaventricular pathology contrasts with dark CSF and is not obscured by proximity to the intense brightness of the ventricular CSF, as occurs in spin-echo T2-weighted studies. These are usually obtained in the sagittal or coronal plane.

5. **Angiographic sequences:** There are many methods, of which 'time-of flight' is one of the more commonly used. This is a very short TR, T1-weighted GE 3D sequence, with sequential presaturation of each partition so that only non-presaturated inflowing blood gives a high signal. Image display is by so-called maximum intensity projection, giving a 3D model of the intracranial vessels. Because it uses the T1 properties, high signal from blood products in the subarachnoid space may reduce the sensitivity to aneurysms. Phase-contrast magnetic resonance angiography (MRA) uses velocity encoding flow and is useful to detect flow in small and tortuous vessels. Contrast-enhanced MRA requires a pump injector and is less susceptible to flow artefacts. Timing of image acquisition is crucial, and it is very useful in neck vessel imaging.

6. **Echoplanar or diffusion-weighted imaging (DWI):** Most units perform DWI on all patients with suspected stroke, vasculitis, encephalitis and abscesses and in the workup of intracranial tumours. DWI examines the free movement, or Brownian motion, of water molecules at a cellular level. In acute infarcts, cytotoxic oedema prevents free movement of water, whereas in tumours, there is no restriction. All DWI should be reviewed together with conventional sequences and apparent diffusion coefficient (ADC) maps. Acute infarcts are hyperintense on DWI and hypointense on ADC.

7. **Non-echoplanar imaging:** This sequence is increasingly used to detect cholesteatoma in the petrous temporal bone. Cholesteatoma appears bright on this sequence in comparison with non-specific granulation or inflammatory tissue. It is especially useful in identifying small areas of recurrence during surveillance imaging because these can be difficult to confirm on a high-resolution CT scan.

Further Reading
Atlas SW. *Magnetic Resonance Imaging of Brain and Spine*. 4th ed. Lippincott Williams & Wilkins; 2009.
Schwartz KM, Lane JI, Bolster BD, et al. The utility of diffusion-weighted imaging for cholesteatoma evaluation. *AJNR Am J Neuroradiol*. 2011;32:430–436.

16

IMAGING OF INTRACRANIAL HAEMORRHAGE

Imaging of suspected ICH is one of the most common requests, usually in the emergency setting. In the acute setting, CT (along with the neurophysiological information available as a result of multidetector technology) is often the first and only modality used to assess these patients. MRI is more often used in situations when the initial workup has been negative and a more sensitive modality is required.

COMPUTED TOMOGRAPHY

A conventional study consists of 1 mm or less contiguous slices from the skull base to vertex. This is the basic MDCT protocol for brain imaging. This is performed without contrast to avoid diagnostic uncertainty in deciding whether a parenchymal abnormality is due to enhancement or blood. Acute blood is typically hyperdense on CT. An exhaustive differential diagnosis for bleeding in different compartments of the brain can be sourced elsewhere, but in general, bleeding can be extraaxial (i.e. epidural, subdural, subarachnoid, intraventricular) or intraaxial. Intraaxial bleeding can be due to head trauma, ruptured aneurysms or arteriovenous malformations, bleeding tumours (either primary disease or secondaries), hypertensive haemorrhages (cortical or striatal) or haemorrhagic transformation of venous or arterial infarcts. In the assessment of SAH and ischaemic stroke, CTA is becoming increasingly used as the screening modality for deciding further intervention. Neurosurgeons are increasingly using CTA as the sole modality for planning microsurgical clipping, particularly in cases in which haematoma is exerting mass effect and needs to be evacuated immediately adjacent to a freshly ruptured intracranial aneurysm. In ischaemic stroke, CTA can localize an acute embolus and its source. CT perfusion imaging can demonstrate the ischaemic core (irreversibly damaged brain) and the ischaemic penumbra (recoverable brain parenchyma) by evaluating the relative cerebral blood flow (rCBF).

MAGNETIC RESONANCE IMAGING

MRI is predominantly used to exclude the presence of an underlying tumour or a cavernoma at an interval after the initial haemorrhage, when there is less perilesional brain swelling and obscuration of the anatomy caused by blood degradation products. It is also used in the setting of subarachnoid bleeding when no aneurysm or arteriovenous malformation is found on CTA or catheter angiography. In these cases, the entire neuraxis must be examined to exclude an 'occult' source of the haemorrhage. If tumour is suspected, MR should be obtained within 48 h after ictus. Diffuse axonal shear injuries in patients with depressed coma scores post head injury in light of a normal-appearing CT scan are best demonstrated on MRI with GE imaging or SWI, looking for a susceptibility artefact caused by 'microbleeds'. Where resources are optimal, MRI can be used as part of the initial imaging pathway in ischaemic stroke, though CT remains the modality of choice in most places. Diffusion imaging can identify an acute infarction as early as 2 h. MR will help determine the volumes of the brain that can be recovered, as well as the presence of early haemorrhage that is not visible on CT, which would contraindicate thrombolysis.

Further Reading

Haacke EM, Mittal S, Wu Z, et al. Susceptibility-weighted imaging: technical aspects and clinical applications, part 1. *AJNR Am J Neuroradiol*. 2009;30(1):19–30.

Mittal S, Wu Z, Neelavalli J, et al. Susceptibility-weighted imaging: technical aspects and clinical applications, part 2. *AJNR Am J Neuroradiol*. 2009;30(2):232–252.

Wada R, Aviv RI, Fox AJ, et al. CT angiography 'spot sign' predicts hematoma expansion in acute intracerebral hemorrhage. *Stroke*. 2007;38(4):1257–1262.

Westerlaan HE, Gravendeel J, Fiore D, et al. Multislice CT angiography in the selection of patients with ruptured intracranial aneurysms suitable for clipping or coiling. *Neuroradiology*. 2007;49(12):997–1007.

IMAGING OF GLIOMAS

Glioma is an all-encompassing term for a diverse group of primary brain tumours. They include astrocytomas, oligodendrogliomas, choroid plexus tumours and ependymomas, amongst others. The most commonly presenting tumour, however, is the World Health Organization grade IV astrocytoma, or glioblastoma multiforme. Other brain tumours are derived from neuronal cell lines, mixed glial–neuronal cell lines, the pineal gland and embryonal cell lines, peripheral cranial nerves (e.g. vestibular schwannoma), meningeal tumours and lymphoma. Appropriate differential diagnoses can be derived from noting the age of the patient, the tumour location (i.e. supra- or infratentorial, cortex or white matter, basal ganglia or brainstem, intra- or extraaxial), its consistency (i.e. cyst formation, mural nodule) and its enhancement characteristics.

COMPUTED TOMOGRAPHY

CT is often the first modality to demonstrate the presence of a brain tumour due to widespread utilization. The indications for scanning can include unrelenting morning headaches, drowsiness, strokelike presentation and seizures. In addition to making the initial diagnosis, MDCT can be used for obtaining high-resolution data sets for image guidance for brain biopsies, with and without stereotactic frames. In the absence of advanced MR neuroimaging software and for patients who are unable to undergo MRI, imaging MDCT can be used to obtain rCBF data for tumour matrix as well as the normal brain. Studies have been performed to correlate ratios of rCBF with tumour grade, assessment of radiation necrosis or dedifferentiation when following up on tumours.

16

MAGNETIC RESONANCE IMAGING

MRI is the preferred modality for detailed assessment of brain tumours. In addition to using conventional imaging parameters to assess volume, location and tumour substance in multiple planes, advanced imaging techniques or 'multimodality' imaging can reveal information about tumour grade and biology. Conventional T1- and T2-weighted images are obtained. DWI and diffusion tractography reveal information about tumour substance and effect on white matter tracts in the brainstem and the cerebrum. Multiple lesions, if present, can be better seen on postcontrast MRI, in which case metastatic disease becomes a consideration in the differential diagnosis. Because grade IV gliomas can have a similar appearance, a search for a primary epithelial neoplasm elsewhere (e.g. in the breast and lung) is indicated. MR spectroscopy is a technique whereby relative amounts of cell metabolites are detected to reflect the biochemical environment in a tumour. N-acetylaspartate, choline, creatine, lactate and myoinositol are a few of the major metabolites assessed. Single voxel techniques are preferable using stimulated echo acquisition mode or point-resolved spectroscopy. Perfusion-weighted imaging can provide information about tumour grade and help differentiate between tumour recurrence and radiation necrosis. It is also used during surveillance imaging of low-grade tumours and in planning biopsies. Susceptibility perfusion imaging is most often used where GE images are obtained of the entire brain during the first pass of gadolinium chelate, and analysis of the collated data using small regions of interest is carried out, looking at the normal brain and the tumour. Magnetization-prepared rapid-acquisition gradient echo volumetric data can also be used postcontrast in image guidance for biopsy or tumour debulking.

Further Reading

Computed Tomography

Jain R. Perfusion CT imaging of brain tumours: an overview. *AJNR Am J Neuroradiol.* 2011;32(9):1570–1577.

Magnetic Resonance Imaging

Al-Okaili RN, Krejza J, Wang S, et al. Advanced MR imaging techniques in the diagnosis of intraaxial brain tumors in adults. *Radiographics.* 2006;26(suppl):S173–S189.

Osborn AG. *Osborn's Brain: Imaging, Pathology, Anatomy.* Amirsys; 2012.

Stadlbauer A, Gruber S, Nimsky C, et al. Preoperative grading of gliomas by using metabolite quantification with high-spatial-resolution proton MR spectroscopic imaging. *Radiology.* 2006;238(3):958–969.

IMAGING OF ACOUSTIC NEUROMAS

MRI is the definitive diagnostic method. The neurophysiological methods, although quite sensitive, produce a large number of false-positive studies.

COMPUTED TOMOGRAPHY

Some departments use 1-mm or less section IV contrast-enhanced CT with bone and soft tissue windowed images for suspected acoustic neuroma to relieve pressure on their MRI services. This approach is usually reserved for older adult patients, mostly to exclude the presence of large lesions that may require debulking or excision. Intracanalicular tumours cannot be shown by this method, but this limitation is considered acceptable because they are unlikely to be addressed surgically in these patients.

MAGNETIC RESONANCE IMAGING

Most imaging departments will have 1.5-T scanner high-resolution heavily T2-weighted MR cisternography sequences, nulling the CSF pulsation artefact and highlighting the appearance of cranial nerves, arteries and veins, which may also contribute to sensorineural deafness and tinnitus. Nulling the pulsation artefact from CSF provides the contrast required, and images as thin as 0.8 mm, with no gap, can be obtained. From these types of data, multiplanar, reformatted images can be reviewed. Postcontrast studies can be obtained if a change in the contour of the nerve is observed or a filling defect is seen in the labyrinthine structures.

Further Reading
Rupa V, Job A, George M, et al. Cost-effective initial screening for vestibular schwannoma: auditory brainstem response or magnetic resonance imaging. *Otolaryngol Head Neck Surg.* 2003;128(6):823–828.

RADIONUCLIDE IMAGING OF THE BRAIN

There are currently two main modalities: regional cerebral blood flow imaging and PET imaging.

REGIONAL CEREBRAL BLOOD FLOW IMAGING

Indications

1. Localization of epileptic foci
2. Mapping of cerebrovascular disease
3. Investigation of dementias, including Huntington's and Alzheimer's diseases
4. Assessment of the effects of treatment regimens
5. Confirmation of brain death

Contraindications

None

Radiopharmaceuticals

1. 99mTc-hexamethylpropyleneamineoxime (HMPAO or exametazime), 500 MBq (5 mSv effective dose (ED)). The most commonly used agent, HMPAO, is a lipophilic complex that crosses the blood–brain barrier and localizes roughly in proportion to cerebral blood flow. It is rapidly extracted by the brain, reaching a peak of 5%–6% of injected activity within 1 min or so, with minimal redistribution (~86% remains in the brain at 24 h).

2. 99mTc-ethyl cysteinate dimer (ECD), 500 MBq (5 mSv ED). This localizes rapidly in proportion to cellular metabolism rather than blood flow, and the distribution has some differences from that of HMPAO, which may need to be taken into consideration for clinical diagnosis.[1,2] It currently has the advantage of greater stability than HMPAO and can be used for up to 6 h after reconstitution, which is of particular benefit for ictal epilepsy studies, in which an injection is only given when a seizure occurs.

Equipment

1. Single-photon emission computed tomography (SPECT) gamma camera, preferably dual-headed
2. SPECT imaging couch with head extension
3. Low-energy high-resolution collimator (or more specialized slant-hole or fan-beam collimator)

Patient Preparation

Because cerebral blood flow is continuously varying with motor activity, sensory stimulation, emotional arousal and other neural activity, it is important to standardize the conditions under which the tracer is administered, especially if serial studies are to be undertaken in the same individual. Familiarization with the procedure to reduce anxiety and injection in a relaxing environment through a previously positioned IV cannula should be considered.

For localization of epileptic foci, ictal studies are much more sensitive than interictal, and if feasible, the patient should be admitted under constant monitoring, with injection as soon as a seizure starts.

Technique

1. Administer 500 MBq of tracer
2. SPECT imaging is performed any time, from 5 min to 2 h after injection with the patient supine

Images

The acquisition protocol will depend upon the system available. Suitable parameters for a modern single-headed gamma-camera might be:

1. 360 degrees circular orbit
2. 60–90 degrees projections or continuous rotation over a 30-min acquisition
3. Combination of matrix size and zoom to give a pixel size of 3–4 mm

Analysis

A cine film of the projections is reviewed before the patient leaves to detect if any significant movement degradation is present. If movement that cannot be rectified by computer motion correction algorithms has occurred, the patient must be rescanned. SPECT reconstructions are made in three planes.

Additional Techniques

1. If blood flow in the carotid and major cerebral arteries is of interest, a dynamic study during injection is performed.
2. 3D mapping of activity distributions onto standard brain atlases and image registration with MRI, CT and quantitative analysis are areas of increasing interest, particularly with the development of SPECT-CT scanners.

Aftercare

Radiation dose may be reduced by administration of a mild laxative on the day after the study and maintenance of good hydration to promote urine output.

Complications

None

POSITRON EMISSION TOMOGRAPHY

Indications

1. Localization of epileptic foci
2. Investigation of dementias
3. Grading of brain tumours

Contraindications

1. Recent chemotherapy: minimum interval of 2–3 weeks recommended
2. Recent radiotherapy: minimum interval of 8–12 weeks recommended
3. Poorly controlled diabetes: for example, serum glucose greater than 8.5 mmol L^{-1} at time of scanning

Radiopharmaceuticals

Fluorine-18 fluorodeoxyglucose (^{18}FDG) is a glucose analogue that is the most commonly used agent for oncological work and is also used for the investigation of dementias. There are other radiopharmaceuticals, such as L-[methyl-^{11}C]methionine ([^{11}C] MET) and 3′-deoxy-3′-[^{18}F] fluorothymidine ([^{18}F] FLT), that have the advantage of little normal cerebral uptake.

Patient Preparation
Fasting for 4–6 h, with plenty of non-sugary fluids

Technique
1. ^{18}FDG up to the UK limit of 400 MBq IV (10 mSv ED) is administered.
2. To reduce muscle uptake of ^{18}FDG, patients should remain in a relaxed environment, such as lying in a darkened room without talking, if the head and neck area are being imaged, between the injection and scan.
3. Image at 1 h postinjection. Later imaging has been reported to enhance tumour conspicuity because of a higher tumour-to-background ratio.
4. If combined with CT scanning:
   (a) Low-dose CT technique
   (b) No IV contrast medium
5. PET imaging of the following:
   (a) Brain
   (b) Whole body, if indicated

16

^{201}THALLIUM BRAIN SCANNING

Indications
1. Central nervous system (and other) tumours:
   (a) Grading
   (b) Differentiation of postsurgical or radiotherapy change from residual or recurrent tumours

This radionuclide procedure has largely been superseded by PET.

Contraindications
None

Radiopharmaceutical
^{201}Thallium 100 MBq (25 mSv ED)

Equipment
1. SPECT gamma camera
2. VerteX High-Resolution (VXHR) gamma camera

Technique
IV injection of radiopharmaceutical

Analysis
SPECT

Aftercare
None

DOPAMINE TRANSPORTER LIGANDS

Indications

Ioflupane, 123-I FP-CIT (DatSCAN, GE Healthcare), contains a dopamine transporter radioligand and can be used to assess striatal uptake in possible Parkinson's disease and differentiate from other movement disorders.

Contraindications

None

Radiopharmaceuticals

^{123}I DatSCAN 185 MBq (4.5 mSv ED)

Equipment

1. SPECT gamma camera
2. VXHR

Patient Preparation

Thyroid blockade (400 mg of potassium perchlorate orally 1 h before scan)

Technique

IV injection of radiopharmaceutical

Images

Image with SPECT at 3–6 h.

Analysis

Diagnosis depends on an assessment of relative uptake in the caudate and putamen.

Aftercare

None

References

Radiopharmaceuticals
1. Asenbaum S, Brücke T, Pirker W, et al. Imaging of cerebral blood flow with technetium-99m-HMPAO and technetium-99m-ECD: a comparison. *J Nucl Med*. 1998;39(4):613–618.
2. Koyama M, Kawashima R, Ito H, et al. SPECT imaging of normal subjects with technetium-99m-HMPAO and technetium-99m-ECD. *J Nucl Med*. 1997;38(4):587–592.

Further Reading

Radionuclide Imaging of the Brain
Freeman LM, Blaufox MD. Functional brain imaging (part 1). *Semin Nucl Med*. 2003;33(1):1–85.

Complications
Murray AD. The brain, salivary and lacrimal glands. In: Sharp PF, Gemmell HG, Murray AD, eds. *Practical Nuclear Medicine*. 3rd ed. Springer-Verlag; 2005.

Aftercare

Hammoud DA, Hoffman JM, Pomper MG. Molecular neuroimaging: from conventional to emerging techniques. *Radiology*. 2007;245(1):21–42.

CEREBRAL ANGIOGRAPHY

16

Indications

1. Intracerebral and SAH
2. Aneurysms presenting as space-occupying lesions
3. Brain arteriovenous shunts, caroticocavernous fistulas (direct and indirect)
4. Cerebral ischaemia, both of extracranial and intracranial origin
5. Preoperative assessment of intracranial tumours

Contraindications

1. Patients with unstable neurology (usually following SAH or stroke) that has changed after ictus
2. Patients unsuitable for surgery
3. Patients in whom vascular access would be impossible or relatively risky
4. Iodine allergy: relative contraindication because angiography could be performed with gadolinium chelates

Equipment

A biplane digital subtraction angiography apparatus is required, with a C-arm allowing unlimited imaging planes, high-quality fluoroscopy and road-mapping facility.

3D rotational angiography is now increasingly available and forms an important part of the analysis of aneurysms during treatment. There should be access to the patient for both the radiologist and the anaesthetist, with appropriate head immobilization.

Preparation

When the patient is able to understand what is proposed, a clear explanation should be given, together with a presentation of the risks and benefits. Most patients do not require sedation for diagnostic procedures, and this would be relatively contraindicated in acute neurological presentations. Children, patients who are excessively anxious, those who cannot cooperate because of confusion and those who would be managed better during the procedure with full ventilation control are examined under general anaesthesia. Neurointerventional studies are done under general anaesthesia. Groin shaving is now regarded as unnecessary. Patients should not be starved unless general anaesthesia is to be used but should nevertheless be restricted to fluid intake and only a light meal.

Technique

Catheter flushing solutions should consist of heparinized saline bolus followed by flush (50–100 units kg^{-1}). Using standard percutaneous catheter introduction techniques, the femoral artery is catheterized. It is a common practice to deliver an access sheath through which catheters are introduced and exchanged if necessary. There is a wide range of catheters available, and there are proponents of many types. In patients up to middle age without major hypertension, there will be little difficulty with any standard catheter, and a simple 4-Fr polythene catheter with a slightly curved tip or 45-degree bend will suffice in the majority. Older patients and those with atherosclerotic disease may need catheters offering greater torque control such as the JB2 or Simmons catheters (Figs. 16.1 and 16.2) as appropriate. Catheter control will be better if passed through an introducer set, and this is also indicated when it is anticipated that catheter exchange may be required. Selective studies of the common carotids and the vertebrals are preferable to superselective studies of the internal and external carotids unless absolutely necessary. The following points should be noted:

1. The hazards of cerebral angiography are largely avoidable; they consist of the complications common to all forms of angiography (see Chapter 11) and those that are particularly related to cerebral angiography.
2. Any on-table ischaemic event has an explanation. Cerebral angiography does not possess an inherently unavoidable complication rate as has been suggested in the past. If an ischaemic

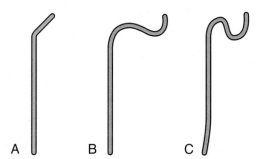

Fig. 16.1 **A,** Vertebrale or Berenstein catheters. **B,** JB2 catheter. **C,** Mani. End holes, 1; side holes, 0.

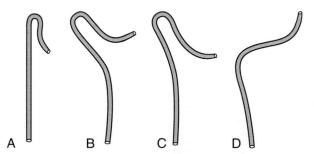

Fig. 16.2 Simmons (sidewinder) catheters. **A,** For narrow aorta. **B,** For moderately narrow aorta. **C,** For wide aorta. **D,** For elongated aorta. End holes, 1; side holes, 0.

event occurs, there has been a complication, and its cause must be identified.

3. The most significant complications are embolic in origin, and the most important emboli are particulate. Air bubbles should be avoided as part of good angiographic practice but are unlikely to cause a severe neurological complication.

4. Emboli may come from the injected solutions. Avoid contamination from glove powder or dried blood or clot on gloves. Take care to avoid blood contamination of the saline or of the contrast medium, which is always dangerous. Avoid exposure of solutions to air. Contrast medium, heparin or saline in an open bowl is bad practice.

5. Emboli may arise from dislodgement of plaque or thrombus. Never pass a catheter or guidewire through a vessel that has not been visualized by preliminary injection of contrast medium. Use appropriate angled, hydrophilic guidewires. Do not try to negotiate excessively acute bends in vessels. The splinting effect of the catheter will cause spasm and arrest the flow in the artery. Dissections could occur, which may lead to occlusion. Newer catheter designs tend to be softer and allow further distal access for more complex procedures. Sharp curves can otherwise be safely negotiated with microcatheters.

6. Emboli may arise from the formation of thrombus within a catheterized vessel. Always ensure that there is free blood flow past the catheter and avoid forceful passage of a guidewire or catheter in such a way that may damage the intima of the vessel and cause thrombus formation.

7. Emboli may arise within the catheter. Do not allow blood to flow back into the catheter, or if it does occur, flush regularly or by continuous infusion. Never allow a guidewire to remain within a catheter for more than 1 min without withdrawal and flushing it and never introduce a guidewire into a contrast-filled catheter but instead fill the catheter with heparinized saline first.

8. Keep study time to a minimum but not at the expense of the diagnostic quality or therapeutic benefit.

Contrast Medium

Non-ionic monomers (e.g. iohexol and iopamidol). The iodine concentration required is equipment dependent, but with modern DSA, 300 mg mL^{-1} is suitable.

Contrast Medium Volume

1. Common carotid: 10 mL by hand in about 1.5–2 s
2. Internal carotid: 7 mL by hand in about 1.5 s
3. Vertebral artery: 7 mL by hand in about 1.5 s, but this volume can be diluted by 2 mL of saline to opacify the contralateral vertebral artery on the same injection

Projections

As required, but basically 20 degrees anteroposterior, Townes, lateral, occipitomental and oblique views as indicated. Multiple projections are especially needed for aneurysm studies to open loops and profile aneurysms; however, with 3D rotational angiography, contrast runs can now be cut down to a minimum, and computer models of aneurysms and vessels can be analyzed instead.

Films

From early arterial to late venous, about 8 s in total in most cases, system acquisitions will be at 2–4 frames s^{-1}, depending on the study. With digital fluoroscopy, acquisitions typically will be 2 frames s^{-1} for 4 s and then 1 frame every 2 s for 4 s.

Aftercare

1. Standard nursing care for the arterial puncture site
2. Most departments adopt the practice of maintaining neurological observation for a period of 4 h or so after the procedure
3. Good hydration should be maintained

ENT
Sofia Otero

Methods of Imaging the Nasolacrimal Drainage Apparatus

1. Conventional or digital subtraction (DS) dacryocystography (DCG)
2. Computed tomography (CT) DCG
3. Magnetic resonance (MR) DCG
4. Dacryoscintigraphy

CONVENTIONAL, DIGITAL SUBTRACTION AND COMPUTED TOMOGRAPHY DACRYOCYSTOGRAPHY

Conventional and DS DCG use fluoroscopy to visualize the lacrimal system during direct injection of contrast media into the canaliculus of the eyelid. Alternatively, low-dose cone-beam computed tomography (CBCT) can be performed immediately after injection to assess local bony anatomy,[1] or higher-dose multidetector computed tomography (MDCT) can be performed to provide additional information about adjacent soft tissue structures. CT can also be acquired after passive administration of contrast drops into the conjunctival sac; this method combined with CBCT in the sitting position is considered to be more physiological.

Indication

Epiphora: to demonstrate the site and degree of obstruction when direct clinical examination and irrigation are insufficient for assessment[2]

Contraindications

Pregnancy, allergy, acute dacryocystitis

Contrast Medium

Low-osmolar contrast medium (LOCM) 300 mg I mL^{-1}, 0.5–2.0 mL per side

Oil-based contrast (e.g. Lipiodol) should be avoided because of the risk of granuloma formation or persistent tissue reaction if accidental extravasation occurs.[3]

Equipment

1. Fluoroscopy unit, CBCT or MDCT
2. Silver punctum or lacrimal dilator and lacrimal probe set
3. Lacrimal cannula or blunt catheter with tubing (e.g. 21- to 30-gauge sialography catheter); the latter can be used to inject contrast on both sides simultaneously

Patient Preparation

0.5% bupivacaine eye drops

Technique

1. For conventional, DS and MDCT DCG, the patient is positioned supine in the occipitomental (OM) position. For CBCT, the patient can be sitting (more physiological) or supine, depending on the unit.
2. The lacrimal sac is massaged to express its contents. The lower eyelid is everted to locate the lower canaliculus at the medial end of the eyelid.
3. The lower punctum measures approximately 0.3 mm in diameter and is gently dilated. The lower eyelid should be drawn laterally to straighten the curve in the canaliculus. To avoid perforation, the cannula is initially positioned perpendicular to the eyelid margin as it enters the punctum. The cannula is then rotated by 90 degrees horizontally along the natural curve of the lower canaliculus.
4. Care is taken not to advance the cannula too far into the canaliculus because proximal stenosis can be missed.
5. The upper canaliculus may be cannulated if there is difficulty accessing the lower canaliculus.
6. For conventional and DS DCG, a control image or mask is obtained. After removal of air bubbles, contrast medium is injected, and a fluoroscopy or DS is run at one image per second is obtained, allowing for a dynamic study in real time.
7. For CT, contrast can be injected directly as above. Alternatively, non-dilute contrast media can be administered into the conjunctival sac (2–3 drops per eye) just before acquisition.

Images

The control and other appropriate images are digitally stored.

Aftercare

Up to 1 h of protection with an eye patch may be necessary in view of the local anaesthetic used.

Complication

Perforation of the canaliculus

References

1. Tschopp M, Bornstein MM, Sendi P, et al. Dacryocystography using cone beam CT in patients with lacrimal drainage system obstruction. *Ophthalmic Plast Reconstr Surg.* 2014;30(6):486–491.

2. Singh S, Ali MJ, Paulsen F. Dacryocystography: from theory to current practice. *Ann Anat.* 2019;224:33–40.

3. Delaney Y, Khooshabeh R. Lipogranuloma following traumatic dacryocystography in a 4-year-old boy. *Eye.* 2001;15:683–684.

17

MAGNETIC RESONANCE IMAGING OF THE LACRIMAL SYSTEM

The lacrimal system can be assessed with MRI (MR DCG), either after topical administration of eye drops containing a dilute gadolinium solution (sterile 0.9% NaCl solution containing 1:100 diluted gadolinium chelate) or by direct injection of a dilute gadolinium solution into the lacrimal canaliculus.[1] The less-invasive, topical administration technique is more widely used. MR can diagnose the level of the obstruction in patients with epiphora while also assessing the adjacent soft tissues. Fat-suppressed and dynamic sequences and dedicated surface coils improve visualization of the lacrimal system. Diagnostic images can also be obtained with heavily T2-weighted fast spin-echo sequences after topical administration of lidocaine or saline drops.[2–4]

References

1. Coskun B, Ilgit E, Onal B, et al. MR dacryocystography in the evaluation of patients with obstructive epiphora treated by means of interventional radiologic procedures. *AJNR Am J Neuroradiol.* 2012;33:141–147.

2. Higashi H, Tamada T, Mizukawa K, et al. MR dacryocystography: comparison with dacryoendoscopy in positional diagnosis of nasolacrimal duct obstruction. *Radiol Med.* 2016;121(7):580–587.

3. Takehara Y, Isoda H, Kurihashi K, et al. Dynamic MR dacryocystography: a new method for evaluating nasolacrimal duct obstructions. *AJR Am J Roentgenol.* 2000;175:469–473.

4. Cubuk R, Tasali N, Aydin S, et al. Dynamic MR dacryocystography in patients with epiphora. *Eur J Radiol.* 2010;73(2):230–233.

DACRYOSCINTIGRAPHY

This provides functional information while mimicking physiological lacrimal flow. A single drop (10 μL) of technetium-99m colloid 20 MBq in 1 mL is delivered to each eye via the conjunctival sac. The patient is imaged sitting up with a head support and chin rest. Imaging is commenced as soon as possible after administration of contrast.[1]

Reference

1. Costa IM, Pereira LR, Jessop M, et al. British Nuclear Medicine Society Professional Standards committee (PSC). Lacrimal scintigraphy BNMS Guidelines. *Nucl Med Commun.* 2021;42(4):459–467.

Methods of Imaging the Salivary Glands

1. Plain film
2. Ultrasound (US)
3. Conventional and DS sialography
4. MRI ± intravenous (IV) contrast medium for the assessment of inflammatory processes and masses; may include MR sialography and MR spectroscopy
5. Thin-section unenhanced CT for diagnosis of sialolithiasis ± IV contrast medium for suspected abscess or tumour
6. Radionuclide imaging (sialoscintigraphy): IV ^{99m}Tc-pertechnetate is taken up by the salivary glands and secreted into the oral cavity. Uptake indicates that there is functional epithelial tissue present and correlates with salivary output.

PLAIN FILM

Mandibular anterior occlusal or orthopantomogram are useful when US has revealed submandibular or sublingual duct dilation but no stone; small (<3 mm) and distal submandibular duct stones may not be seen with US.[1,2]

References

1. Terraz S, Poletti PA, Dulguerov P, et al. How reliable is sonography in the assessment of sialolithiasis? *AJR Am J Roentgenol.* 2013;201(1):W104–W109.
2. Goncalves M, Schapher M, Iro H, et al. Value of sonography in the diagnosis of sialolithiasis: comparison with the reference standard of direct stone identification. *J Ultrasound Med.* 2017;36(11):2227–2235.

ULTRASOUND

High-frequency linear array US is the first-line investigation for salivary obstruction to assess the presence, level and degree of obstruction; its cause (e.g. stone or stricture); and associated parenchymal changes. Oral sialagogue (e.g. citric acid or citrus sweets) can help to reveal occult stones and strictures and may also demonstrate mobility of a stone within a duct, which may influence its management. A stone is seen as a hyperechoic focus that casts an acoustic shadow; stones smaller than 3 mm in size may not cast an acoustic shadow and may not be seen on US. Stones within the distal third of the duct can also be difficult to see because of acoustic shadowing from the mandible; if an anterior stone is suspected, a mandibular occlusal radiograph may reveal it. US is also the first-line investigation for a salivary gland mass and for diffuse salivary inflammation. A medium-frequency small, curved array transducer should be used to assess large lesions and the deep lobe of the parotid gland. Where required, focal lesions can be targeted with US-guided fine-needle aspiration biopsy (FNAB) or core biopsy. Local anaesthesia with up to 5 mL of 1% lidocaine is advised for core biopsy and sometimes used for FNAB.

FNAB is a low-risk, well-tolerated and highly accurate procedure,[1,2] often performed using capillary action technique.

References
1. Sharma G, Jung AS, Maceri DR, et al. US-guided fine-needle aspiration of major salivary gland masses and adjacent lymph nodes: accuracy and impact on clinical decision making. *Radiology.* 2011;259(2):471–478.
2. Rivera Rolon M, Schnadig VJ, Faiz S, et al. Salivary gland fine-needle aspiration cytology with the application of the Milan system for risk stratification and histological correlation: a retrospective 6-year study. *Diagn Cytopathol.* 2020;48(11):1067–1074.

17

CONVENTIONAL AND DIGITAL SUBTRACTION SIALOGRAPHY

Fluoroscopic sialography is the gold standard test for duct evaluation.[1]

Indications
1. Positive US findings for salivary obstruction: may not be appropriate for patients with known distal submandibular duct stones because the stone could be washed back into the gland during sialography
2. Persistent symptoms of salivary obstruction with negative US findings
3. Planning endoluminal interventional procedures such as basket retrieval of stones and balloon dilation of strictures
4. Therapeutic: duct washout[2,3]

Contraindications
Pregnancy, allergy, clinically active infection or inflammation

Contrast Medium
LOCM 240–370 mg I mL^{-1}

Equipment
Equipment varies, depending on operator preference, but typically:

1. Fluoroscopy unit
2. Nettleship punctum dilator or silver lacrimal dilator and probe set (size 0–2)
3. Sialography catheter with blunt tip (21–30 gauge)
4. Focused light with or without magnifying glasses
5. Lubricant gel (e.g. Instillagel) may be helpful for introducing the catheter.

Patient Preparation
Any radiopaque artefacts are removed (e.g. false teeth).

Preliminary Images

Next are listed some of the commonly used projections, although the selection and number of control images is operator dependent and reliant on the suspected pathology (e.g. stone or stricture).

Parotid gland

- Lateral, centred to the angle of the mandible with 3× magnification
- If a distal stone is suspected, an OM or oblique view turned away from the side of interest may also be helpful to view the anterior duct. For strictures, extra views are not helpful.

Submandibular gland

- Lateral or oblique lateral centred 1 cm anterior to the angle of the mandible with 3× magnification
- Mandibular occlusal
- Orthopantomogram

Technique

1. The orifice of the parotid duct is adjacent to the crown of the second upper molar and may be obscured by a mucosal bite ridge. Gentle abduction of the cheek using the thumb and index finger assists identification and cannulation of the parotid duct.
2. The orifice of the submandibular duct is on or near the sublingual papilla next to the lingual frenulum. It is smaller than the parotid duct orifice and is more difficult to identify and cannulate. Raising the tip of the tongue to touch the hard palate puts tension on the papilla.
3. If the orifice is not visible, the gland can be massaged to extrude saliva, or a sialagogue (e.g. citric acid) can be placed in the mouth to promote secretion from the gland and render the orifice visible. The orifice is gently dilated, if necessary, using the dilator or probe, and the catheter is introduced into the duct. Care must be taken when advancing the catheter into the submandibular duct because of the risk of painless perforation into the floor of the mouth.
4. Alternatively, modified Seldinger technique can be used; a 0.018-in guidewire is placed within the duct, and a 22-gauge polythene catheter is advanced over the wire.
5. The catheter is held in place by the patient closing their lips firmly onto the catheter tubing. They should avoid biting the tubing because this may block contrast from passing through. Up to 2 mL of contrast medium is injected; all air bubbles must be eliminated from the catheter before injection as these can mimic stones or mucus plugs. The injection is terminated immediately if any pain is experienced or extravasation is witnessed on the images. The duct and acini should not be overfilled because this may obscure duct pathology.

Images

1. Dynamic images can be acquired during the injection at 2 frames/s, with or without DS. DS is helpful in eliminating large dense superimposed objects such as teeth and restorations but is usually not required.[4]

2. A full exposure should be taken at the end of the run while maintaining gentle pressure on the syringe to more clearly delineate the ducts. If a distal parotid duct stricture is suspected, oblique images can be acquired to better assess the most anterior part of the duct, as this turns approximately 90 degrees towards the buccal mucosa.

3. Single fluoroscopic images are saved immediately after removal of the catheter and after 1 min to assess drainage from the gland. If contrast persists within the gland at that stage, massage of the gland can be undertaken to attempt to extrude the contrast followed by a final fluoroscopic image.

17

Aftercare

None

Complications

1. Local pain
2. Damage to the duct orifice or ductal perforation with or without extravasation of contrast
3. Infection should be suspected if local pain persists 24 h after the procedure; the patient should be evaluated for any requirement of antibiotic therapy.

References
1. iRefer Guidelines: Making the best use of clinical radiology. Version 8.0.1. Royal College of Radlologlsts; 2022.
2. Tucci FM, Roma R, Bianchi A, et al. Juvenile recurrent parotitis: diagnostic and therapeutic effectiveness of sialography. Retrospective study on 110 children. *Int J Pediatr Otorhinolaryngol.* 2019;124:179–184.
3. Kim JE, Lee SS, Lee C, et al. Therapeutic effect of intraductal saline irrigation in chronic obstructive sialadenitis. *BMC Oral Health.* 2020;20(1):86.
4. Brown AL, Shepherd D, Buckenham TM. Per oral balloon sialoplasty: results in the treatment of salivary duct stenosis. *Cardiovasc Intervent Radiol.* 1997;20(5):337–342.

IMAGE-GUIDED BASKET RETRIEVAL OF STONES AND BALLOON DILATION OF STRICTURES

Both of these gland-preserving techniques are most often done under fluoroscopic guidance. Occasionally, stones can be retrieved with a basket using US guidance, although sialography is recommended before intervention to exclude a distal stricture, which could limit access with a basket and which could increase the risk of a complication from the procedure if not known about in advance.

Indications

1. Stones up to 7 mm in size within the extraglandular ducts are amenable to basket retrieval (stones >4 mm may be difficult to retrieve by a less experienced operator). About 80% of stones occur within the submandibular system.[1] Be aware that strictures

distal to the stone may require balloon dilation before basket retrieval is attempted.

2. Strictures of the extraglandular ducts, which are point, multiple (known as sialadochitis) or diffuse, can be stretched with a balloon. About 75% of strictures occur within the parotid system.[2] The experience of the operator usually determines the length and position of stricture that can be treated.

Contraindications

Pregnancy, allergy and clinically active infection or inflammation

Contrast Medium

LOCM 240–370 mg I mL^{-1}

Equipment

As for sialogram:

1. Local anaesthetic for injection (lidocaine hydrochloride 2% and adrenaline 1:80,000 or lidocaine 1%)
2. For stone retrieval: an end-grabbing or Dormia basket. A salivary access introducer set and guidewire may be used.
3. For balloon dilatation: salivary or cardiac balloon catheter (usually 2 cm in length and 2.5–4 mm in diameter when inflated, slightly wider than the normal duct lumen). A salivary access introducer set and guidewire may be used.

Patient Preparation

Any radiopaque artefacts are removed (e.g. false teeth).

Techniques

Stone retrieval

1. A preliminary sialogram is performed to assess the location, size and mobility of the stone.
   a. For submandibular stones, local anaesthetic is injected adjacent to the submandibular duct papilla and in the ipsilateral floor of mouth. Anaesthetic can also be injected adjacent to the second mandibular molar for a lingual nerve block or as inferior dental nerve block. For parotid stones, local anaesthetic is injected adjacent to the papilla and anterior duct. Local anaesthetic is often also instilled into the duct via a salivary catheter.
   b. Fluoroscopy (more often) or US can be used to guide the basket into position.
   c. If required, a guidewire and salivary access introducer set can be used to provide access for the basket.
   d. A Dormia basket is positioned proximal to the stone, opened and trawled distally to collect the stone. The basket can be rotated as it comes into contact with the stone to secure the stone within it. An end-grabbing basket is opened, advanced onto the stone and

closed to trap the stone before pulling the stone distally towards the duct orifice. It is easier to trap the stone within a Dormia basket; however, it has the disadvantage that the stone cannot be released, and the basket cannot be collapsed if the apparatus were to become stuck within the duct.

e. A small papillotomy may be required to release the basket containing the stone. Sutures are not usually required.

Balloon dilation of strictures

1. A preliminary sialogram is performed to assess the location and length of the stricture.
2. Anaesthesia is as for stone retrieval.
3. If required, a guidewire and salivary access introducer set can be used to provide access for the balloon.
4. Under fluoroscopic guidance, the balloon is advanced just beyond the most proximal part of the stricture and inflated for 1–2 min at a pressure of 10–15 atm. The balloon can be decompressed and reinflated several times in the same position until adequate distension has been achieved. For multiple or long strictures, the balloon is gradually pulled distally and reinflated as required.
5. A postoperative sialogram is recommended to confirm successful elimination of the stricture.

Aftercare

Operators may choose to prescribe oral antibiotics (those secreted in saliva, such as cephalosporins) or steroids (or both) in cases when there has been extensive manipulation.

Complications

1. Local pain and swelling (usually self-limiting and resolves after 24–48 h)
2. Infection
3. Perforation of the floor of mouth or duct
4. The basket and stone may become impacted, in some cases requiring surgical release.
5. Postprocedure restenosis[3]

References

1. Kraaij S, Karagozoglu KH, Forouzanfar T, et al. Salivary stones: symptoms, aetiology, biochemical composition and treatment. *Br Dent J.* 2014;217(11):E23.
2. Ngu RK, Brown JE, Whaites EJ, et al. Salivary duct strictures: nature and incidence in benign salivary obstruction. *Dentomaxillofac Radiol.* 2007;36(2):63–67.
3. McGurk M, Brown J. Alternatives for the treatment of salivary duct obstruction. *Otolaryngol Clin North Am.* 2009;42(6):1073–1085.

MAGNETIC RESONANCE IMAGING SIALOGRAPHY

MR sialography is a non-invasive technique that can be used when the duct cannot be cannulated or when the patient declines or cannot have conventional sialography. It can be used safely in acute and subacute sialadenitis. It also eliminates the risks associated with conventional sialography, including duct injury, postprocedure stricture and ionizing radiation. A heavily T2-weighted three-dimensional sequence enables visualization of hyperintense saliva within the ductal system.[1,2] Patients fast for 4 h before imaging, and an oral sialagogue can be used during the study, although patients must be told to minimize tongue movement and swallowing during image acquisition. MR sialography is a reliable technique to detect glandular anomalies in patients with Sjögren's syndrome and can be a valuable diagnostic aid.[3] It has good sensitivity and specificity for diagnosing chronic sialadenitis and sialolithiasis, but it is inferior to conventional and DS sialography.[4]

References

1. Becker M, Marchal F, Becker CD, et al. Sialolithiasis and salivary ductal stenosis: diagnostic accuracy of MR sialography with a three-dimensional extended-phase conjugate-symmetry rapid spin-echo sequence. *Radiology.* 2000;217(2):347–358.
2. Tassart M, Zeitoun D, Iffenecker C, et al. SIALO-IRM [MR sialography]. *J Radiol.* 2003;84(1):15–26.
3. André R, Becker M, Lombardi T, et al. Comparison of clinical characteristics and magnetic resonance imaging of salivary glands with magnetic resonance sialography in Sjögren's syndrome. *Laryngoscope.* 2021;131(1):E83–E89.
4. Kalinowski M, Heverhagen JT, Rehberg E, et al. Comparative study of MR sialography and digital subtraction sialography for benign salivary gland disorders. *AJNR Am J Neuroradiol.* 2002;23(9):1485–1492.

COMPUTED TOMOGRAPHY AND CONE-BEAM COMPUTED TOMOGRAPHY SIALOGRAPHY

This is performed in the same way as conventional sialography. CBCT has the advantages of a low radiation dose, limited field of view and elimination of the soft tissue components from the image, rendering the duct system more conspicuous. However, CBCT may be less sensitive in the identification of strictures than plain radiography.[1] Because there is a delay between injection of the contrast media into the duct system and image acquisition, there is also the potential for duct distension to be suboptimal using this method.

Reference

1. Jadu FM, Lam EW. A comparative study of the diagnostic capabilities of 2D plain radiograph and 3D cone beam CT sialography. *Dentomaxillofac Radiol.* 2013;42(1):20110319.

CONTRAST-ENHANCED MAGNETIC RESONANCE IMAGING AND COMPUTED TOMOGRAPHY

Contrast-enhanced MRI and CT are used to evaluate salivary gland infection, inflammatory conditions and the anatomical relations of salivary gland masses. CT is more readily available and quicker to obtain in the acute setting. Novel multiplanar or volumetric high-resolution, fat-suppressed and contrast-enhanced MRI sequences effectively demonstrate the relationship of a mass to the parotid duct and facial nerve[1-3] and perineural spread.[4,5] Diffusion-weighted imaging,[6] dynamic contrast-enhanced MRI[7,8] and MR spectroscopy[9] have been used to differentiate between benign and malignant salivary gland tumours.

17

References

1. Kim Y, Jeong HS, Kim HJ, et al. Three-dimensional double-echo steady-state with water excitation magnetic resonance imaging to localize the intraparotid facial nerve in patients with deep-seated parotid tumors. *Neuroradiology.* 2021;63(5):731–739.
2. Guenette JP, Ben-Shlomo N, Jayender J, et al. MR imaging of the extracranial facial nerve with the CISS sequence. *AJNR Am J Neuroradiol.* 2019;40(11):1954–1959.
3. Fujii H, Fujita A, Kanazawa H, et al. Localization of parotid gland tumors in relation to the intraparotid facial nerve on 3D double-echo steady-state with water excitation sequence. *AJNR Am J Neuroradiol.* 2019;40(6):1037–1042.
4. Seitz J, Held P, Strotzer M, et al. MR imaging of cranial nerve lesions using six different high-resolution T1- and T2(*)-weighted 3D and 2D sequences. *Acta Radiol.* 2002;43(4):349–353.
5. Freling N, Crippa F, Maroldi R. Staging and follow-up of high-grade malignant salivary gland tumours: the role of traditional versus functional imaging approaches: a review. *Oral Oncol.* 2016;60:157–166.
6. Yuan Y, Tang W, Tao X. Parotid gland lesions: separate and combined diagnostic value of conventional MRI, diffusion-weighted imaging and dynamic contrast-enhanced MRI. *Br J Radiol.* 2016;89(1060):20150912.
7. Lam PD, Kuribayashi A, Imaizumi A, et al. Differentiating benign and malignant salivary gland tumours: diagnostic criteria and the accuracy of dynamic contrast-enhanced MRI with high temporal resolution. *Br J Radiol.* 2015;88(1049):20140685.
8. Mogen JL, Block KT, Bansal NK, et al. Dynamic contrast-enhanced MRI to differentiate parotid neoplasms using golden-angle radial sparse parallel imaging. *AJNR Am J Neuroradiol.* 2019;40(6):1029–1036.
9. Law BKH, King AD, Ai QY, et al. Head and neck tumors: amide proton transfer MRI. *Radiology.* 2018;288(3):782–790.

Methods of Imaging the Thyroid and Parathyroid Glands

1. US
2. CT
3. MRI
4. Radionuclide imaging, including positron emission tomography (PET)

ULTRASOUND OF THE THYROID GLAND

Indications

1. Palpable thyroid mass
2. Screening high-risk patients
3. Suspected thyroid tumour
4. 'Cold spot' on scintigraphy or increased avidity on PET
5. Suspected retrosternal extension of thyroid
6. Guided aspiration or biopsy
7. Thyroid pain

Contraindications

None

Patient Preparation

None

Equipment

1. 10- to 15-MHz high-frequency linear array transducer
2. 3- to 10-MHz medium-frequency small, curved array transducer for large patients or when there is a large goitre to assess the full extent of the thyroid

For FNA:

1. Local anaesthesia: 1% lidocaine
2. Choice of needle: 22- to 25-gauge, hollow bore or with stylet
3. 5-mL syringe: may be needed to dispense sample from syringe onto slides
4. Glass slides with or without fixative

Technique

The patient is supine with the neck extended (a pillow under the shoulders can be helpful). Both lobes of the thyroid and the isthmus are scanned in the transverse and longitudinal planes. Nodules are assessed for features that help to distinguish benign from indeterminate or malignant nodules (including size, echogenicity, outline and vascularity).[1–5] The thyroid parenchyma is also assessed for evidence of thyroiditis, which is usually diffuse but may be heterogeneous or unilateral (e.g. granulomatous thyroiditis).[6] If there is retrosternal extension, angling downward and scanning during swallowing may enable the lowest extent of the thyroid to be visualized. Tracheal size and deviation can also be commented on. The neck should routinely be assessed for the presence of metastatic lymph nodes.

Ideally, US should be undertaken with the facility to proceed to FNAB or core biopsy available if required. Consideration should be given to pausing or changing anticoagulation or antiplatelet therapy before core biopsy or FNAB when there is significant clotting derangement. Core biopsy is performed with local anaesthesia (1% lidocaine) infiltrated down to the capsule; FNAB can be performed with or without local anaesthesia, depending on operator and patient choice. For FNAB, a hollow-bore or stylet needle may be used, and the sample is most often collected via capillary action. For core biopsy, an 18-gauge needle is usually appropriate with one or two passes. Manual compression of the neck after the procedure helps to prevent haematoma formation.

Slides are prepared by placing a small drop of the sample at one end of the slide. A second slide is placed parallel at 45 degrees to the sample, slowly lowered and dragged across the slide to make a flame-shaped spread. Fixative may or not be used, depending on local laboratory protocols.

For thyroid cyst aspiration, the process is similar to FNAB, although a larger bore needle and extension tubing with a three-way tap may be helpful, depending on the size of the cyst and viscosity of the contents. There is a risk of haemorrhage into the cystic part of a nodule after aspiration; although the reported rates are highly variable,[7,8] this is probably a rare occurrence. Nevertheless patients should be warned that excessive postprocedure neck swelling or pain should prompt attendance to the emergency department.

References

1. Perros P, Boelaert K, Colley S, et al. British Thyroid Association. Guidelines for the management of thyroid cancer. *Clin Endocrinol.* 2014;81(suppl 1):1–122.
2. Tessler FN, Middleton WD, Grant EG, et al. ACR Thyroid Imaging, Reporting and Data System (TI-RADS): white paper of the ACR TI-RADS Committee. *J Am Coll Radiol.* 2017;14(5):587–595.
3. Russ G, Bonnema SJ, Erdogan MF, et al. European Thyroid Association guidelines for ultrasound malignancy risk stratification of thyroid nodules in adults: the EU-TIRADS. *Eur Thyroid J.* 2017;6(5):225–237.
4. Shin JH, Baek JH, Chung J, et al. Korean Society of Thyroid Radiology (KSThR) and Korean Society of Radiology. Ultrasonography diagnosis and imaging-based management of thyroid nodules: revised Korean Society of Thyroid Radiology consensus statement and recommendations. *Korean J Radiol.* 2016;17(3):370–395.
5. Haugen BR, Alexander EK, Bible KC, et al. American Thyroid Association management guidelines for adult patients with thyroid nodules and differentiated thyroid cancer: the American Thyroid Association guidelines task force on thyroid nodules and differentiated thyroid cancer. *Thyroid.* 2016;26:1–133.
6. Park SY, Kim EK, Kim MJ, et al. Ultrasonographic characteristics of subacute granulomatous thyroiditis. *Korean J Radiol.* 2006;7(4):229–234.
7. Braga M, Cavalcanti TC, Collaço LM, et al. Efficacy of ultrasound-guided fine-needle aspiration biopsy in the diagnosis of complex thyroid nodules. *J Clin Endocrinol Metab.* 2001;86(9):4089–4091.
8. Cappelli C, Pirola I, Castellano M, et al. Fine needle cytology of complex thyroid nodules. *Eur J Endocrinol.* 2007;157(4):529–532.

ULTRASOUND OF THE PARATHYROID GLANDS

Normal parathyroid glands cannot be seen with US because of their small size and similar echotexture to surrounding adipose tissue.[1] For the detection of enlarged (>1 cm) parathyroid glands by hyperplasia, adenomas and carcinoma, US is performed using a similar technique to that used for the thyroid. Scanning with the patient's head in extreme lateral extension and a small, curved array transducer can help to visualize deeper glands. Visible glands are usually ovoid and hypoechoic compared with the thyroid parenchyma, although some glands undergo cystic change. Colour Doppler imaging will usually show polar vascularity and can help to distinguish a parathyroid adenoma from a lymph node or thyroid nodule.[2] Scanning for ectopic glands should include the neck from the hyoid to the superior mediastinum and laterally to the carotid sheaths.

References

1. Ha TK, Kim DW, Jung SJ. Ultrasound detection of normal parathyroid glands: a preliminary study. *Radiol Med.* 2017;122(11):866–870.
2. Rickes S, Sitzy J, Neye H, et al. High-resolution ultrasound in combination with colour-Doppler sonography for preoperative localization of parathyroid adenomas in patients with primary hyperparathyroidism. *Ultraschall Med.* 2003;24(2):85–89.

COMPUTED TOMOGRAPHY AND MAGNETIC RESONANCE IMAGING OF THE THYROID AND PARATHYROID GLANDS

Indications

1. Staging of known thyroid malignancy in specific cases
2. To assess the extent of a substernal goitre and tracheal compromise
3. Localization of parathyroid glands in hyperparathyroidism

IV contrast should be avoided, when possible, if treatment with radioactive iodine is planned within 8 weeks. Particular care must be taken if iodinated IV contrast is administered to hyperthyroid patients (see Chapter 2).[1] For MRI, gadolinium-based IV contrast agents can be used without compromise. Because of its iodine content, the thyroid is usually hyperdense on unenhanced CT. In parathyroid disease, contrast-enhanced CT and occasionally MRI are used to localize adenomas that are ectopic or occult on other imaging modalities and in patients with persistent or recurrent hyperparathyroidism after neck exploration. Increasingly, parathyroid protocol CT (unenhanced, arterial and delayed phase) is used to localize adenomas before minimally invasive parathyroidectomy; there is evidence that CT alone is as accurate as US and sestamibi and that CT in addition to US is more accurate.[2]

References

1. Bednarczuk T, Brix TH, Schima W, et al. European Thyroid Association Guidelines for the management of iodine-based contrast media-induced thyroid dysfunction. *Eur Thyroid J.* 2021;10(4):269–284.
2. de Jong MC, Jamal K, Morley S, et al. The use of computed tomography as a first-line imaging modality in patients with primary hyperparathyroidism. *Hormones (Athens).* 2021;20(3):499–506.

RADIONUCLIDE THYROID IMAGING

Indications
1. Assessment of functionality of thyroid nodules
2. Assessment of goitre, including hyperthyroid goitre
3. Assessment of uptake function before radioiodine treatment
4. Assessment of ectopic thyroid tissue
5. Assessment of suspected thyroiditis
6. Assessment of neonatal hypothyroidism
7. Assessment and follow-up of differentiated thyroid malignancy (papillary, follicular and Hürthle cell). Medullary thyroid cancer cells do not absorb iodine; therefore, radioiodine scans are not used for this type of cancer.

17

Contraindications
Pregnancy, allergy

Radiopharmaceuticals
^{99m}Tc-pertechnetate, 80 MBq maximum (1 mSv effective dose (ED)). Pertechnetate ions are trapped in the thyroid by an active transport mechanism but are not organified. Cheap and readily available, it is an acceptable alternative to ^{123}I.

1. ^{123}I-sodium iodide, 20 MBq maximum (4 mSv ED). Iodide ions are trapped by the thyroid in the same way as ^{99m}Tc-pertechnetate but are also organified, allowing overall assessment of thyroid function. ^{123}I is the agent of choice, but as a cyclotron product, it is thus relatively expensive with limited availability. (^{131}I-sodium iodide can also be used for imaging but is associated with a significantly higher radiation dose, so it is generally used in the context of whole-body imaging after ^{131}I ablation.)

Equipment
1. Gamma camera
2. Pinhole, converging or high-resolution parallel hole collimator

Patient Preparation
None, but uptake may be reduced by antithyroid drugs, iodine-based preparations and radiographic iodinated contrast media

Technique
^{99m}Tc-pertechnetate
1. IV injection of ^{99m}Tc-pertechnetate
2. After 15 min, immediately before imaging, the patient is given a drink of water to clear ^{99m}Tc-pertechnetate-labelled saliva from the oesophagus.
3. Start imaging 20 min after injection when the target-to-background ratio is maximum.

4. The patient lies supine with the neck slightly extended and the camera anterior. For a pinhole collimator, the pinhole should be positioned to give the maximum magnification for the camera field of view (usually 7–10 cm from the neck).
5. The patient should be asked not to swallow or talk during imaging. An image is acquired with markers on the suprasternal notch, clavicles, edges of the neck and any palpable nodules.
6. The injection site should be imaged if quantification is to be performed.

^{123}I-sodium iodide

The technique is similar to that for ^{99m}Tc-pertechnetate, except for the following:

1. Sodium iodide may be given IV or orally
2. Imaging is performed 3–4 h after IV administration or 24 h after an oral dose
3. A drink of water is not necessary because ^{123}I is not secreted into saliva in any significant quantity

Images

^{99m}Tc-pertechnetate: 100–200 kilocount image
$\quad$ ^{123}I-sodium iodide: 50–100 kilocount image

1. Anterior to include the salivary glands and suprasternal notch marker
2. Left anterior oblique and right anterior oblique views as required, especially for assessment of multinodular disease, and if a nodule is suspected but not seen on the anterior view
3. Large field of view image if retrosternal extension or ectopic thyroid tissue is suspected

Analysis

The percentage thyroid uptake may be estimated by comparing the background-subtracted attenuation-corrected organ counts with the full syringe counts measured under standard conditions before injection.

Additional Techniques

1. Metastatic thyroid cancer can be evaluated using diagnostic ^{123}I or therapeutic ^{131}I whole-body scans. Whole-body ^{131}I imaging is often performed after thyroidectomy and ^{131}I ablation for thyroid cancer to locate sites of metastasis. In this application single-photon emission computed tomography (SPECT)-CT imaging is frequently undertaken to improve tumour detection around the thyroid bed and neck. When the scan results are negative but serum thyroglobulin is raised, fluorodeoxyglucose (FDG) PET-CT results are often positive.
2. Perchlorate discharge tests can be performed after imaging with ^{123}I-sodium iodide to assess possible organification defects, particularly in congenital hypothyroidism.

Metastatic medullary carcinoma of the thyroid can be imaged with either pentavalent dimercaptosuccinic acid, indium-labelled octreotide, MIBG (meta-iodobenzylguanidine), or more recently, FDG PET-CT. These techniques are discussed in Chapter 13.

Aftercare
None

Complications
None

17

RADIONUCLIDE PARATHYROID IMAGING

Indications
Preoperative localization of parathyroid adenomas and hyperplastic glands

Contraindications
Pregnancy, allergy

Radiopharmaceuticals
^{99m}Tc-methoxyisobutylisonitrile (MIBI or sestamibi), 500 MBq typical, 900 MBq maximum (11 mSv ED), and ^{99m}Tc-pertechnetate, 80 MBq maximum (1 mSv ED). Both MIBI and pertechnetate are trapped by the thyroid, but only MIBI accumulates in hyperactive parathyroid tissue. With computer subtraction of ^{99m}Tc-pertechnetate from MIBI images, abnormal accumulation of MIBI may be seen. MIBI also washes out of normal thyroid tissue faster than parathyroid, so delayed images (1–4 h) can highlight abnormal parathyroid activity.

^{99m}Tc-tetrofosmin (Myoview) can be used as an alternative to MIBI and is as effective if the subtraction technique is used but is not as good for delayed imaging since differential washout is not as good as for MIBI.

1. ^{201}Tl-thallous chloride (80 MBq maximum, 18 mSv ED) was previously used in conjunction with ^{99m}Tc-pertechnetate but is increasingly being replaced by the technetium agents because of their superior imaging quality and lower radiation doses.
2. ^{11}C-choline has been shown to be highly sensitive and specific for the localization of parathyroid adenomas in small series,[1] but its effect on patient outcomes compared with MIBI SPECT-CT is unknown, and it is currently three to four times more expensive.[2]

Equipment
1. Gamma camera (small field of view preferable for thyroid images; large field of view for chest images)

2. High-resolution parallel hole collimator is preferred to a pinhole collimator, which may result in repositioning magnification errors and compromise subtraction techniques
3. Imaging computer capable of image registration and subtraction

Patient Preparation

None, but uptake may be modified by antithyroid drugs and iodine-based medications, skin preparations and recent iodinated contrast media.

Technique

A variety of imaging protocols have been used, with either ^{99m}Tc-pertechnetate or MIBI administered first, with subtraction and possibly additional delayed imaging, and using MIBI alone with early and delayed imaging. Subtraction techniques are most sensitive, but additional delayed imaging may increase sensitivity slightly and improve confidence in the result. The advantage of administering ^{99m}Tc-pertechnetate first is that MIBI injection can follow within 30 min, with the patient still in position to minimize movement, and if subtraction shows a clearly positive result, the patient does not need to stay for delayed imaging. With MIBI injected first, ^{99m}Tc-pertechnetate can only be administered after several hours when washout has occurred:

1. 80 MBq ^{99m}Tc-pertechnetate is administered IV through a cannula that is left in place for the second injection.
2. After 15 min, the patient is given a drink of water immediately before imaging to wash away ^{99m}Tc-pertechnetate secreted into saliva.
3. The patient lies supine with the neck slightly extended, and the camera is positioned anteriorly over the thyroid.
4. The patient should be asked to not move during imaging. Head-immobilizing devices may be useful, and marker sources may aid repositioning.
5. Twenty minutes after injection, a 10-min 128 × 128 image is acquired.
6. Without moving the patient, 500 MBq ^{99m}Tc-MIBI is injected IV through the previously positioned cannula (to avoid a second venepuncture, which might cause patient movement).
7. Ten minutes after injection, a further 10-min 128 × 128 image is acquired.
8. A chest and neck image should then be acquired on a large field of view camera to detect ectopic parathyroid tissue.
9. Computer image registration and normalization is performed and the pertechnetate image subtracted from the 10-min MIBI image.
10. If a lesion is clearly visible in the subtracted image, the patient can leave.
11. If the lesion is not obvious, late MIBI imaging can be performed at hourly intervals up to 4 h, if necessary, to look for differential washout.
12. SPECT-CT imaging is increasingly performed. This enables correlation of foci of uptake with CT features increasing sensitivity and specificity and allowing more accurate presurgical localization.

Additional Techniques

1. In patients in whom ^{99m}Tc-pertechnetate thyroid uptake is suppressed (e.g. with use of iodine-containing contrast media or skin preparations), oral ^{123}I (20 MBq) administered several hours before MIBI may be considered.
2. Dynamic imaging with motion correction may reduce motion artefact.

Aftercare

None

Complications

None

References

1. Parvinian A, Martin-Macintosh EL, Goenka AH, et al. ^{11}C-choline PET/CT for detection and localization of parathyroid adenomas. *AJR Am J Roentgenol.* 2018;210(2):418–422.
2. Quak E, Lasne Cardon A, Ciappuccini R, et al. Upfront F18-choline PET/CT versus Tc99m-sestaMIBI SPECT/CT guided surgery in primary hyperparathyroidism: the randomized phase III diagnostic trial APACH2. *BMC Endocr Disord.* 2021;21(1):3.

Further Reading

Agrawal K, Esmail AA, Gnanasegaran G, et al. Pitfalls and limitations of radionuclide imaging in endocrinology. *Semin Nucl Med.* 2015;45(5):440–457.
Hindié E, Zanotti-Fregonara P, Tabarin A, et al. The role of radionuclide imaging in the surgical management of primary hyperparathyroidism. *J Nucl Med.* 2015;56(5):737–744.

THYROID RADIOFREQUENCY ABLATION

Indications

1. To reduce the size of benign thyroid nodules
2. To treat autonomously functioning thyroid nodules

Contraindications

Indeterminate, suspicious or malignant cytology

Equipment

1. US machine and high-frequency linear array transducer (10–15 MHz)
2. Radiofrequency generator, dispersive electrodes and cooling pump
3. Internally cooled monopolar 18-gauge electrode with an active tip of 0.7 or 1 cm

Patient Preparation

1. Consideration should be given to pausing or changing anticoagulant or antiplatelet therapy before the procedure.
2. Two benign FNABs from the nodule to be treated

Technique

1. Patient supine with neck extended (pillow under shoulders can help), sterile drapes and skin cleaned with antiseptic solution
2. A mixture of long- and shorter-acting local anaesthetic in a 1:1 ratio (0.5% bupivacaine:1% lidocaine) infiltrated at the electrode skin entry point down to the thyroid capsule in the midline to facilitate a transisthmic approach
3. Cystic contents aspirated before ablation
4. Moving shot technique under US-guidance: The electrode is placed into the most inferior and lateral part of the nodule and gradually withdrawn while each small volume of tissue is ablated. Ablation is continued in layers, treating inferior to superior, lateral to medial and deep to superficial until the whole nodule has been ablated
5. Care is taken not to ablate close to the 'danger triangle' at the medial aspect of the thyroid, which includes the recurrent laryngeal nerve and cervical oesophagus or within 5 mm of the capsule

Aftercare

After the procedure, a cool pack is placed on the neck, and the patient is monitored for up to 1 h.

Complications

1. Local pain and swelling during and after the procedure and referred pain during the procedure
2. Haematoma
3. Infection
4. Hoarse voice: most often temporary
5. Skin burn or pigmentation
6. Temporary or long-tern thyroid hormone dysregulation
7. Nodule rupture: This is a delayed phenomenon, occurring 6–8 weeks after the procedure.

Further Reading

Jawad S, Morley S, Otero S, et al. Ultrasound-guided radiofrequency ablation (RFA) of benign symptomatic thyroid nodules—initial UK experience. *Br J Radiol.* 2019;92(1098):20190026.

Kim JH, Baek JH, Lim HK, et al. Guideline Committee for the Korean Society of Thyroid Radiology (KSThR) and Korean Society of Radiology. 2017 Thyroid Radiofrequency Ablation Guideline: Korean Society of Thyroid Radiology. *Korean J Radiol.* 2018;19(4):632–655.

THYROID ETHANOL ABLATION

This is done for confirmed benign cystic nodules in the thyroid that recur after aspiration, ethanol injection into the cyst can result in permanent tissue damage with subsequent necrosis, fibrosis and thrombosis of the cyst wall blood vessels.

Indications

Purely or predominantly (>50%) cystic thyroid nodules

Contraindications

Indeterminate, suspicious or malignant cytology

Equipment

1. Needle, syringe and, if required, tubing and a three-way tap for aspiration of the cyst before injection
2. Needle and syringe containing ethanol for injection

17

Technique

1. With or without injection of local anaesthetic to the thyroid capsule, the cyst is aspirated as completely as possible, while the tip of the needle is still visualized within the cyst.
2. Immediately after aspiration, ethanol is injected into the cyst (up to 50% of the volume aspirated).
3. Depending on operator preference, the ethanol can be left within the cyst for several minutes and then aspirated completely, partially aspirated leaving some ethanol within the cyst, or a smaller amount is injected, and the entire amount is left within the cyst.

Aftercare

None

Complications

1. Pain
2. Haemorrhage into the cyst
3. Hoarseness
4. Transient hyperthyroidism

Breast

Megan Bydder and Simon Lowes

OVERVIEW OF BREAST IMAGING

Imaging Pathways

Breast imaging is carried out for a variety of indications, both benign and malignant. The two main routes by which patients enter breast imaging pathways are:

- Symptomatic
  - When women (and men) with breast symptoms are referred via their general practitioners to a one-stop breast clinic under the 2-week pathway
- Screening, including
  - The NHS Breast Screening Programme (NHS BSP) for asymptomatic women aged 50–70 years (by invitation)
  - The NHS BSP for asymptomatic women aged over 70 years (by self-referral)
  - Screening for women at 'moderate', 'high' or 'very high' risk of breast cancer, which typically starts at an earlier age

Triple Assessment

Patients who present with breast symptoms undergo 'triple assessment', which consists of clinical assessment, imaging and (when appropriate) needle biopsy (Fig. 18.1). Imaging in each case is determined by symptoms, clinical findings and age. In women aged younger than 40 years, ultrasound (US) is the first-line modality of choice, and in women aged 40 years and older, mammography is the first-line modality of choice, in combination with US if there are focal symptoms or signs.

The level of suspicion for malignancy is recorded using the British Society of Breast Radiology (BSBR) imaging classification (1 = normal, 2 = benign, 3 = indeterminate, 4 = suspicious, 5 = highly suspicious, with prefix M for mammography and U for ultrasound).[1] Similarly, clinical assessment and needle biopsy are scored using a P1–P5 and B1–B5 scoring system, respectively. All patients undergoing triple assessment are subsequently discussed at a multidisciplinary team (MDT) meeting where concordance between the three components of triple assessment is sought and recommendations for management are made.

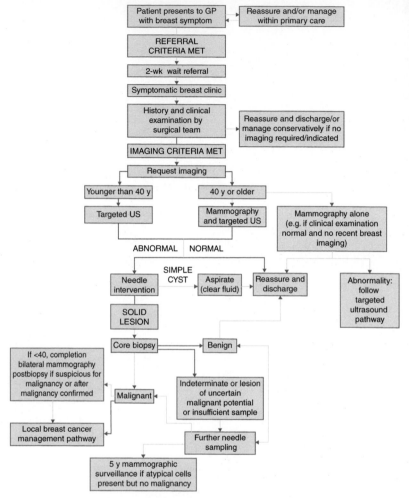

Fig. 18.1 Pathway showing investigation and management of patients presenting with breast symptoms. (*GP,* general practitioner; *US,* ultrasound).

Figure 18.1 outlines the typical approach to investigation and management of patients presenting with breast symptoms.

Screening

Women aged 50–70+ years undergo screening via the NHS BSP with mammography every 3 years. Women at moderate, high risk or very high risk of breast cancer are screened from a younger age and at more frequent intervals, and this may involve mammography, breast magnetic resonance imaging (MRI) or both depending on their risk category.

Those with abnormal screening findings are recalled for triple assessment, which consists of clinical examination, further imaging (additional mammographic views, US or both) and needle biopsy if indicated.

Imaging in Breast Cancer

Breast imaging also plays a major role in the preoperative workup of patients with breast cancer and posttreatment follow-up. Most breast cancers are diagnosed using a combination of mammography and US, together with image-guided needle biopsy. US, in addition to assessing the breast, assesses the axilla to complete locoregional staging of breast cancers. In most cases, this combination of imaging techniques is all that is required for pretreatment planning. Although first-line mammography is usually only carried out in women aged 40 years and older, completion bilateral mammography is performed in younger women when breast cancer is strongly suspected or proven.

18

The mainstay of breast cancer treatment is surgery, either breast-conserving surgery (wide local excision or lumpectomy) or mastectomy, with most patients undergoing breast conservation. Around 90% of patients will proceed directly to surgery as their primary treatment, and around 10% will undergo neoadjuvant chemotherapy (NAC) before surgery to downstage their disease.

For some patients, additional imaging may be indicated preoperatively. For example, patients having NAC typically undergo serial MRI scanning to monitor response to treatment. Other indications for preoperative MRI include invasive lobular carcinoma, which comprises around 15% of breast cancers and is often mammographically subtle, and mammographically occult breast cancer.

Breast-conserving surgery necessitates accurate preoperative staging of breast cancer, but because most breast cancers are either impalpable or poorly palpable, it also requires effective preoperative localization of disease so that the surgeon can precisely excise the cancer without taking excess tissue or leaving disease behind. Thus, the breast imaging team plays a critical role in image-guided tumour localization.

Guidance

Key guidance for appropriate use of breast imaging is provided via several sources, including

- The Royal College of Radiologists (RCR)
- British Society of Breast Radiology (BSBR)
- The NHS Breast Screening Programme (NHS BSP)
- National Institute for Health and Care Excellence (NICE)

Reference
1. Bydder M, Cornford E, Cox J, et al. *Guidance on screening and symptomatic breast imaging*. Fourth edition. The Royal College of Radiologists; 2019. <https://www.rcr.ac.uk/system/files/publication/field_publication_files/bfcr199-guidance-on-screening-and-symptomatic-breast-imaging.pdf>.

MAMMOGRAPHY

Indications

1. Focal breast symptoms or signs in women aged 40 years and older in the context of triple assessment at a specialist, multidisciplinary, diagnostic breast clinic
2. All patients with strongly suspected or confirmed malignancy, irrespective of age
3. Breast cancer follow-up, typically annually for 5 years
4. Men aged 50 years and older with unexplained or suspicious unilateral breast enlargement or when there is clinical uncertainty in differentiating between true gynaecomastia and fatty breast enlargement
5. Axillary lump without clinical breast abnormality in patients aged 40 years and older
6. NHS BSP population screening of asymptomatic women or trans or non-binary individuals with breasts, with 3-yearly screening by invitation (aged 50–70 years) or self-referral (older than 70 years)
7. Screening for women at 'moderate', 'high' or 'very high' risk of breast because of a significant family history of breast cancer, the presence of a pathogenic gene variant such as *BRCA1/2* or previous history of mantle radiotherapy for Hodgkin lymphoma[1]
8. Investigation in women with metastatic malignancy of unknown origin
9. Selected patients undergoing aesthetic surgery, including asymptomatic women aged 40 years and older with no prior mammography in the preceding 12 months[2]

Not Indicated

1. Symptomatic women younger than 40 years unless breast cancer is strongly suspected or confirmed
2. Screening in women younger than 50 years unless at 'moderate', 'high' or 'very high' risk of breast cancer
3. Investigation of generalized signs or symptoms such as cyclical mastalgia or non-focal pain or lumpiness
4. To assess the integrity of silicone implants
5. Individuals affected by ataxia-telangiectasia mutated gene mutation with resultant high sensitivity to radiation exposure, including medical x-rays
6. Routine investigation of gynaecomastia

Equipment

Conventional film-screen mammographic technology has been superseded by full-field digital mammography (FFDM), which has a higher sensitivity in younger women and those with dense breasts, which contain a high proportion of fibroglandular tissue compared with fatty tissue.[3]

Advances in FFDM include the following:

1. Digital breast tomosynthesis (DBT), which creates a stack of 'slices' through the breast volume by combining data from a series of two-dimensional projections acquired during a single sweep of the x-ray tube. DBT has a significant increased accuracy in the diagnostic

evaluation of masses and parenchymal distortions, irrespective of breast density. Further studies suggest the potential, within the screening setting, to increase sensitivity by around 30% with a concomitant reduction in recall rate of 15%, as well as a potential radiation dose reduction of up to 50% compared with the current two-view mammography.[4] It is now possible to carry out x-ray–guided biopsy using tomosynthesis to identify the 'slice' most accurately demonstrating the target lesion, thus avoiding the requirement to carry out stereotactic, paired images for depth localization.

2. Contrast-enhanced spectral mammography (CESM) combines mammography with intravenous (IV) iodinated contrast to improve cancer detection. A dual-energy technique produces a low-energy image (similar to a conventional mammogram) and a high-energy image, which on its own is non-diagnostic. The recombined subtracted images highlight areas of contrast uptake within the breast. CESM can be a valuable tool in the diagnosis and local staging of breast cancer, particularly when MRI is contraindicated.

3. Computer-aided detection (CAD) software can assist mammogram reading by placing prompts over areas of potential mammographic concern. In the screening setting, single reading in association with CAD may offer sensitivities and specificities comparable to that of double reading.[5] Artificial intelligence in breast imaging, as in other areas of radiology, is a rapidly emerging adjunct.[6]

18

Technique

Standard mammographic examination comprises imaging of both breasts in two views, namely the mediolateral oblique (MLO) (which is angled to include the axillary tail) and craniocaudal (CC) positions. Screening methodology is bilateral, two-view (MLO and CC) mammography at all screening rounds.

Additional views may be required to provide adequate visualization of all breast tissue:

1. Laterally and medially extended CC
2. True lateral view
3. Eklund 'implant-displaced' view in patients with breast implants'

Compression of the breast is an integral part of mammographic imaging resulting in:

1. Reduction in radiation dose
2. Immobilization of the breast, thus reducing blurring
3. Uniformity of breast thickness, allowing even penetration
4. Reduction in breast thickness, thus reducing scatter and noise, achieving higher resolution

Adaptation of the technique can provide additional information:

1. Spot compression to reduce the impact of overlapping composite tissue

2. Magnification (smaller focal spot combined with a raised table to bring the breast closer to the x-ray source, thus geometrically magnifying the image), to permit detailed analysis, particularly of the morphology and distribution of microcalcification

References

1. Hancock SL, Tucker MA, Hoppe RT. Breast cancer after treatment of Hodgkin's disease. *J Natl Cancer Inst*. 1993;85:25–31.
2. Lowes S, MacNeill F, Martin L, et al. Breast Imaging for Aesthetic Surgery: Best Practice Guidance from the British Society of Breast Radiology (BSBR), Association of Breast Surgery (ABS), and the British Association of Plastic Reconstructive and Aesthetic Surgeons (BAPRAS). *J Plast Reconstr Aesthet Surg*. 2018;71(11):1521–1531.
3. Pisano ED, Gatsonis C, Hendrick E, et al. Diagnostic performance of digital versus film mammography for breast cancer screening. *N Engl J Med*. 2005;353:1773–1783.
4. Skaane P, Bados AI, Gullien R, et al. Comparison of digital mammography alone and digital mammography plus tomosynthesis in a population-based screening program. *Radiology*. 2013;267:47–56.
5. Gilbert FJ, Astley SM, McGee MA, et al. Single reading with computer-aided detection and double reading of screening mammograms in the United Kingdom National Breast Screening Program. *Radiology*. 2006;241:47–53.
6. Le EPV, Wang Y, Huang Y, et al. Artificial intelligence in breast imaging. *Clin Radiol*. 2019;74(5):357–366.
7. Eklund GW, Busby RC, Miller SH, et al. Improved imaging of the augmented breast. *AJR Am J Roentgenol*. 1988;151:469–473.

Further Reading

Mackenzie A, Bydder M. *National Breast Imaging Academy e-Learning for Healthcare programme*. <https://portal.e-lfh.org.uk/Component/Details/662955>.

Moyle P, Given-Wilson R, Dumonteil S. *National Breast Imaging Academy e-Learning for Healthcare programme*. <https://portal.e-lfh.org.uk/Component/Details/642877>.

National Institute for Health and Care Excellence. NICE Clinical Guidelines. Familial breast cancer: classification, care and managing breast cancer and related risks in people with a family history of breast cancer (CG 164). 2013. <https://www.nice.org.uk/guidance/cg164>.

ULTRASOUND

Indications

1. Evaluation of focal breast symptoms in women of all ages in the context of triple assessment at a specialist, multidisciplinary diagnostic breast clinic
2. Men with unexplained or suspicious unilateral breast enlargement or clinical uncertainty in differentiating between true gynaecomastia and fatty breast enlargement
3. Evaluation of axillary lymph nodes in patients with suspected or confirmed breast cancer as part of locoregional staging
4. Image-guided diagnostic biopsy of breast and axillary abnormalities
5. Image-guided excision of breast abnormalities
6. Image-guided preoperative localization of both palpable and impalpable breast lesions
7. Diagnosis and guidance of drainage of fluid collections within the breast, including seroma and abscess

8. Assessment of implant integrity

Not Indicated

1. In the investigation of generalized signs or symptoms such as cyclical breast pain or non-focal pain or lumpiness
2. In the routine investigation of gynaecomastia

Equipment

Handheld, high-frequency (18-MHz) contact US is widely used in breast imaging, with concomitant advantages of cost, accessibility and safety. Proprietary standoff gels can be useful when assessing superficial lesions and the nipple–areolar complex.

18

Technique

1. The patient lies on the examination couch with the upper clothing removed and the ipsilateral arm behind the head.
2. Positioning is supine for examination of the medial breast and lateral oblique for examination of the lateral breast, axillary tail and axilla.

Additional Techniques

Elastography is a non-invasive US technique that measures the elasticity or stiffness of tissue by evaluating its transformation when pressure is applied. It provides a visual representation of the stiffness of tissue and is increasingly being used as an adjunct to greyscale imaging to assist in benign–malignant differentiation of solid masses.[1] Malignant lesions tend to show increased stiffness, with stiffness correlating with increasing size and histological grade, so elastography can be particularly useful in high-grade cancers that may have deceptively benign greyscale appearances.

Contrast-enhanced US using microbubbles has the potential to improve the diagnostic accuracy of preoperative axillary staging by allowing accurate identification of the sentinel lymph node and thereby enabling targeted core biopsy.[2]

References
1. Navarro B, Ubeda B, Vallespi M, et al. Role of elastography in the assessment of breast lesions—preliminary results. *J Ultrasound Med.* 2011;30:313–321.
2. Sever AR, Mills P, Weeks J, et al. Preoperative needle biopsy of sentinel lymph nodes using intradermal microbubbles and contrast-enhanced ultrasound in patients with breast cancer. *AJR Am J Roentgenol.* 2012;199:465–470.

Further Reading
Evans A, Lowes S. Advanced ultrasound techniques 1: elastography. *National Breast Imaging Academy e-Learning for Healthcare programme.* <https://portal.e-lfh.org.uk/Component/Details/647859>.
Jenkins F, Lowes S. Axillary staging in breast cancer patients. *National Breast Imaging Academy e-Learning for Healthcare programme.* <https://portal.e-lfh.org.uk/Component/Details/635120>.
Nash J, Leaver A. Principles of ultrasound-guided intervention. *National Breast Imaging Academy e-Learning for Healthcare programme.* <https://portal.e-lfh.org.uk/Component/Details/662517>.

Sever A, Lowes S. Advanced ultrasound techniques 2: microbubbles. *National Breast Imaging Academy e-Learning for Healthcare programme.* <https://portal.e-lfh.org.uk/Component/Details/662904>.

Stavros AT. *Breast Ultrasound.* Lippincott, Williams & Wilkins; 2003.

Verheuvel NC, van den Hoven I, Ooms HW, et al. The role of ultrasound-guided lymph node biopsy in the axillary staging of invasive breast cancer in the post-ACOSOG Z0011 trial era. *Ann Surg Oncol.* 2015;22:409–415.

MAGNETIC RESONANCE IMAGING

Breast MRI has two main applications: the investigation of breast cancer and the assessment of implant integrity.

In the context of breast cancer, there are specific indications for MRI. As such, it is not used as a routine investigation for the preoperative assessment of all breast cancers.[1,2] The indications can, however, vary slightly between different sets of guidance and in different countries. A representative overview is given here.

Indications in the Context of Malignancy

1. If breast conservation is being considered in:
   - Cases in which sizing is uncertain on clinical examination and conventional imaging (mammography and US)[1,2]
   - Cancers with a lobular component (invasive lobular carcinoma or mixed carcinomas with a lobular component)[1,2]
   - Paget's disease of the nipple[2]
2. In cases of occult disease, including:
   - Mammographically occult tumours
   - Patients presenting with axillary node metastases in whom conventional breast imaging fails to detect a primary tumour[1,2]
   - In carefully selected cases to clarify suspicious clinical findings when conventional breast imaging shows no abnormality
3. When there is suspicion of multifocal disease unconfirmed on conventional imaging[2]
4. Monitoring response to neoadjuvant chemotherapy. Typically baseline and posttreatment MRI studies ae carried out, though some centres may also use an interim scan (after two or three cycles).[2]
5. Posttreatment surveillance in carefully selected cases for the detection or exclusion of recurrent malignant disease in the conserved breast 6 months or more after surgery
6. Combined with mammography as a screening tool in women deemed to be at very high risk of developing breast cancer (see the section on mammography)
7. MRI may also have a role in the preoperative evaluation of the extent of high-grade ductal carcinoma in situ

Indications in Assessing Implant Integrity

1. MRI should be limited to cases in which there are equivocal findings on US; a normal US has a high negative predictive value for implant

rupture, and further investigation to establish implant integrity is not normally required. Similarly, unequivocal signs of rupture on US do not mandate further imaging.[2]

Technique

1. Contraindications are the same as for standard MRI examinations. Caution should be exercised in pregnancy; although MRI itself is safe, the use of gadolinium-based contrast agents is discouraged because their safety for the foetus has not yet been established.
2. Minimum field strength for breast MRI should be equivalent to 1.5 T.
3. The patient lies prone, with breasts placed in a dedicated minimum 8-channel diagnostic breast coil. Open MRI scanners are not recommended.
4. Tumour protocols necessitate IV contrast, so venous access is required. Images are obtained pre- and postcontrast (0.1 mmol kg^{-1} gadolinium chelate, given IV via pump injector).[3]
5. The current RCR guidance recommends:
   - High-resolution T2-weighted imaging with or without fat saturation
   - Diffusion-weighted imaging
   - Dynamic contrast-enhanced acquisition: each acquisition time period not to exceed 60 s (preferably not >45 s), out to 5 min
6. High-resolution 3D T1-weighted fat-suppressed gradient echo with isotropic voxels in either axial fat suppression or coronal subtraction sequences. The presence, degree, speed and morphology of the pattern of enhancement are analyzed.[2] Other breast cancer protocols such as abbreviated MRI are also in use in some centres but are currently not approved for use in screening assessment and should only be used in the context of research.[2]
7. Implant protocols typically comprise T2-weighted imaging, silicone only and silicone-suppressed sequences. IV contrast is not required.

18

References

1. National Institute for Health and Care Excellence. Early and locally advanced breast cancer: diagnosis and management (NICE guideline NG101); 2018. <https://www.nice.org.uk/guidance/ng101>.
2. Bydder M, Cornford E, Cox J, et al. *Guidance on screening and symptomatic breast imaging.* Fourth edition. London: The Royal College of Radiologists; 2019. <https://www.rcr.ac.uk/system/files/publication/field_publication_files/bfcr199-guidance-on-screening-and-symptomatic-breast-imaging.pdf>.
3. Mann RM, Cho N, Moy L. Breast MRI: state of the art. *Radiology.* 2019;292(3): 520–536.

Further Reading

American Society of Breast Surgeons. *Consensus Guideline on Diagnostic and Screening Magnetic Resonance Imaging of the Breast.* 2018. <https://www.breastsurgeons.org/docs/statements/Consensus-Guideline-on-Diagnostic-and-Screening-Magnetic-Resonance-Imaging-of-the-Breast.pdf>.

Sardanelli F, Boates C, Borisch B, et al. Magnetic resonance imaging of the breast: recommendations from the EUSOMA working group. *Eur J Cancer.* 2010;46:1296–1316.

RADIONUCLIDE TECHNIQUES

Intraoperative Sentinel Node Identification

A sentinel lymph node is the first node to which malignant cells are likely to spread from the primary tumour. The lower axillary sentinel lymph node(s) can be identified at operation after injection of a combination of radioisotope ^{99m}Tc colloidal albumin, particle size 3–80 nm and blue dye. Subareolar injection of the radioisotope in the same quadrant as the cancer allows rapid uptake to lymph nodes via the plexus of Sappey.

^{99m}Tc-Methylene Diphosphonate Bone Scintigraphy

^{99m}Tc-methylene diphosphonate (MDP) bone scintigraphy may be used to assess bony metastases in advanced breast cancer, though metastatic disease is overall uncommon as a proportion of all breast cancers, and as such, systemic imaging in not needed in the majority of patients diagnosed with breast cancer. The modality of choice in most cases in staging advanced breast cancer, including assessing the skeleton, is contrast-enhanced computed tomography (CT) of the chest, abdomen and pelvis, incorporating the supraclavicular fossae and proximal femora. This is more accurate than conventional chest radiography combined with liver US and MDP bone scintigraphy.[1] In the absence of bone symptoms, MDP scintigraphy is not routinely indicated in addition to CT.[1–3]

MDP scintigraphy may be used in the initial diagnosis of symptomatic bony metastatic disease but does not perform well in follow-up and for monitoring treatment response, in which PET-CT (see later discussion) should be considered.[1]

Positron Emission Tomography Scanning

Hybrid positron emission tomography (PET)-CT scanning with ^{18}F-fluorodeoxyglucose (FDG) may provide additional information in carefully selected cases in which restaging of disease, monitoring response to treatment or the detection of distant metastases are required. As part of systemic staging, FDG PET-CT can be used as problem-solving tool when other imaging modalities are indeterminate.[4]

In inflammatory breast cancer, PET-CT has an incremental detection rate of distant metastases over CT of approximately 25%, so its use in patients with inflammatory breast cancers should also be considered.[1]

References

1. Bydder. M, Cornford E, Cox J, et al. *Guidance on screening and symptomatic breast imaging.* Fourth edition. London: The Royal College of Radiologists; 2019. <https://www.rcr.ac.uk/system/files/publication/field_publication_files/bfcr199-guidance-on-screening-and-symptomatic-breast-imaging.pdf>.

2. Chang CY, Gill CM, Simeone FJ, et al. Comparison of the diagnostic accuracy of 99 m-Tc-MDP bone scintigraphy and 18 F-FDG PET/CT for the detection of skeletal metastases. *Acta Radiol.* 2016;57(1):58–65.
3. Bansal GJ, Vinayan Changaradil D. Planar bone scan versus computerized tomography in staging locally advanced breast cancer in asymptomatic patients: does bone scan change patient management over computerized tomography? *J Comput Assist Tomogr.* 2018;42(1):19–24.
4. Groheux D, Espié M, Giacchetti S, et al. Performance of FDG PET/CT in the clinical management of breast cancer. *Radiology.* 2013;266(2):388–405.

Further Reading
Clarke D, Khonji NI, Mansel RE. Sentinel node biopsy in breast cancer: ALMANAC trial. *World J Surg.* 2001;25:819–822.

18

IMAGE-GUIDED BIOPSY OF THE BREAST AND AXILLA

Indications

The purpose of an image-guided breast biopsy is to obtain a tissue diagnosis when the imaging findings are either indeterminate or suspicious for malignancy. There are different approaches depending upon the type of target lesion seen on imaging. Most breast biopsies (and all axillary biopsies) are done under US guidance. A smaller proportion are done under stereotactic x-ray guidance, and these mainly comprise microcalcifications, which are often not possible to discern on US. Breast biopsies can also be guided using other imaging modalities, including MRI and CESM, but these are more specialist interventions and not available at all centres.

- **Sonographically visible targets** (e.g. masses, other soft tissue abnormalities, lymph nodes): These should be biopsied under US guidance using a 14-gauge core biopsy device. In general, the only solid masses that it is not necessary to biopsy are typical fibroadenomas in women younger than 25 years old,[1] though there is evidence to suggest it is safe to increase the threshold to women up to 29 years old[2] and, if elastography is used as an adjunct, up to 39 years old.[3]
- **Targets visible only on mammography:** These tend to be microcalcifications, which are generally difficult or impossible to see on mammography, particularly if they are not associated with a mass lesion. Other entities that may only be seen on mammography include parenchymal distortions (differential diagnoses include radial scar or malignancy) and small, poorly defined opacities. These are biopsied under stereotactic x-ray guidance using either a standard core biopsy needle (14 or 12 gauge) or a vacuum-assisted biopsy (VAB) device (available in a range of needle bores but typically in the 10- to 7-gauge range), which gives a significantly larger volume of tissue.

Biopsy Outcomes

In most cases, the initial biopsy is diagnostic, and the patient will require no further needle sampling before either discharge (if

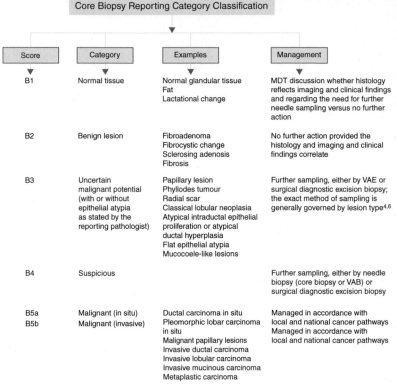

Score	Category	Examples	Management
B1	Normal tissue	Normal glandular tissue Fat Lactational change	MDT discussion whether histology reflects imaging and clinical findings and regarding the need for further needle sampling versus no further action
B2	Benign lesion	Fibroadenoma Fibrocystic change Sclerosing adenosis Fibrosis	No further action provided the histology and imaging and clinical findings correlate
B3	Uncertain malignant potential (with or without epithelial atypia as stated by the reporting pathologist)	Papillary lesion Phyllodes tumour Radial scar Classical lobular neoplasia Atypical intraductal epithelial proliferation or atypical ductal hyperplasia Flat epithelial atypia Mucocoele-like lesions	Further sampling, either by VAE or surgical diagnostic excision biopsy; the exact method of sampling is generally governed by lesion type[4,6]
B4	Suspicious		Further sampling, either by needle biopsy (core biopsy or VAB) or surgical diagnostic excision biopsy
B5a B5b	Malignant (in situ) Malignant (invasive)	Ductal carcinoma in situ Pleomorphic lobar carcinoma in situ Malignant papillary lesions Invasive ductal carcinoma Invasive lobular carcinoma Invasive mucinous carcinoma Metaplastic carcinoma	Managed in accordance with local and national cancer pathways Managed in accordance with local and national cancer pathways

MDT, Multidisciplinary team; *VAB*, vacuum-assisted biopsy; *VAE*, vacuum-assisted excision.

definitively benign) or treatment (if malignant). In a smaller number of cases, patients will undergo further needle sampling. The indications for this are given later. All breast biopsy results should be discussed at a specialist breast MDT meeting where the histopathology results can be discussed in correlation with the radiological and clinical findings to ensure concordance. This helps ensure the appropriate management.

As well as providing a histological diagnosis of the biopsy sample, the reporting pathologist assigns a B score to aid in deciding the outcome.[4]

- **B1** indicates a core of normal tissue. Because core biopsies are targeted to entities that do not correspond to what is perceived as normal tissue on imaging, a B1 outcome should be approached with caution because it may indicate that the lesion has not been sampled. However, in the case of certain benign lesions, such as hamartomas and lipomas, apparently normal histological features would be expected on core biopsy.[4] Correlation between histopathology results, imaging and clinical findings at the breast MDT meeting will decide whether further sampling is needed.
- **B2** indicates a benign abnormality, and provided the histological entity correlates with the imaging appearances and clinical findings, no further action is usually indicated.

- **B3** lesions are a heterogenous group of histological entities that carry an increased risk of associated malignancy. This risk varies with lesion type and whether there are associated atypical cells. If a B3 lesion is diagnosed on initial core biopsy, further sampling is indicated. The management of B3 lesions is covered later.
- **B4** lesions are suspicious for malignancy, and technical problems such as crushed or poorly fixed cores that contain probable carcinoma but cannot provide the definitive diagnosis tend to be assigned this. B4 results are uncommon. Further sampling, either with VAB or surgical diagnostic excision, is indicated.
- **B5** lesions are malignant. There are different subcategories, but the commonest are B5a (in situ malignancy) and B5b (invasive malignancy). A metastatic lymph node is assigned a score of B5.

Management of B3 Lesions

Lesions falling into the category 'uncertain malignant potential' (B3) are histologically diverse, and as such, the management is dependent upon the lesion type, though there are common themes.[5]

Most lesions are sampled using vacuum-assisted excision (VAE) under either US or stereotactic guidance. VAE is in principle the same as VAB in terms of equipment and approach, with the exception that VAE aims to excise rather than biopsy the lesion, and for B3 lesions, the recommendation is that about 4 g of tissue is excised.[4] VAE is recommended for atypical intraductal epithelial proliferation, flat epithelial atypia, classical lobular neoplasia, papilloma without epithelial atypia, radial scars and mucocoele-like lesions. A simplified overview is given in Figure 18.2.

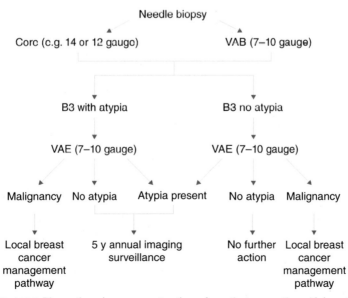

Fig. 18.2 Diagnostic and management pathway for patients presenting with breast symptoms. *VAB,* Vacuum-assisted biopsy; *VAE,* vacuum-assisted excision.

Diagnostic surgical excision is usually recommended for papillomas with epithelial atypia, cellular fibroepithelial lesions (incorporating phyllodes tumours), spindle cell lesions and certain vascular lesions.

For reporting purposes, the VAE specimen is treated like a surgical biopsy, and a B code is not appropriate.[4]

VAE can also be used for therapeutic excision of benign and malignant lesions. Many centres offer therapeutic VAE of biopsy-proven fibroadenomas. Therapeutic VAE of invasive breast cancers as an alternative to open surgery is also gaining momentum but currently only in the context of research and in certain patient groups.

Equipment

1. Requires either:
   (a) US guidance, using a handheld, high-frequency (18-MHz) probe. When possible, this is the preferred method because it allows the patient to lie in a comfortable position, there is no breast compression (as there is for stereotactic biopsy), there is no radiation burden and the sampling is visualized in real time, giving confidence to the operator that the lesion has been adequately targeted.
   (b) X-ray guidance: applying the principle of stereotaxis whereby imaging a static object from two known angles from a known zero point can provide data from which the x, y and z coordinates can be calculated. Small-field digital stereotactic equipment can be purchased as an add-on to conventional mammography machines, thus providing the most common approach to x-ray–guided biopsy, namely with the patient in the seated, upright position. Less commonly, the small-field digital stereotactic system is attached to a prone table (dedicated to biopsy use), with resultant increased accessibility for posteriorly sited lesions and reduction in syncopal episodes; advantages can be reproduced by the use of an appropriate biopsy chair, allowing the adoption of the lateral decubitus position in conjunction with an upright imaging system. The technique can now also be carried out under x-ray guidance using tomosynthesis to identify the plane optimally demonstrating the target lesion and thus identifying the depth to target. This negates the requirement to carry out paired stereotactic images, thus increasing the accuracy of the technique as well as reducing procedure time and radiation.
2. Automated biopsy device: The choice of needle depends on the nature of the imaging abnormality and the imaging modality being used. For US-guided biopsy of masses, a 14-gauge biopsy needle is adequate. For stereotactic biopsy of microcalcification and poorly defined opacities, a 14- or 12-gauge needle may be used, but larger volume VAB needles up to 7-gauge can also be used, which give larger sample volumes. Sparser microcalcification and subtle parenchymal distortions may benefit from VAB. There is currently mixed evidence regarding the diagnostic accuracy of 14-gauge core versus larger-bore VAB as a first-line biopsy,[7,8] but data suggest that for certain high-risk lesions,

the subsequent upgrade rate to malignancy is higher in patients undergoing first-line core biopsy versus VAB.[9]

Patient Preparation

1. Consent:
   - Whether this is verbal or written will depend upon local policy.
   - The common risks are bleeding or bruising and discomfort.
   - Infection should also be mentioned, though with appropriate, aseptic technique, this is uncommon.
   - Damage to adjacent structures such as pectoral muscles or axillary vasculature is possible but should be avoidable in experienced hands. There is also a theoretical small risk of pneumothorax, but this is exceptionally rare and should be avoidable.
   - Women with implants should also be counselled on the small risk of damage to the implant. Again, in experienced hands, this is rare.
   - In lactating women, there is a small risk of causing a milk fistula.
   - For larger-gauge VABs and VAEs (e.g. 10 and 7 gauge), consideration should be given to the site of the lesion in relation to the overlying skin and the nipple because there may be a small risk of causing damage to these structures when the tissue is drawn in by the vacuum.
2. For patients receiving anticoagulant treatment, a benefit-to-risk discussion should underpin decisions for each patient before proceeding to biopsy. A summary adapted from the current guidance from the BSBR is given in Table 18.1.[10]

Table 18.1   British Society of Breast Radiology. Guidelines for Performing Breast and Axillary Biopsies in Patients on Anticoagulant and Antiplatelet Therapy[10]

Medication	FNA	Core Biopsy (14 Gauge)	VAB or VAE	Restart Treatment (if Stopped)
Warfarin	Continue medication	If INR[1] ≤4.0: proceed	If INR[1] ≤2.5: proceed (≤2.0 for VAE)[2]	6–8 h after procedure
		If INR[1] >4.0: consult haematologist or cardiologist to consider discontinuing warfarin	If INR[1] >2.5(>2.0 for VAE): consult haematologist or cardiologist to consider discontinuing warfarin	24 h after procedure for VAE
DOACs, e.g. rivaroxaban, apixaban, dabigatran): no known renal function abnormality	Continue medication	Continue medication[3]	Stop 12–24 h before procedure for VAB. Stop 48 h before procedure for VAE	6–8 h after procedure for VAB. 24 h after procedure for VAE

Continued

Table 18.1   British Society of Breast Radiology. Guidelines for Performing Breast and Axillary Biopsies in Patients on Anticoagulant and Antiplatelet Therapy—cont'd

Medication	FNA	Core Biopsy (14 Gauge)	VAB or VAE	Restart Treatment (if Stopped)
DOACs: known renal function abnormality CrCl <50 mL/min	Continue medication	Continue medication[4]	Stop 48 hours before procedure	24 h after procedure
Aspirin, clopidogrel and other antiplatelet agents (e.g. ticagrelor, prasugrel)	Continue medication	Continue medication	If patient on dual therapy, consider discontinuing clopidogrel or ticagrelor 5 d before or prasugrel 7 d before procedure (with cardiology approval)	6–h hours after procedure 24 h after procedure for VAE
LMWH	Continue medication	Continue medication	Stop 12 h before biopsy (prophylactic dose) Stop 24 h before procedure (treatment dose)	6–8 h after procedure (prophylactic dose) 24 h after procedure (treatment dose)

CrCl, Creatine clearance; *DOAC,* direct oral anticoagulant; *INR,* international normalized ratio; *LMWH,* low-molecular-weight heparin; *VAB,* vacuum-assisted biopsy; *VAE,* vacuum-assisted excision.

Notes
1. Patients taking warfarin usually have their anticoagulation clinic cards with them. A recent international normalized ratio (INR) result (ideally within 5 days but longer if INR is stable over a prolonged period) should be known before proceeding with biopsy. Some patients must not stop taking their warfarin (e.g. those with mechanical mitral prosthetic heart valves or those with a venous thrombosis within 3 months). There should be prior discussion with a haematologist or cardiologist (as appropriate) if the INR is outside these limits as bridging heparin therapy may be advised.
2. Diagnostic VAB (especially as a first-line procedure for microcalcification) is regarded as having a moderate risk of bleeding, whereas VAE (e.g. for second-line large volume sampling of B3 lesions or therapeutic excision of fibro adenomas) is best regarded as high risk.
3. Direct anticoagulant agents (e.g. rivaroxaban, apixaban, dabigatran) are not monitored by INR level but require cessation for 24 hours to remove the anticoagulant effect in patients with normal renal function. There is no reversal agent. It is considered generally safe to proceed with core biopsy, but prolonged compression of the biopsy site may need to be applied.
4. There is a higher risk of bleeding in patients on direct anticoagulant agents who have reduced renal function (creatinine clearance it is considered generally safe to proceed with core biopsy, but prolonged compression of the biopsy site may need to be applied).

Technique

1. Standard skin cleansing: Local anaesthetic is infiltrated into the skin and into the deeper tissues around and beyond the target lesion.
2. A biopsy needle is introduced via a small nick in the skin and deployed through the target lesion.
3. For stereotactic guidance, x-ray images are taken during insertion to ensure adequate needle placement relative to the target. For US guidance, real-time visualization of the needle relative to the target allows accurate sampling. The needle should be visible at all times, including during firing of the biopsy device. Most biopsy needles have a 'throw' when deployed, so it is important to account for this when planning sampling to ensure that the needle will not contact important structures such as the chest wall or axillary vasculature when fired. It is also important for this reason to ensure that local anaesthetic is infiltrated beyond the lesion during preparation for the biopsy. Planning a trajectory that is parallel to the probe and the chest wall ensures better needle visualization and minimize risk of contacting the chest wall.
4. For both VAB and VAE, generally more local anaesthetic is used than for a standard core biopsy. For US-guided VAB and VAE, it is especially important to ensure continual visualization of the needle, the target lesion and the surrounding tissues during sampling. VAB and VAE needles have a cutting edge on the side of the needle tip, and for US-guided sampling, the needle is placed underneath the target lesion; during sampling, the lesion is drawn into the needle using the vacuum and the cutting edge excises the tissue. Care must be taken to ensure that the overlying skin (or nipple if in close proximity) is not drawn into the needle.
5. At the time of biopsy, for subtle abnormalities, when the target may be completely removed or obscured either by diagnostic biopsy (e.g. small masses on US or small clusters of microcalcification on mammography) or for lesions undergoing VAE or to confirm concordance of the target site with other imaging modalities, a tiny metallic marker (typically a titanium alloy) can be deployed either via an introducer or the large-volume biopsy needle. There are many different types of marker clip available, and the choice of marker is largely down to user preference. All metallic markers are radiopaque and hence visible on mammography. To aid their visibility on US, some tissue markers are shaped to increase their specular surface, and some include a surrounding gel component. Other indications for inserting marker clips are preneoadjuvant chemotherapy, so if the patient has a complete radiological response and there is no residual tumour, the marker clip can be identified in the tumour bed and targeted with a localization device preoperatively.
6. Confirmatory imaging should accompany all cases:
   - For biopsy of calcification, x-rays of the samples should be taken to confirm the presence of calcification.
   - If marker clips are deployed postbiopsy, postprocedure mammograms are usually carried out to confirm marker position.

18

References

1. Maxwell AJ, Pearson JM. Criteria for the safe avoidance of needle sampling in young women with solid breast masses. *Clin Radiol.* 2010;65(3):218–222.
2. Taylor K, Lowes S, Stanley E, et al. Evidence for avoiding the biopsy of typical fibroadenomas in women aged 25-29 years. *Clin Radiol.* 2019;74(9):676–681.
3. Evans A, Sim YT, Lawson B, et al. Audit of eliminating biopsy for presumed fibroadenomas with benign ultrasound greyscale and shear-wave elastography findings in women aged 25–39 years. *Clin Radiol.* 2020;75(11):880.e1–880.e3.
4. The Royal College of Pathologists. Guidelines for non-operative diagnostic procedures and reporting in breast cancer screening; 2021. <https://www.rcpath.org/uploads/assets/4b16f19c-f7bd-456c-b212f557f8040f66/G150-Non-op-reporting-breast-cancer-screening.pdf>.
5. Forester ND, Lowes S, Mitchell E, et al. High risk (B3) breast lesions: what is the incidence of malignancy for individual lesion subtypes? A systematic review and meta-analysis. *Eur J Surg Oncol.* 2019;45(4):519–527.
6. Pinder SE, Shaaban A, Deb R, et al. NHS breast screening multidisciplinary working group guidelines for the diagnosis and management of breast lesions of uncertain malignant potential on core biopsy (B3 lesions). *Clin Radiol.* 2018;73(8):682–692.
7. Ames V, Britton PD. Stereotactically guided breast biopsy: a review. *Insights Imaging.* 2011;2(2):171–176.
8. Bundred SM, Maxwell AJ, Morris J, et al. Randomized controlled trial of stereotactic 11-G vacuum-assisted core biopsy for the diagnosis and management of mammographic microcalcification. *Br J Radiol.* 2016;89(1058):20150504.
9. Liu RQ, Chen L, Padilla-Thornton A, et al. Upstage rate of radial scar/complex sclerosing lesion identified on core needle biopsy. *Am J Surg.* 2021;221(6):1177–1181.
10. British Society of Breast Radiology. Guidelines for performing breast and axillary biopsies in patients on anticoagulant and antiplatelet therapy. <https://breastradiology.org/media/1022/bsbr-anticoag-guidelines-august-2018.pdf>.

PREOPERATIVE TUMOUR LOCALIZATION

For most breast cancers, the primary treatment is surgical excision. When appropriate, there is a strong emphasis on breast conservation over mastectomy. Because of earlier detection through breast screening and increased breast awareness, many breast cancers are impalpable or poorly palpable. Preoperative tumour localization is commonly required to allow the surgeon to confidently locate the lesion intraoperatively to ensure the cancer is adequately excised without leaving disease behind or removing too much normal tissue.

Pivotal to the success of this technique is close MDT working at preoperative discussion and planning, accurate communication between the imaging department and theatre and postoperative confirmation of adequacy of surgery at the MDT meeting.

For many years, the standard method of tumour localization involved percutaneous insertion of a guidewire under image guidance using local anaesthetic. The tip of the wire is passed through the lesion; small hooks at the tip of the wire then transfix the lesion. The patient is left with a length of wire protruding from the breast, which is usually fixed to the skin using an adhesive dressing to minimize movement and potential dislodgement. The wire then guides the surgeon to the lesion intraoperatively. Multiple wires can be inserted if there is more than one lesion, or if a large contiguous area of disease (e.g. large field of malignant microcalcification) is being excised, this will need to be 'bracketed'. Image-guided percutaneous insertion of guidewire is still used in the majority of centres and remains very effective at localizing breast lesions and is low in cost. Disadvantages are that it is done on the morning of surgery, meaning that patients have an extra procedure to undergo on an already stressful day and that careful coordination is needed between radiology and surgery to ensure that theatre start times are not delayed because of unexpected difficulties from the localization procedure.

18

In recent years, a number of non-guidewire localization methods have been introduced, and as their safety and effectiveness have become more established, they are gradually becoming incorporated into routine clinical practice.

Non-guidewire methods typically comprise small implantable devices that are inserted in a similar way to a guidewire (image-guided using local anaesthetic) but have the advantage that they are not visible or palpable to the patient and can typically be inserted days or weeks (or in some cases, months) before surgery, which is more relaxing for the patient and helps to decouple radiology and surgery, placing less pressure on surgical planning. Many centres now exclusively use non-guidewire localization devices, and in the future, it is possible this method will entirely replace guidewires.

Non-guidewire methods include:

- Radioactive iodine seeds[1]
- Magnetic seeds[2]
- Radiofrequency ID (RFID) tags[3]
- Radar reflectors[4]

Each has its own advantages and disadvantages, but all so far are effective, and adoption of a particular method appears to be largely due to user preference (see References).

Equipment

1. Localization device of choice
2. Antiseptic swab or solution for cleansing the skin, local anaesthetic and a scalpel for making small skin nick depending on device type
3. Non-allergenic adhesive to fix the wire to adjacent skin if using wires; otherwise a small non-allergenic dressing to cover the puncture site
4. Image guidance:

- Case selection for localization should be discussed with the surgical team. Lesions that are easily palpable may not need any preoperative localization. Lesions that are poorly palpable may need preoperative localization, but sometimes US with a mark drawn on the skin overlying the lesion (done on the morning of surgery) may be adequate.
- Localization devices can be inserted either by US or under x-ray or stereotactic guidance. The avoidance of radiation and accessibility of the technique results in US being the method of image guidance of choice, particularly if the original diagnostic biopsy was achieved via US guidance. For lesions sampled stereotactically, if a sonographically visible marker was deployed at the time of biopsy (and is in a good representative position), then localization can be done using US guidance. Even if the marker clip is not ultrasonically visible, often the biopsy cavity or haematoma from the stereotactic VAB can be seen on US and targeted.

Patient Preparation
As for image-guided biopsy

Technique
1. Standard skin cleansing and local anaesthetic infiltration
2. Guidewires come preloaded in needles. The needle is usually inserted using a direct puncture through the anaesthetized skin. If using US guidance, the needle tip is passed through the lesion so it passes through the other side. The needle is then carefully withdrawn, leaving the hooks transfixing the target.
3. The non-guidewire localization devices also come preloaded in needles. The device size (and hence needle bore) varies between devices, and it may be necessary to make a small skin nick before inserting. The precise technique for deploying the device varies slightly, but essentially, it is the same as inserting a tissue marker after biopsy. Certain devices have special considerations such as radioactive iodine seeds, which require specific regulatory approvals for their insertion and excision.
4. After device placement, mammograms (orthogonal views) indicating the precise position of device (or tip of the localizing wire) are taken. These must be available to the surgeon at the time of operation.
5. After excision, x-rays of the surgical specimen are usually undertaken to confirm excision of the mammographic lesion and any associated marker clips.

References
1. Milligan R, Pieri A, Critchley A, et al. Radioactive seed localization compared with wire-guided localization of non-palpable breast carcinoma in breast conservation surgery- the first experience in the United Kingdom. *Br J Radiol.* 2018;91(1081):20170268.

2. Harvey JR, Lim Y, Murphy J, et al. Safety and feasibility of breast lesion localization using magnetic seeds (Magseed): a multi-centre, open-label cohort study. *Breast Cancer Res Treat*. 2018;169(3):531–536.
3. Lowes S, Bell A, Milligan R, et al. Use of Hologic LOCalizer radiofrequency identification (RFID) tags to localise impalpable breast lesions and axillary nodes: experience of the first 150 cases in a UK breast unit. *Clin Radiol*. 2020;75(12):942–949.
4. Kasem I, Mokbel K. Savi Scout Radar localisation of non-palpable breast lesions: systematic review and pooled analysis of 842 Cases. *Anticancer Res*. 2020;40(7):3633–3643.

18

Role of the radiographer and the nurse in interventional radiology

Dawn Hopkins, Nick Watson and Emma Ross

Interventional radiology (IR) is a constantly expanding field, with an increasing number and variety of procedures. These are continually becoming more innovative and complex, performed by multidisciplinary teams (MDTs) whose core members include radiologists and radiographic and nursing staff.

Radiological procedures now range from straightforward diagnostic biopsies and aspirations performed under local anaesthetic through to advanced therapeutic interventions with critically ill patients who previously would have undergone major surgery.

Radiographers and nurses play a vital role in IR and need specialist skills as integral members of the interventional team.

ROLE OF THE RADIOGRAPHER IN INTERVENTIONAL RADIOLOGY

As the scope of IR broadens and procedures become more complex, the need for a well-trained and integrated team becomes increasingly important. Most patients are conscious for their procedures in interventional suites, so a harmonious environment with a cohesive team approach is vital to ensure the best possible patient experience. Radiographers are a core part of this team, providing guidance on optimizing image quality while ensuring that current radiation protection laws are adhered to and patients are safely examined.

Preprocedural Role

It is common practice in some centres for the interventional suite to be coordinated by a superintendent radiographer who monitors incoming requests and books procedures. Many patients visiting the interventional suite are on a 2-week wait for suspected cancer or a 31-day decision-to-treat pathways. To ensure that the interventional suite is compliant with these (and other) waiting time initiatives, careful monitoring of patient bookings is required, with identification and appropriate management of potential breaches.

Procedure requests are usually first vetted by a radiologist to determine suitability and urgency. After these factors are confirmed and a procedure date decided, the patient is weaned off anticoagulant and antiplatelet therapy, if necessary, and preprocedural blood tests are performed. The liaison with the patient and their team can mostly be performed by the senior radiography or nursing team, reducing the burden on the interventional radiologist. This includes the discussion and booking of simple cases, in accordance with each centre's standard operating procedure (SOP) for scheduling. More complex or unusual procedures continue to need discussion between the patient's team and the interventionalist.

Each interventional procedure should have a corresponding SOP, which includes pre-prescribed parameters for blood results and stopping times for anticoagulant and antiplatelet drugs if necessary. These SOPs enable the radiographer and nursing team to check the pathology results and liaise with the patient's team to achieve any required correction before the day of the procedure.

Many trusts now have multiple sites and rotating radiologists, so the radiographer and nursing team provide a fixed point of contact within the IR department. This helps ensure continuity of care and a robust line of communication for patients and medical teams.

Further liaison with the clinical team is essential to ensure beds are booked, patients are informed and preprocedural tests are carried out in a timely manner. Clearly delineated communication pathways minimize clinical risk and reduce delays.

In addition to the elective work, there is increasing delivery of IR as out-of-hours emergency procedures; therefore, the radiographer service must provide comprehensive on-call cover. The on-call team must consist of suitably trained radiographers who are able to manage the increasingly complex acute cases seen in many centres outside the standard working day (e.g. embolization in acute trauma bleeding, emergency management of thoracic and abdominal aortic aneurysms, acute neurointervention for stroke). The advent of the image exchange portal has facilitated the straightforward transfer of images between hospitals, particularly for emergencies and out of hours, and the radiographer and nursing team can play an important role in accelerating this process. The interventional MDT can then assess whether the patient is suitable for treatment and transfer.

Communicating with one's own team is significantly easier if a daily safety briefing is held, attended by the whole team. This is designed to identify and preempt potential issues to avoid delay in treatment and unnecessary clinical risk.

In the Interventional Suite

After the patient has been fully prepared and is ready to enter the interventional suite, the radiographer is able to advise on optimizing the imaging and minimizing the dose to the patient. It is important to emphasize that the radiation dose to staff members in the rooms is composed almost entirely of scattered radiation. Working with the table at the highest point that is comfortable for the interventionalist dramatically decreases the skin entry dose and decreases backscatter from the table; similarly, the detector should be positioned as close to the patient as possible. Isocentres are best avoided because of the low working table height and resulting higher skin entry doses. The frame rate for digital acquisitions should be reduced, if possible; remember that a compliant patient 'makes or breaks' an examination—a good explanation and a trial run of any breathing instructions can significantly improve the chances of quality imaging on the first run. Careful monitoring of the fluoroscopic images by the radiographer is important during examinations, particularly when working with junior radiologists. It is easy for fingers to 'creep' into the main beam of the images, and these often go unnoticed by the interventionalist because they are concentrating on the end of the catheter or the wire. The radiographer must be alert to such events and be confident enough to guide the radiologist.

19

Additionally, while also decreasing the radiation dose, tightly collimated radiation beams and soft filters improve the diagnostic quality of the images, particularly on older equipment, which is less forgiving than newer 'state-of-the-art' digital equipment. Radiographers should also have a practical knowledge of the use of positioning aids, which can greatly help with image quality and the patient's comfort levels.

The radiographer will be able to give advice on the correct use of personal protective equipment, such as lead aprons and glasses, additional shielding, new emerging personal protection methods and adherence to the hospital's last menstrual period policy. The superintendent radiographer may well be the radiation protection supervisor (RPS) and will additionally be able to advise any staff who also think they may be pregnant or help with dosimetry. IR(99) dictates that the individual is responsible for wearing and changing their dosimeter badges. However, the badges can potentially be worn incorrectly, not returned in time or omitted completely. Advice from the RPS can be helpful in increasing compliance; it is helpful to remember that careful monitoring of one's lifetime dose is an essential part of radiation protection.

Close liaison between the radiographers and physicists is vital for robust radiation protection, helping to pinpoint where any improvements in radiation protection or dose can be sought. Physicists should be involved in the setting up of new equipment and lead the quality assurance team, set the dose reference levels (DRLs) and create local rules. The radiographers act as monitors for the local rules and DRLs, reporting any excessive doses to the physicists. The radiographer should also give patients an information leaflet on how to care for their skin if a high radiation dose is received.

The safe use of equipment within the interventional suites is paramount, and radiographers should be trained to safely use high-pressure injectors and to set up pressure bags for the monitoring of intra-arterial and venous pressures. In addition, most angiographic equipment has diagnostic tools and advanced processing features, such as rotational angiography and computed tomography (CT) guidance. These tools are exceptionally user dependent and require careful training to ensure accurate and reproducible results. Similarly, the radiographer needs to be trained to postprocess the images using the available tools, such as annotation, remasking and pixel shifting. This ensures that the images accurately reflect the work that has been performed and again allows for reproducible results in future examinations.

Depending on the structure of the individual department, when interventional procedures take place outside of the angiographic suite, there may not be a nurse to assist the procedure. Therefore, in addition to radiographic duties, the radiographer should be able to set up a basic sterile trolley using an aseptic non-touch technique (ANTT), apply basic monitoring to the patient and record observations.

As a final note, advanced practitioner radiographers are now performing some of the simpler diagnostic procedures within the intervention phase, such as peripheral angiograms, nerve root injections and line insertions. With adequate training, these procedures are safely performed by the radiographer and help departments provide resilient cover for procedures.

ROLE OF THE NURSE IN INTERVENTIONAL RADIOLOGY

Nurses are key members of the IR MDT and have a vital role in contributing to patient care and safety. This role involves not only the delivery of procedural care but also the creation and maintenance of a safe clinical environment informed by the most up-to-date evidence base. It is the responsibility of the IR nurse to foster a culture of collaborative teamwork while promoting ongoing education and continuing professional development.

Skilled nursing support is essential for the safe and successful management of patients within imaging departments. Radiology nurses have a broad knowledge base and skillset, combining the expertise of ward and theatre-based nurses while demonstrating an understanding of radiological techniques and radiation protection.

Procedures are mostly carried out within the imaging department in dedicated settings, including IR suites, ultrasound, CT or magnetic resonance imaging (MRI). However, on occasions when patients are too unstable to be transferred, nurses must also be adaptable and able to perform their role effectively when delivering interventions at the patient's bedside. In addition, although much of procedural radiology is delivered as elective daytime work, up to one-third of interventions are carried out as emergency out-of-hours procedures, usually involving the most critically ill patients. Therefore, it is imperative that nurses have the skills to perform a significant portion of their role outside the radiology department and outside of normal hours while maintaining the highest standards of clinical care.

The Royal College of Nursing (RCN) has identified six core competencies that form the framework underlying best practice in IR[1]:

1. Preparing patients effectively for imaging procedures
2. Supporting patients through imaging procedures
3. Safely caring for patients after their procedures
4. Assisting with imaging procedures
5. Maintaining a safe environment
6. Carrying out specific interventions

This document is supported by guidelines created jointly by the RCN and Royal College of Radiologists. These describe the role of the nurse within the imaging department while emphasizing the need for collaborative team working between the radiologist, radiographer and nurse.

Nursing involvement is evident at many levels in the radiology department, from the undertaking of basic patient observation and care to assisting with increasingly complex procedures. The role of the nurse in radiology can be further developed to include advanced, autonomous practice. This may consist of obtaining consent, nurse-led sedation and performing certain procedures such as barium examinations, hysterosalpingography, diagnostic arteriography, central line insertion and peritoneal drainage. It is essential that the nurse has appropriate training to develop the necessary skills and knowledge to fulfill their role at each level.

Although direct patient care is at the forefront of the core competencies laid out by the RCN, the nurse also plays a key role in liaising with ward staff and is often instrumental in communication with patients and their caregivers and families.

The IR nurse has a myriad of skills and roles vital to the delivery of effective, safe patient-centred care. Based on the six broad competencies outlined by the RCN, these include[1-4]:

1. Preparing patients effectively for imaging procedures:
   - Allaying anxieties and concerns of patients and their families and carers before the procedure, a role underpinned by thorough understanding of the planned intervention, possible complications and postprocedural care
   - Nurses may have advanced practice roles and be involved in consent clinics.
   - Nurses communicate any preprocedural requirements such as fasting and so on to the patient or, in the case of an inpatient, the ward staff.
   - The positive identification of patients upon their arrival to the radiology department, in accordance with local guidelines.
   - To review patient documentation from the ward or outpatient clinic. Assess comorbidities, particularly relating to current drug therapies, drug (or other) allergies, pregnancy status, renal function status, current use of anticoagulant or antiplatelet drugs and up-to-date clotting indices.

- Obtain baseline vital observations and record findings appropriately.
- The nurse may be the person leading and recording the preprocedural World Health Organization checklist process and has a very important role in ensuring the whole interventional team, including the radiologist, radiographer, further nurses, and when appropriate, other involved staff, such as assistant practitioners, operating department personnel anaesthetists and so on are fully informed.

2. Supporting patients through imaging procedures:
   - Carrying out and recording clinical observations of patient: vital signs, pain score and so on
   - Alleviating anxiety and concerns in the conscious patient
   - Assessing sedation requirements of the patient, including the airway assessment of patients undergoing nurse-led sedation
   - Assisting anaesthetists in the care of the patient under general anaesthetic
   - Administering intravenous fluids, blood products and drugs as prescribed

3. Safely caring for patients after their procedures:
   - Postprocedural recording of vital signs
   - Wound inspection and applying secure dressings
   - Assessing patient comfort and administering prescribed analgesia as required
   - Having knowledge of and recognizing complications of procedures and instituting first-line actions if these occur
   - Completing appropriate documentation and undertaking handover back to the ward nurses or care or observation of patients on day-case units and subsequent preparation or discharge of the patient

4. Assisting with imaging procedures:
   - Knowledge of exactly what equipment is required for all interventional procedures performed at your individual trust
   - Preparing equipment trolleys with the appropriate procedural equipment, adhering to strict ANTT and ensuring additional equipment is available if required
   - Acting as a scrub practitioner and assistant during the procedure. Maintaining a sterile field. Nurses therefore require a high-level knowledge of the procedures and the use of guidewires, catheters, intravascular devices, drugs and so on used during procedures.
   - Ensuring specimens are managed appropriately after the procedure

5. Maintaining a safe environment:
   - Nurses play a key role in creating and maintaining a clinically safe environment for both elective and emergency procedures to be undertaken, not only within the imaging department and within hours but also when interventions are undertaken elsewhere within the hospital or out of hours.

- Nurses must have up-to-date knowledge of a broad range of topics relating to nursing within the modern radiology department. These include radiation protection issues (IR(ME) R 2020 regulations), MRI safety, consent processes, emergency resuscitation and so on.
- Nurses are central to delivery of effective infection control within the imaging department, both in the creation of policies and procedural documentation and in the delivery of staff training, equipment auditing and maintaining the sterile field during procedures.
- Nurses have a key role in contributing to the development of evidence-based care plans, policies and procedural guidelines, reflecting the highest level of patient care and current best practice.
- Nurses should be integral to the creation of patient care plans; documentation, including patient information leaflets, safety checklists and so on; and liaising when necessary with other groups within the hospital, including ward nursing staff, theatre nurses and operating department practitioners, infection control nurses and so on.
- Collaboration with company representatives to ensure equipment used in procedures is kept updated to achieve optimal therapeutic effect. This may include trialling new equipment and arranging staff training and support to facilitate this.
- Carrying out risk assessments and equipment checks
- Ensure drug safety: safe storage and administration of drugs, involvement in developing patient group directions and so on
- Participation in clinical governance and audit relating to the radiology department

6. Carrying out specific interventions:
- While assisting the interventional radiologist, the nurse may be undertaking tasks, including flushing catheters; postprocedural arterial compression; and administering drugs such as sedatives, heparin, and infusions and so on.
- In some institutions, the advanced practitioner nurse may be working autonomously, carrying out procedures such as administering and monitoring patient sedation and undertaking interventions such as peripheral diagnostic angiography, central line insertion, hysterosalpingography, ascitic drainage and so on.

19

The roles of the radiographer and nurse are essential to the provision of safe, effective patient-centred care in IR. They are integral members of the IR team and as such play an important part in the enhancement of the patient experience as radiological interventional practice evolves.

References

1. Royal College of Nursing. *RCN Competencies—Core Competencies for Imaging Nurses*. Publication Code: 004; 2012:265.

2. Royal College of Nursing and the Royal College of Radiologists. *Guidelines for Nursing Care in Interventional Radiology.* 2nd ed. Reference No. *BFCR.* 2014;7(14). [rev 2017].
3. Deichelbohrer L. The role of the advanced practice nursing interventional radiology. *J Radiol Nurs.* 2004;23(2):51.
4. The Royal College of Nursing. *Patients Undergoing Minor Interventional Procedures such as Biopsy, Drain Insertion and Aspiration. Best practice Guidance for Nursing staff.* Publication RCN 2014.

Further Reading

Grossman VA. *Fast Facts for the Radiology Nurse: An Orientation and Nursing Care Guide in a Nutshell (Fast Facts).* 2nd ed. Springer; 2020.
Royal College of Radiologists. *IR(ME)R: Implications for Clinical Practice in Diagnostic Imaging, Interventional Radiology and Diagnostic Nuclear Medicine.* Reference No. BFCR(20)3. The Royal College of Radiologists; 2020.

Consent

Nick Watson

The current General Medical Council (GMC) guidance on consent, *Decision making and consent*, came into effect in November 2020.[1] The fundamental principles and processes underlying obtaining informed consent with 'patients and doctors making decisions together' are in essence unchanged from the previous version,[2] but following landmark legal rulings, the new guidance reemphasizes the primary importance of the nature, content and documentation of the discussion between doctor and patient when consent is sought.

As previously, all patients 'have the right to be involved in decisions about their treatment and care and to make informed decisions if they can', but the content of the dialogue and discussion are now even more overtly patient-centred rather than a matter of medical judgement alone. The guidance sets out a framework for decision making that covers all forms of patient treatments; therefore, radiologists need to use their judgement in applying these principles to the specifics of interventional radiological procedures and in some invasive radiological investigations. Although the Royal College of Radiologists (RCR) now defers to the GMC guidance in matters of consent, its *Standards for patient consent particular to radiology* document from 2012 still provides useful advice specific to procedural radiological practice.[2]

Decision Making and Consent

The latest guidance sets out seven underlying principles of decision making and consent:

From the GMC guidance, the seven principles of decision making and consent are as follows:[1]

1. All patients have the right to be involved in decisions about their treatment and care and be supported to make informed decisions if they are able.
2. Decision making is an ongoing process focused on meaningful dialogue: the exchange of relevant information specific to the individual patient.
3. All patients have the right to be listened to, and to be given the information they need to make a decision and the time and support they need to understand it
4. Doctors must try to find out what matters to patients so they can share relevant information about the benefits and harms of proposed options and reasonable alternatives, including the option to take no action.

5. Doctors must start from the presumption that all adult patients have capacity to make decisions about their treatment and care. A patient can only be judged to lack capacity to make a specific decision at a specific time, and only after assessment in line with legal requirements.

6. The choice of treatment or care for patients who lack capacity must be of overall benefit to them, and decisions should be made in consultation with those who are close to them or advocating for them.

7. Patients whose right to consent is affected by law should be supported to be involved in the decision-making process, and to exercise choice if possible.

The guidance provides a pragmatic approach reflecting factors that include the nature and severity of the patient's condition, how quickly the treatment must be made, the complexity of the decision being made, the range of choices available and the level of risk or degree of uncertainty associated with any of them, the impact of the potential outcome on the patient's individual circumstances, and the patient's wishes. It does not set out to define how the process is undertaken but guides the practitioner to make appropriate judgements relating to the consent process.

The guidance suggests that obtaining a patient signature on a consent form is not always required, particularly for minimally or non-invasive interventions, but this does not remove the practitioner's obligation to clearly explain the nature of and reason for a particular intervention and make it clear that the patient has ability to refuse the intervention both at the beginning and even during the procedure itself and that while obtaining consent, the doctor must be mindful of any signs indicating the patient might not fully understand or is unhappy about what is being discussed.

Content of the Consent Discussion

The GMC makes it clear that to make an informed decision, a patient needs to be given appropriate information. In radiological procedures, this includes not only a description of the procedure itself and the potential risks involved but, importantly, also a discussion of alternative diagnostic or therapeutic options, including the consequences of not undertaking a particular procedure. It is important that the risks of the procedure (including not just complications) are explained objectively but also that uncertainties relating to these risks and to the outcomes of an intervention (e.g. failure rate of a procedure) are shared and clearly understood by the patient.

Doctors need to mindful of how their own personal preferences might have an impact upon their discussions with patients and ensure the information and recommendations given remain objective and that the rationale for a proposed treatment option is clearly explained and understood by the patient. The patient should be given the opportunity to ask any questions, raise any concerns or request clarification, and these should be actively explored and discussed.

Formally obtaining a patient's signature on a consent form is appropriate for more invasive procedures but represents only a part of the process. The consent form offers a standardized way to record what has been discussed and act as a prompt to the content of the discussion. However, appropriately documenting within the patient's notes or records the details of the discussion of consent with the patient, evidencing that the relevant information has been shared with the patient and the patient's questions and priorities have been explored is as, if not more, important than the signature of consent. This is particularly pertinent after a relatively recent and significant legal ruling, *Montgomery v. Lanarkshire Health Board* (2015) *UKSC11*, which places a far greater emphasis on the patient's, rather than doctor's, views and has superseded the use of the Bolam test in informing aspects of the consent process.[3] This precedent is reflected in the GMC guidance when *judging what to discuss* when obtaining consent, which specifically states:

'You should not rely on assumptions about:

20

a) the information a patient might want or need
b) the factors a patient might consider significant
c) the importance a patient might attach to different outcomes'.

The Bolam test is often used in cases of alleged negligence against doctors: a doctor cannot be held negligent if they are shown to have upheld a reasonable standard of care. It defines this standard of care as one that would be supported by a reasonable body of medical professionals. In the past, this has also been used in relation to claims of negligence on the part of the doctor for inadequate disclosure during the consent process and would be tested against the standard provided by what a reasonable body of other experts would have done in the same situation.

In the *Montgomery v. LHB* case, the Supreme Court overturned the initial court ruling that the consent process was deemed appropriate because it aligned to what other medical practitioners would have undertaken. There had been non-disclosure of specific risks to avoid worsening the patient's anxiety, and successful application of the Bolam test had been initially used to support the doctor's actions and disprove negligence. The Supreme Court, however, rejected this ruling and found there had been a failure (a) to fully inform the patient of the consequences and risks involved and specifically (b) to inform the patient of other treatment options available.

The judges stated:

'An adult person of sound mind is entitled to decide which, if any, of the available forms of treatment to undergo, and her consent must be obtained before treatment interfering with her bodily integrity is undertaken. The doctor is therefore under a duty to take reasonable care to ensure that the patient is aware of any material risks involved in any recommended treatment, and of any reasonable alternative or variant treatments.'

Montgomery v. Lanarkshire Health Board (2015)[3]

The ruling separated the use of the Bolam test in matters related to alleged negligence of doctors' actions (e.g. diagnosis, actions, treatment) and for the use in cases of alleged negligence related to consent processes. Although it acknowledged that a doctor needs skill and judgement in explaining the risks of a procedure, these skills were considered not dependant on medical expertise, and therefore the Bolam test did not apply. Importantly, it emphasized that the test of materiality in consent is not doctor-related, that is, not what a reasonable body of doctors would deem appropriate to discuss with a patient, but, importantly, is patient-centred; what a reasonable person in that patient's situation would deem important to be made aware of and an awareness on the part of the doctor, as to the significance that the individual patient would place upon those risks.

The GMC takes a pragmatic approach and suggests that it not necessary or appropriate for a doctor to discuss every possible risk and potential complication of a procedure but that the discussion should be tailored to include any risks and complications that patients themselves would consider to be important and significant to them. It is therefore important, particularly with higher risk procedures, that patients are encouraged to discuss what they value and deem to be important so there is clearer understanding of the personal impact a possible complication may have on their life. With more complex, more hazardous medical interventions, this would include not only exploring what risks a patient would be prepared to take but also the outcomes they would not be willing to risk. The person seeking consent should not make assumptions as to the importance that a patient might place upon a particular risk. Regardless, any risk of serious adverse outcome, particularly those that might have significant impact (including pain and disability) on their personal life or ability to carry out their roles such as occupation, for instance, however unlikely, must be discussed.

The emphasis is very clearly not upon the end point of having obtained consent but upon the undertaking of the decision-making process with dialogue and information sharing of matters that the doctor has determined the patient considers relevant and important to them.

Withholding Information

There are very limited situations when a doctor may choose not to share all relevant information during the decision-making process. This is clearly the case if the patient has expressly indicated they would prefer not to discuss such matters but only exceptionally, in other circumstances. Specifically, when a doctor believes that sharing information might cause a patient serious harm, it may be acceptable to not undertake an appropriate full discussion.

Doctors cannot withhold information because of a request from a relative or someone close to the patient. A doctor's concern that disclosure of particular risks might cause a patient to become upset, decide to refuse treatment or choose an alternative approach would also not be considered reasonable justification for withholding information.

Obtaining Consent

It is acceptable to delegate the responsibility for obtaining consent, particularly for more straightforward procedures, to others provided they have appropriate knowledge of the procedure, including its benefits and harms and alternative treatment options, and have the skills to undertake the dialogue with the patient.

With more complex interventional procedures, particularly if there is uncertainty about the outcome or there are particular aspects of the patient's condition that are of concern, it would be appropriate for the senior person undertaking the procedure to have the discussion with the patient and obtain consent themselves.

Ideally, unless in an emergency situation, the conversation with the patient and the obtaining of consent should be sought away from the environment of the procedural room and preferably take place at a time before the planned procedure, giving the patient time to consider the information and, if they wish, consult with others. This is particularly important with higher-risk procedures.

The use of standardized patient information leaflets that the patient can take away with them and share with friends or relatives is recommended wherever possible, particularly for more complex or riskier interventions or when specific patient preparation or aftercare is an important part of the procedure. Most departments have these for many procedures, often based upon national body or subspecialty group guidelines[4] (see GMC[5]). Leaflets may help ensure consistency in the information that is shared and can be reviewed at leisure by the patient away from the clinical setting, but the doctor must still be mindful during the consent process that patients may interpret the information differently, reflecting their individual clinical needs, concerns and expectations as well as the values and priorities within their lives.

When the consent discussion has taken place a significant time before the procedure, it will need to be reviewed by the person undertaking the intervention before the procedure can commence. This gives the opportunity to confirm that neither the patient's condition nor the planned procedure have changed and that the patient has the opportunity to ask any further questions and reconfirm their consent for the procedure to take place.

Capacity

Each jurisdiction of the United Kingdom has its own legislation and codes of practice relating to mental capacity, but the GMC guidance offers an overarching framework. However, departments and

20

individuals need to be aware of the specific legislation relevant to their geographical location (see GMC[5]).

The Mental Capacity Act (MCA) 2005 of England is underpinned by five statutory principles:[6]

- All persons are assumed to have capacity unless the contrary is demonstrated.
- All practicable steps must be taken to assist the person in making a decision.
- The person should not be considered to lack capacity if they choose to make an unwise decision.
- Any decision made or act done under this act on behalf of a person lacking capacity should be in that person's best interests.
- Any act done or decision made should be the least restrictive possible that would ensure a good outcome.

The Adults with Incapacity (Scotland) Act has similar requirements and includes an expectation that interested parties should be consulted and that incapacitated people are encouraged to use existing skills.

Northern Ireland is introducing the Mental Capacity Act (Northern Ireland) 2016, but this is not yet in full force, so treatment and care currently remains aligned to common law principles.[6]

The legislation together with the GMC guidelines require doctors to assume that patients have the capacity to accept or decline a treatment or intervention unless the doctor has demonstrated and documented that the person lacks capacity.

ASSESSMENT OF CAPACITY

It is important to remember that capacity is not generalized. Capacity assessments aim to establish whether the person in question has the capacity to make a specific decision related to a specific matter at a specific time. Someone may have the capacity to consent to have their nightclothes changed on the ward but not to the siting of a percutaneous intravenous central catheter because the process of the latter is more complex and requires greater mental processing abilities to evaluate risks and benefits.

To undertake a capacity assessment, a two-stage test of capacity should occur.

1. Does the person have an impairment (of mind or brain), or is there a disturbance affecting the way their mind or brain works?
2. If so, does the impairment mean that the person is unable to make the relevant decision at the time needed?

An assessment of capacity need only be undertaken if there is doubt about the person's mental functioning at the time. Assessing capacity is a core clinical skill that forms part of the dialogue with the patient and not one that usually requires a specialist (e.g. psychiatric) opinion.

To assess capacity, the following aspects need to be evaluated:

- Does the person have a general understanding of what decision they need to make and why they need to make it?
- Does the person have a general understanding of the likely consequences of making or not making this decision?
- Is the person able to understand, retain, use and weigh up the information relevant to this decision?
- Can the person communicate their decision (by talking, using sign language or other means)? Would the services of a professional (e.g. a speech and language therapist) be helpful?
- In more complex or serious decisions, is there a need for a more thorough assessment (perhaps by involving another professional expert)?

Patients are deemed to lack capacity if they cannot:

20

- Understand information about the decision to be made (the Act calls this 'relevant information')
- Retain this information in their minds
- Use or weigh that information as part of the decision-making process
- Communicate their decision (by talking, using sign language or any other means)

Only one of these items listed needs to be absent for the person to lack capacity, although more than one is often present.

Capacity to consent is best established by the clinicians offering the proposed intervention, sometimes in conjunction with medical professionals caring for the patient because they have more specialist knowledge of the patient's condition, risks and benefits involved. For more complex procedures or when there is an underlying illness contributing to difficulties in reasoning (e.g. dementia), it may be of benefit to work in collaboration with expert colleagues (e.g. psychiatrists).

SUPPORTING PATIENTS IN DECISION MAKING

Before a patient can be deemed to lack capacity to consent to a procedure, all practicable steps should be taken to support the person to make the decision. Making use of images or visual aids and involving family members, interpreters or other professionals may be beneficial. When a treatment can safely be delayed to allow the person to regain capacity, this should be done.

Doctors may encounter patients who choose not to undergo treatments or procedures offered to them even though doing so may result in significant morbidity or death. Patients have the right to make unwise decisions, and doctors should guard against coercion.[5]

In these cases, all discussions with the patient should be documented with a comprehensive and contemporaneous record of the capacity assessment and the consent procedure entered into the patient's medical notes. The RCR recommends that in these cases the notes are witnessed by a third party.[2] If this patient later loses the capacity to consent to a procedure, clinicians must not then perform the intervention in the patient's best interests under the MCA; this would be considered a criminal offence of ill-treatment.

ACTING FOR A PERSON WHO LACKS CAPACITY

When it has been established that a person lacks capacity to decide on the treatment offered, the treating clinician may lawfully treat the patient in their best interests. Before proceeding, the clinician should take into consideration any previously expressed wishes. These may be formalized in advanced statements or may be ascertained from other sources (family, caregivers or other professionals involved in providing care to the person previously).

Clinicians should establish if any proxy decision makers have been appointed. Under English law, a person may have designated a Lasting Power of Attorney (LPA) to make health and welfare decisions on their behalf after they no longer have mental capacity.

Note, however:

- Within the health and welfare LPA agreement, there is an explicit declaration made determining whether the attorney is empowered to give or refuse consent for treatments specifically deemed to be life-sustaining, so clarification should be sought.
- Separate LPA arrangements can also be made for property and financial decisions, but these alone do not confer any power for the attorney to make health-related decisions on behalf of the patient.
- Similarly, any older Enduring Power of Attorney arrangements still in force (made pre-2007) allow only proxy financial, not health or welfare, decisions to be made.
- Scottish law makes no distinction between differing powers of attorney.

When acting in a person's best interests, clinicians should do so in the least restrictive manner possible. If less invasive alternatives to the proposed intervention exist, then these should be attempted first.

In an emergency situation when consent cannot be obtained, clinicians can act in the patient's best interest to administer emergency treatment. Treatment should be immediate and necessary to prevent further deterioration. No further treatment may be given until a capacity and, if necessary, a 'best interests' assessment has been undertaken.

Clinicians are directed to the MCA 2005 and Adults with Incapacity (Scotland) Act 2000 Codes of Practice for details on the jurisdiction of powers of attorney. These can be stored as PDF documents on computers or smartphones. Seeking legal advice from employment lawyers or protection societies is recommended if clinicians are unclear on how to proceed. The GMC has recently developed a helpful online decision-making tool to guide the process if the clinician is in any doubt.

DOCUMENTING ASSESSMENT OF CAPACITY

Most hospitals have standardized preprinted consent forms for patients who lack capacity. In addition to completion of these forms, the authors recommend contemporaneous documentation of the assessment of capacity in the patient's notes or the relevant radiology report. Documentation should include the following information:

- Full patient details
- The details of the intended intervention
- The specific reason the patient has been deemed to lack capacity and how this judgement was reached (as noted previously)
- Attempts that have been made to assist the patient to make his or her own decision and why these were unsuccessful
- The likelihood that the patient may regain capacity and the reason the intervention needs to be performed before this can occur
- The steps taken to establish the patient's previously expressed wishes, including the names of the family members consulted
- The names and designation of clinical colleagues consulted in deciding on the proposed intervention
- The name of the clinician responsible for performing the procedure
- The name and designation of any clinician who has provided a second opinion.

20

SHARED DECISION MAKING

As part of the 'Liberating the NHS' white paper published in May 2011, there has been an increasing requirement for clinicians to involve patients in decisions about their care. 'No decision about me without me' requires clinicians to agree on treatment plans in partnership with their patients. There is a growing expectation from the public for doctors to provide sufficient information for patients to allow them to make their own decisions. This fundamental ethos has been repeatedly reemphasized in subsequent iterations of the GMC's guidance on consent matters. This is particularly important in procedures where there is a lack of consensus and a perceived variance of risk between the clinician and the patient. In these cases, clear documentation of all information given and the agreed upon decision arrived at should be made. This documentation of the consent process might also involve including the patient in any correspondence with other clinicians, so that they have a written copy available to them.

References

1. General Medical Council. *Decision Making and Consent*; 2020 <https://www.gmc-k.org/ethical-guidance/ethical-guidance-for-doctors/decision-making-and-consent>.
2. The Royal College of Radiologists. *Standards for Patient Consent Particular to Radiology*. 2nd ed. The Royal College of Radiologists; July 2012.
3. *Montgomery v Lanarkshire Health Board* [2015] UKSC11. *Med Law Rev.* 2015;23:455–466.
4. British Society of Interventional Radiology. *Patient Information Leaflets.* <https://www.bsir.org/patients/patient-information-leaflets>.
5. General Medical Council. *Factsheet: key legislation and case law relating to Decision making and consent.* <https://www.gmc-uk.org/-/media/documents/factsheet—key-legislation-and-case-law-relating-to-decision-making-and-consent-84176182.pdf>.
6. Department of Health. *Mental Capacity Act.* HMSO; 2005. <https://www.legislation.gov.uk/ukpga/2005/9/contents>.

Sedation and monitoring

Matthew Bridge

SEDATION

Sedation is the use of a drug or drugs to produce a state of depression of the central nervous system (CNS) that enables interventional procedures or treatment to be performed. Sedative drugs may be combined with drugs used for pain relief (analgesia). Sedation is only part of a 'package' of care comprising preassessment, properly informed consent, adequate facilities, good techniques and risk avoidance.[1]

Over the recent years, the number and complexity of diagnostic imaging and image-guided interventional procedures in radiology departments have increased; often these patients are frail, medically unfit and unable to cooperate or lie still. The relief of anxiety, discomfort and pain allows patients to tolerate these procedures. Some drugs, such as benzodiazepines, have purely sedative effects, but others, such as opioids, have combined sedative and analgesic effects. Although sedative and analgesic agents are generally safe, catastrophic complications related to their use can occur, often as a result of incorrect drug administration or inadequate patient monitoring.[2] The incidence of adverse outcomes is reduced by improved understanding of the pharmacology of drugs used, appropriate monitoring of sedated patients and recognizing those at increased risk of adverse events.

There is a continuum between the main types of sedation (Fig. 21.1) defined in the following way:

1. Anxiolysis: The patient is alert and calm.
2. Conscious sedation: a state of depression of the CNS that enables diagnostic and therapeutic procedures to be carried out but during which the patient remains conscious, retains protective reflexes and is able to understand and respond to verbal commands
3. Deep sedation in which these criteria are not fulfilled and airway or ventilation intervention may be required. Deep sedation requires the presence of an anaesthetist.
4. General anaesthesia

The joint Royal College of Radiologists/Royal College of Anaesthetists Working Party on Sedation and Anaesthesia in Radiology

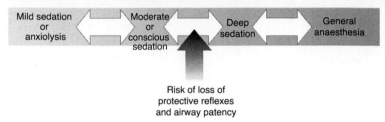

Fig. 21.1 The continuum of patient conscious level from mild sedation to general anaesthesia.

recommended establishment of local guidelines for sedation in radiology.[3] These include the following:

1. Each patient must have a preprocedural evaluation to assess their suitability for sedation.
2. The operator must not supervise the sedation.
3. Nurses and technicians should not administer drugs without medical supervision.
4. All staff carrying out sedation should have undertaken training in sedation and resuscitation and should have knowledge and experience of the sedative drugs, monitoring and resuscitation equipment.
5. There should be periodic retraining and assessment of staff.
6. There should be an appropriate recovery area.
7. Resuscitation equipment and appropriate reversal drugs must be immediately available.

Preparation

Sympathetic patient management with an explanation of the procedure may reduce anxiety and remove the need for any medication. Sedation should be explained and consent obtained. Patients who are to be given intravenous (IV) sedation should undergo a period of fasting before the procedure: 6 h fasting for solid food and 2 h for clear liquids.

Resuscitation and monitoring equipment and oxygen delivery devices should be checked and venous access established.

Equipment

1. Appropriate drugs, including reversal agents
2. Monitoring equipment
3. Resuscitation equipment

Preassessment

It is essential to anticipate and reduce the risk of potential problems before the procedure. Preassessment must include:

1. Evaluation of the patient's airway
2. Full assessment of the patient's medical, drug and allergy history
3. Cardiorespiratory reserve assessment

DRUGS

As part of a sedation protocol, the following may be used:

1. Combination of a sedative drug and an analgesic drug (e.g. IV midazolam and IV opiate). IV analgesic and sedative drugs have a synergistic sedative effect, and the dose of each drug must be reduced by up to 70% when administered together. It is best to give the IV analgesic first and then titrate the dose of IV sedative.
2. Analgesic drug alone (e.g. IV opiate)
3. Sedative drug alone (e.g. IV midazolam)

Analgesic Drugs

Analgesic drugs are used for pain control and to improve patient comfort. For some procedures, local anaesthesia or oral analgesia (using paracetamol 1 g or ibuprofen 400 mg taken 1–2 h before the procedure) is appropriate. For more invasive interventional radiology procedures, the use of IV analgesia may be required.

LOCAL ANAESTHESIA

21

For recommended doses, see Table 21.1.

Commonly used local anaesthetics for subcutaneous infiltration are the following:

1. Lidocaine 1% may be used in combination with adrenaline (epinephrine) and is supplied in premixed ampoules for this purpose. Adrenaline causes local vasoconstriction, decreases drug absorption and increases the intensity and duration of action of lidocaine. Lidocaine is also available as a 2% solution.
2. Bupivacaine 0.25% has a slower onset but longer duration of action than does lidocaine. The effects of adrenaline on the duration and intensity of bupivacaine are much less pronounced. Bupivacaine is also available as a 0.5% solution.

INHALATIONAL ANALGESIA

A mixture of 50% nitrous oxide and 50% oxygen (Entonox) may be used. This has both analgesic and sedative properties.

INTRAVENOUS ANALGESIA

These drugs are used for pain control but also have a dose-dependent sedative effect. The most commonly used are the opioid drugs morphine, pethidine and fentanyl. These drugs must be given in small, divided doses and dose titrated to the patient's need. It is extremely important to titrate the dosage to effect rather than assume a fixed dose based on body weight. The maximum recommended dose must

Table 21.1   Recommended Doses of Local Anaesthetic Drugs

Drug	Onset of Effect (min)	Duration of Effect (h)	Maximum Total Recommended Dose	Route of Administration
Lidocaine 1% (1% = 10 mg mL^{-1})	10–15	1–2	*Without adrenaline:* 3 mg kg^{-1} (maximum, 200 mg) *With adrenaline:* 7 mg kg^{-1} (max 500 mg)	SC injection
Bupivacaine 0.25% (0.25% = 2.5 mg mL^{-1})	15–30	2–3	2 mg kg^{-1} (maximum, 150 mg)	SC injection

SC, Subcutaneous.

Table 21.2   Recommended Doses of Intravenous Analgesic Drugs[a]

Drug	Maximum Total Recommended Dose	Onset of Effect (min)	Duration of Effect (h)	Route of Administration
Morphine	100 µg kg^{-1} body weight	5–10	4–5	IV injection
Pethidine	1 mg kg^{-1} body weight	5	1–2	IV injection
Fentanyl	1 µg kg^{-1} body weight	1	0.5–1	IV injection

IV, Intravenous.
[a]These drugs should be used in divided doses, and the maximum total dose must not be exceeded. It is always important to titrate the dosage of medication to effect rather than assume a fixed dose based on body weight.

not be exceeded because of the risk of adverse events, particularly respiratory depression. For recommended doses, see Table 21.2.

The opioid drugs can cause:

1. Nausea and vomiting
2. Hypotension
3. Respiratory depression
4. Bradycardia

Effects of opioids can be reversed by the competitive antagonist naloxone (dose 0.4–2 mg). Naloxone should be administered intravenously in a solution containing 0.4 mg in 10 mL and given in 1-mL increments. It has peak effect at 1–2 min, with duration of 20–60 min.

As a result of the relatively short duration of action, repeated doses of naloxone may be necessary.

SEDATIVE DRUGS

For conscious sedation in the radiology department, the water-soluble benzodiazepine midazolam is the drug of choice. Midazolam has superseded diazepam because the latter has active metabolites and longer duration of effect.

Midazolam produces:

1. Dose-dependent anxiolysis
2. Intense amnesia (for 20–30 min)
3. Sedation
4. Muscle relaxation

Midazolam is given IV It has a rapid onset of effect, within 1–5 min, and a variable duration of effect of 1–4 h. The sedative dose is 70 µg kg^{-1} body weight (for an average adult, ~4–5 mg), and the sleep dose is 100–200 µg kg^{-1} (>7 mg). Typically, 2–2.5 mg is administered IV over 30–120 s, with further 0.5-mg doses titrated as required. Only rarely are total doses of more than 5 mg required. In older adults, smaller doses of 1–3 mg must be used.

The effects of midazolam can be reversed by the competitive antagonist flumazenil; onset of flumazenil is within 1–3 min, with a half-life of 7–15 min. The dose of flumazenil should be titrated every 1–2 min, starting with 200 µg up to a maximum of 1 mg. The clinical effect depends on the dose of flumazenil and sedative given. Note that the half-life of flumazenil is shorter than that of midazolam; therefore, resedation effects can occur.

Remifentanil is a potent ultra-short-acting synthetic opioid analgesic drug. The sedative dose range by IV infusion is 0.025–0.1 µg kg^{-1} min^{-1}; at higher doses, it can cause marked respiratory depression. Dexmedetomidine is an agonist of α_2-adrenergic receptors; it can provide sedation, analgesia and anxiolysis without respiratory depression when given as an IV infusion at 0.2–1 µg kg^{-1} h^{-1}. The use of IV anaesthetic agents, such as ketamine and propofol, can result in the patient's moving quickly from a state of sedation to anaesthesia with concomitant risks. These drugs should only be used by those who have undergone appropriate specialist training. However, the risk of oversedation and subsequent loss of airway reflexes is possible with all sedative drugs.

Sedation of Children

See Chapter 3.

Complications of Sedation

Early recognition and treatment of complications are essential to reduce morbidity and mortality from sedation in all patients.

Minor complications include:

1. Syncope
2. Phlebitis
3. Emesis
4. Agitation
5. Rash

Major complications are rare, but include:

1. Bradycardia
2. Hypotension
3. Hypoxia
4. Death

Sedation causes a reduction in muscle tone of the oropharynx, and at deeper levels of sedation the glottic reflexes may fail. Major complications of sedation are most often caused by airway obstruction and respiratory depression. The following patient groups are at high risk:

1. Older adults: Old age is an independent risk factor for sedation. The effects of sedative drugs are more pronounced and prolonged in older adults. Small incremental doses of sedatives are required.
2. Chronic obstructive pulmonary disease: These patients have a blunted ventilator drive. Supine position impairs chest wall function and oxygenation. Patients may need supplemental oxygen and bronchodilators. Local anaesthesia should be used for pain whenever possible, and sedative drugs should be used sparingly.
3. Coronary artery disease: Undersedation will increase cardiac oxygen demand, but oversedation can cause hypotension and hypoxaemia and decrease myocardial oxygen delivery, leading to myocardial ischaemia. Patients should be given supplemental oxygen.
4. Hepatic dysfunction or renal failure: Altered drug metabolism in renal and liver disease increases the risk of overdose when using opioids and benzodiazepines. These drugs should be used in reduced doses. In children, similarly, triclofos should be avoided in those with end-stage liver failure and used with caution in those with cholestasis. In renal impairment, dose reduction should be considered.
5. Those with drug dependency (including alcohol, opiates or recreational drugs) may exhibit unpredictable requirements. Local anaesthetics and short-acting benzodiazepines are preferred; reversal agents should be avoided.

References
1. Royal College of Radiologists. *Safe Sedation, Analgesia and Anaesthesia Within the Radiology Department*. The Royal College of Radiologists; 2003. <https://www.rcr.ac.uk/publication/safe-sedation-analgesia-and-anaesthesia-within-radiology-department>.

2. Martin ML, Lennox PH. Sedation and analgesia in the interventional radiology department. *J Vasc Interv Radiol.* 2003;14(9 Pt 1):1119–1128.
3. Royal Radiologists/Royal College of College of Anaesthetists Joint Publication. *Sedation and Anaesthesia in Radiology.* The Royal College of Radiologists; 1992.

Further Reading
American College of Radiology. *ACR-SIR Practice Guideline for Sedation/Analgesia.* <http://www.acr.org/~/media/F194CBB800AB43048B997A75938AB482.pdf>.
Patatas K, Koukkoulli A. The use of sedation in the radiology department. *Clin Radiol.* 2009;64:655–663.
Royal College of Anaesthetists. *Guidance on the Provision of Sedation Services.* <http://www.rcoa.ac.uk/document-store/guidance-the-provision-of-sedation-services-2016>.

MONITORING

Monitoring should be used:

1. In all patients receiving any form of sedation
2. For those at risk of haemorrhage
3. In all prolonged or complicated procedures

21

The purposes are to observe and assess the response of the patient to any psychological or physiological stress imposed by the procedure or sedative agents administered and allow appropriate therapeutic action to be taken.

Equipment

1. Pulse oximetry: This is the most sensitive monitoring method to detect hypoxaemia. It is the minimum requirement for safe monitoring and may suffice as the sole monitoring device in young and fit patients. It accurately measures the oxygen saturation of blood and provides information on pulse rate and adequacy of the circulation. The oxygen saturation should be maintained at or above 95%. Most pulse oximeters have a short lag time in demonstrating desaturation. Because of the nature of the oxygen dissociation curve, patients may rapidly desaturate from 90% to 70%. Oxygen saturation of 90% is an emergency, and corrective action should be taken immediately. The pulse oximeter signal may be affected by interference from nail polish, light, movement, cold extremities and skin pigmentation. Ensure an oxygen saturation signal is present before administering sedation.
2. Electrocardiography: A continuous electrocardiography monitor provides information on pulse rate and rhythm, presence of arrhythmia and signs of ischaemia but does not monitor circulation or cardiac output.
3. Automated blood pressure monitor: Minimum acceptable mean arterial pressure is 60 mmHg, but patients with cardiac disease or

hypertension require higher pressures. Falsely high arterial pressure readings are obtained with cuffs that are too small. Manual blood pressure measurements are inconvenient and inconsistent. The blood pressure monitor may impede function of the pulse oximeter and thus should not be on the same arm. The monitor should be set to 5-min recording intervals; nerve damage has been reported with prolonged use.

Monitor alarms may be the first signal of an adverse event and should not be silenced. If there is any doubt, repeat measurement should be performed.

Technique

Monitoring should include assessment of:

1. The patient's level of consciousness
2. Ability to maintain airway
3. Adequacy of respiratory function: respiratory rate and pattern
4. Adequacy of cardiac function: pulse and skin colour
5. Pain level
6. Side effects or complications of any drugs administered
7. Hydration and urine output during prolonged procedures

The patient should be monitored by a trained professional who should have no other role at the time of the procedure than to continuously monitor these parameters. The radiologist performing the procedure should not monitor the patient.

Vital signs (pulse, blood pressure and respiratory rate) should be regularly measured. All adverse events must be fully recorded in the patient's notes. Monitoring should continue into the recovery period.

SEDATION AND MONITORING FOR MAGNETIC RESONANCE IMAGING

Sedation should be given in a quiet area close to the scanner, and there should be an appropriate recovery area available.

The magnetic resonance imaging (MRI) scan room is a challenging environment in which to monitor the patient. The scanner is noisy and potentially claustrophobic, and patients inside the scanner are relatively inaccessible.

All equipment used for monitoring and all anaesthetic equipment must be MR compatible (e.g. MR-compatible pulse oximeters with fibreoptic cabling). Potential problems include effects from the gradient field and radiofrequency fields. Heat induction in conducting loops formed by electrocardiogram leads can cause superficial burns, and induced current in monitoring equipment may produce unreliable readings or malfunction of syringe drivers, resulting in incorrect drug-dose delivery. Responsibility for safe use of MRI monitoring equipment should be allocated to a small number of experienced and appropriately trained staff.

RECOVERY AND DISCHARGE CRITERIA

The effects of most agents used for sedation and analgesia last longer than the duration of the procedure; therefore, monitoring of the patient must continue into the recovery period. When the patient is alert and orientated and vital signs have returned to their baseline values or acceptable levels, the patient can be considered fit to be moved from the radiology department. The overall responsibility for the patient's care until discharge is with the consultant radiologist or main operator, and every unit should have written guidelines for discharge criteria.

Further Reading

American Society of Anesthesiologists Committee on Standards and Practice Parameters and the Task Force on Anesthetic Care for Magnetic Resonance Imaging. Practice advisory on anesthetic care for magnetic resonance imaging: an updated report by the American Society of Anesthesiologists Task force on anesthetic care for magnetic resonance imaging. *Anesthesiology.* 2015;122:495–520.

21

Medical emergencies

Matthew Bridge

Medical emergencies occurring in the radiology department may be caused by:

1. Medication or radiographic contrast given
2. Procedure-related complications
3. Deterioration of pre-existing morbidities

Patients may develop cardiac arrhythmias, hypotension, inadequate ventilation or adverse drug or radiographic contrast reactions. Complications arise from sedative drug administration, invasive procedures and human error; poor monitoring and organizational failings may contribute. Specific consideration should also be made in imaging departments where cardiac imaging (computed tomography (CT), magnetic resonance imaging (MRI) and nuclear medicine) is undertaken; see the Cardiovascular Emergencies section.

If a complication occurs, rapid recognition of the problem and effective management are essential. A call must be made to summon the hospital medical emergency or cardiac arrest team for any medical emergency event that is not immediately reversed or if ongoing care will be required.

The basic principles are summarized in the ABCs of resuscitating acutely ill patients:

1. Airway: ensuring a patent airway
2. Breathing: providing supplemental oxygen and adequate ventilation
3. Circulation: restoration of circulating volume

These early interventions should proceed in parallel with diagnosis and definitive treatment of the underlying cause. If cardiac arrest is suspected, the adult advanced life support algorithm in Figure 22.1 should be followed.

EQUIPMENT

A resuscitation trolley which is regularly checked and restocked should be kept in the radiology department and contain:

1. A defibrillator
2. A positive-pressure breathing device (Ambu bag) and mask

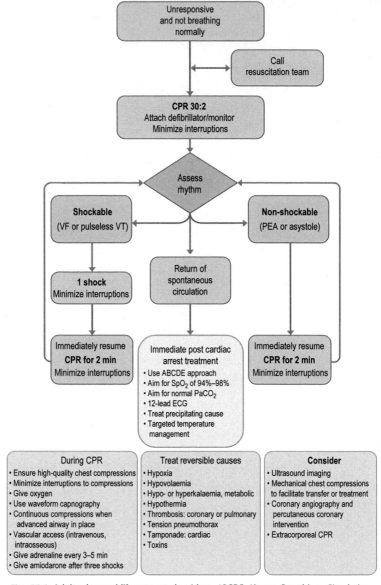

Fig. 22.1 Adult advanced life support algorithm. *ABCDE,* Airway, Breathing, Circulation, Disability, Exposure; *CPR,* cardiopulmonary resuscitation; *ECG,* electrocardiogram; *PEA,* pulseless electrical activity; *VF,* ventricular fibrillation; *VT,* ventricular tachycardia. (Reproduced with the kind permission of the Resuscitation Council (UK).)

3. Supplemental oxygen and oxygen delivery devices
4. Suction equipment
5. An intubation tray with airways, laryngoscopes and endotracheal tubes
6. Intravenous (IV) cannulas and IV fluids

7. Drugs:
   (a) Sedative reversal drugs, including naloxone and flumazenil
   (b) Resuscitation drugs, including adrenaline (epinephrine), atropine and hydrocortisone
8. Pulse oximeter
9. Non-invasive blood pressure device and appropriately sized brachial cuffs
10. An electrocardiograph
11. Capnography

RESPIRATORY EMERGENCIES

In all cases, it is essential to call for urgent anaesthetic assistance if the medical emergency event is not immediately reversed.

RESPIRATORY DEPRESSION

Sedative and analgesic drugs can cause depression of respiratory drive and compromise of the airway leading to hypoxia and hypercapnia. The clinical signs are:

1. Decreased, shallow, laboured breathing
2. Decreased oxygen saturations
3. In partial airway obstruction, snoring and paradoxical chest wall movement

22

The patient should immediately be placed in the supine position. If the airway is compromised, it can be maintained by opening the mouth, tilting and extending the head and lifting the chin or by a jaw thrust manoeuvre; insertion of an oropharyngeal airway may also be of benefit. Supplemental oxygen must be provided. If respiratory depression is caused by sedative drugs, then reversal agents should be considered.

LARYNGOSPASM

This is airway obstruction caused by tonic contractions of laryngeal and pharyngeal muscles. Risk factors include excessive secretions and mechanical irritation:

1. In partial obstruction, stridor is present. Partial airway obstruction can be treated with oxygen, coughing and calming measures.
2. In complete obstruction, there is chest wall movement but no air movement. Immediate anaesthetic assistance is required.

BRONCHOSPASM

This is constriction of bronchial airways by increased smooth muscle tone leading to small airway obstruction. Risk factors are pre-existing asthma, airway irritation, histamine release and smoking. The signs include:

1. Wheeze
2. Tachypnoea and dyspnoea
3. Decreased oxygen saturations
4. Use of accessory respiratory muscles
5. Tachycardia
6. Silent chest

Treatment includes high-flow oxygen, nebulized salbutamol 2.5–5 mg, nebulized ipratropium bromide 0.25–0.5 mg and IV hydrocortisone 100–200 mg.

ASPIRATION

Aspiration of blood or gastric contents into the lungs occurs when protective reflexes are lost and, if severe, can cause hypoxia, requiring mechanical ventilation. Risk factors are:

1. Postprocedure nausea and vomiting
2. Obesity
3. Hiatus hernia
4. Non-adherence to fasting guidelines
5. Deep levels of sedation

The patient should be placed on their side in the head-down position; high-flow oxygen should be administered, airway adjuncts should be removed and the airway should be suctioned.

PNEUMOTHORAX

This is likely to be related to a procedure such as lung biopsy (see also Chapter 9). Presentation is with unilateral pleuritic chest pain and dyspnoea:

1. For asymptomatic small pneumothorax, the patient should be observed.
2. For symptomatic small pneumothorax, simple aspiration should be performed and the patient subsequently observed.
3. If the pneumothorax is greater than 2 cm in depth (which is equivalent to 49% of the volume of the hemithorax), an intercostal chest drain should be inserted.
4. If the dyspnoea increases rapidly and the patient becomes cyanosed, tension pneumothorax should be suspected, and air should be aspirated immediately by insertion of a 16-gauge cannula through the second intercostal space in the midclavicular line.

CARDIOVASCULAR EMERGENCIES

In all cases, it is essential to call for urgent anaesthetic assistance if the medical emergency event is not immediately reversed.

It is particularly important in departments where cardiac imaging is performed that the side effects of all administered cardioactive drugs are fully understood. Drugs commonly administered in cardiac imaging include beta-blockers (in cardiac CT) and dobutamine and adenosine (in MR or isotope stress imaging). Clearly, many of the patients undergoing such investigations potentially have significant cardiovascular disease, and particularly in the in-patient setting, may already be unstable. It is therefore vital that appropriate clinical assessment and monitoring before, during and after the test is undertaken and that appropriate drugs to reverse reactions are readily available.

HYPOTENSION

This is defined as a decrease of greater than 25% from the patient's preprocedure systolic blood pressure. Hypotension may be a manifestation of shock, which is a state of circulatory failure resulting in inadequate tissue perfusion to vital organs. The signs of hypotension are pallor, faints, tachycardia and reduction in capillary refill and oliguria. The common causes are:

1. Pharmacological vasodilatation
2. Myocardial depression
3. Hypovolaemia caused by procedure-related haemorrhage or haematoma
4. Sepsis
5. Vasovagal event

The treatment depends on the cause; pressure should be applied to any developing haematoma, the patient placed in the Trendelenburg position and oxygen administered. In the case of haemorrhage or haematoma, normalization of blood pressure is not the initial priority until bleeding is controlled. Patients with hypotension are treated at first by the administration of an IV fluid bolus such as Hartmann's solution 10 mL kg^{-1}, and patients are immediately reassessed. Major haemorrhage protocols should be available in all hospital settings and activated as appropriate.

TACHYCARDIA

This is classified as a heart rate greater than 100 beats min^{-1} and is associated with stimulation of the sympathetic nervous system caused by:

1. Undersedation
2. Pain
3. Hypotension
4. Hypoxia

Heart rates of up to 160 beats min^{-1} are generally well tolerated, but tachycardia-induced hypotension or myocardial ischaemia require urgent treatment.

BRADYCARDIA

This is classified as a heart rate less than 60 beats min^{-1} and may be caused by sedative depressant effect, vasovagal or secondary to hypoxia or pain. Management is as follows:

1. If the patient is non-symptomatic, monitor closely.
2. If hypotension or bradycardia less than 40 beats min^{-1} is present, an anticholinergic drug such as atropine 0.3–0.6 mg may be given IV.
3. If the patient develops asystole, pulseless electric activity or ventricular fibrillation, then confirm the diagnosis—unconscious, apnoeic, absent carotid pulse. Call for help (defibrillator and cardiac arrest team) and follow the advanced life support algorithm outlined in Figure 22.1.

ADVERSE DRUG REACTIONS

CONTRAST MEDIA REACTION

This is also discussed in detail in Chapter 2. Suggested management is as follows:

1. Nausea or vomiting: Provide patient reassurance. Retain IV access and observe.
2. Urticaria: Retain IV access and observe. If troublesome, give an antihistamine by slow IV injection (e.g. chlorphenamine maleate 10–20 mg). If the patient has severe urticaria, add IV hydrocortisone 100 mg.
3. Hypotension with bradycardia (vasovagal reaction)
4. Mild wheeze (discussed previously)
5. Anaphylaxis: rare, most often mild, but may be life threatening. Iodinated IV contrast media are the commonest sources of anaphylaxis in the radiology department; however, other possible causes include gadolinium agents, opioid drugs, antibiotics, aspirin, latex and local anaesthetics. Anaphylaxis is a hypersensitivity reaction that causes a range of symptoms and signs, including oedema of the face and airway, wheeze, cyanosis, tachycardia, hypotension, erythema and urticaria. Traditionally, anaphylaxis is considered likely when all of the following three criteria are met:
   (a) Sudden onset and rapid progression of symptoms
   (b) Life-threatening airway ± breathing ± circulation problems
   (c) Skin or mucosal changes (flushing, urticaria, angio-oedema). It should be noted, however, that skin or mucosal changes alone do not indicate anaphylactic reaction and that these changes are subtle or absent in up to 20% of anaphylactic reactions.
   The Royal College of Anaesthetist National Audit Project 6 (NAP 6) is the largest-ever prospective study on anaphylaxis and found

that hypotension was the presenting feature in 48% of cases and was present in all episodes. Persistent hypotension should therefore raise the suspicion of anaphylaxis.

The recommended management plan for anaphylaxis is the UK Resuscitation Council algorithm in Figure 22.2.

6. Unconscious, unresponsive, pulseless, collapse; see Figure 22.1

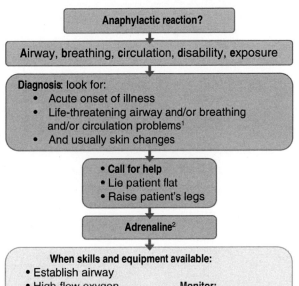

Anaphylactic reaction?

Airway, breathing, circulation, disability, exposure

Diagnosis: look for:
- Acute onset of illness
- Life-threatening airway and/or breathing and/or circulation problems[1]
- And usually skin changes

- **Call for help**
- Lie patient flat
- Raise patient's legs

Adrenaline[2]

When skills and equipment available:
- Establish airway
- High-flow oxygen
- IV fluid challenge[3]
- Chlorphenamine[4]
- Hydrocortisone[5]

Monitor:
- Pulse oximetry
- ECG
- Blood pressure

22

1 **Life-threatening problems:**
Airway: Swelling, hoarseness, stridor
Breathing: Rapid breathing, wheeze, fatigue, cyanosis, SpO$_2$ < 92%, confusion
Circulation: Pale, clammy, low blood pressure, faintness, drowsy or coma

2 **Adrenaline** *(give IM unless experienced with IV adrenaline)*
IM doses of 1:1000 adrenaline (repeat after 5 min if no better)

• Adult:	500 µg IM (0.5 mL)
• Child older than 12 y	500 µg IM (0.5 mL)
• Child 6–12 y	300 µg IM (0.3 mL)
• Child younger than 6 y	150 µg IM (0.15 mL)

Adrenaline IV to be given only by experienced specialists
Titrate: adults, 50 µg; children, 1 µg/kg

3 **IV fluid challenge:**
Adult: 500–1000 mL
Child: crystalloid 20 mL/kg

Stop IV colloid
if this might be the cause
of anaphylaxis

	4 Chlorphenamine (IM or slow IV)	5 Hydrocortisone (IM or slow IV)
Adult or child older than 12 y	10 mg	200 mg
Child 6–12 y	5 mg	100 mg
Child 6 months to 6 y	2.5 mg	50 mg
Child younger than 6 mo	250 µg/kg	25 mg

Fig. 22.2 Anaphylaxis algorithm. *ECG*, Electrocardiogram; *IM*, intramuscular; *IV*, intravenous. (Reproduced with the kind permission of the Resuscitation Council (UK).)

LOCAL ANAESTHETIC TOXICITY

Accidental IV injection of local anaesthetic or systemic absorption can result in toxicity due to membrane effects on the heart and central nervous system:

1. Early signs of toxicity are tingling around mouth and tongue, lightheadedness, agitation and tremor.
2. More severe reactions include sudden loss of consciousness, with or without tonic–clonic convulsions and cardiovascular collapse.

The immediate management includes stopping injection, calling for help, maintaining airway (including securing the airway with intubation if required), giving 100% oxygen, ensuring adequate IV access, ensuring ventilator and cardiovascular support and controlling seizures. The toxicity can be reversed by IV administration of 20% lipid emulsion (intralipid).[1] In the event of a cardiac arrest, resuscitation should be prolonged.

Reference

1. National Institute for Health and Care Excellence. Severe local anaesthetic-induced cardiovascular-toxicity. <https://bnf.nice.org.uk/treatment-summaries/severe-local-anaesthetic-induced-cardiovascular-toxicity>.

Dose limits: from The Ionising Radiations Regulations 2017[1]

Body Part etc.	Dose Limit (mSv)		
	Employees 18 y or Older	Special Circumstances[a]	Trainees Aged 16–18 y
Effective dose in any calendar year	20	50 (not more than 100 mSv averaged over 5 y)	6
Equivalent dose for the skin in a calendar year as applied to the dose averaged over any area of 1 cm², regardless of the area exposed	500	500	150
Equivalent dose for hands, forearms, feet and ankles in a calendar year			
Equivalent dose for the lens of the eye in a calendar year	20	Not more than 100 mSv in any period of 5 consecutive years subject to a maximum of 50 mSv in any single year	15

Other Persons (Including Any Person Younger Than 16 y)
1 (5[b])
50
15

Continued

Body Part etc.	Dose Limit (mSv)			
	Employees 18 y or Older	Special Circumstances[a]	Trainees Aged 16–18 y	Other Persons (Including Any Person Younger Than 16 y)
Equivalent dose for the abdomen of a woman of reproductive capacity at work, being the equivalent dose from exposure to ionizing radiation averaged throughout the abdomen in any consecutive 3-mo period	13	13	N/A	N/A

[a]If an employer demonstrates to the Health and Safety Executive (HSE) that it cannot meet the 20 mSv/calendar year limit, it may apply this limit after notifying HSE, the employees concerned and the approved dosimetry service.
[b]The dose limit for persons who are exposed to ionizing radiation from a medical exposure of another person but are not 'comforters or carers' is 5 mSv in any period of 5 consecutive calendar years. (A 'comforter and carer' is defined in The Ionising Radiations Regulations (IRR) 2017 as an individual who [other than as part of his occupation] knowingly and willingly incurs an exposure to ionizing radiation resulting from the support and comfort of another person who is undergoing or who has undergone any medical exposure).
N/A, Not Applicable.

Reference
1. The Ionizing Radiations Regulations 2017, Schedule 3, Dose Limits.

Appendix II

The Ionising Radiation (Medical Exposure) Regulations 2017 with the Ionising Radiation (Medical Exposure) (Amendment) Regulations 2018 and the Ionising Radiation (Medical Exposure) (Amendment) Regulations 2011[1]

These Regulations, together with the Ionising Radiations Regulations 1999 (S.I. 1999/3232), partially implement, as respects Great Britain, Council Directive 97/43/Euratom (OJ No. L180, 9.7.97, p. 22) laying down basic measures for the health protection of individuals against dangers of ionizing radiation in relation to medical exposure. The regulations impose duties on those responsible for administering ionizing radiation to protect persons undergoing medical exposure whether as part of their own medical diagnosis or treatment or as part of occupational health surveillance, health screening, voluntary participation in research or medico-legal procedures.

They replaced The Ionising Radiation (Protection of Persons Undergoing Medical Examination or Treatment) Regulations 1988.

1. Commencement

These regulations came into force on 6 February 2018.

2. Glossary of (Some of the) Terms

"accidental exposure" means an exposure of an individual as a result of an accident;

"adequate training" means training which satisfies the requirements of Schedule 3 and the expression "adequately trained" is to be construed accordingly;

"assessment" means prior determination of amount, parameter or method;

"carers and comforters" means individuals knowingly and willingly incurring an exposure to ionising radiation by helping, other than as part of their occupation, in the support and comfort of individuals undergoing or having undergone an exposure;

"clinical audit" means a systematic examination or review of medical radiological procedures which seeks to improve the quality and outcome of patient care through structured review, whereby medical radiological practices, procedures and results are examined against agreed standards for good medical radiological procedures, with modification of practices, where indicated, and the application of new standards if necessary;

"diagnostic reference levels" means dose levels in medical radiodiagnostic or interventional radiology practices, or, in the case of radio-pharmaceuticals, levels of activity, for typical examinations for groups of standard-sized individuals or standard phantoms for broadly defined types of equipment;

"dose constraint" means a restriction set on the prospective doses of individuals which may result from a given radiation source;

"employer" means any person who, in the course of a trade, business or other undertaking, carries out (other than as an employee), or engages others to carry out, those exposures described in regulation 3 or practical aspects, at a given radiological installation;

"employer's procedures" means the procedures established by an employer pursuant to regulation 6(1);

"equipment" means equipment which—

(a) delivers ionising radiation to a person undergoing exposure; or

(b) which directly controls or influences the extent of such exposure;

"evaluation" means interpretation of the outcome and implications of, and of the information resulting from, an exposure;

"health screening" means a procedure for early diagnosis in population groups at risk;

"interventional radiology" means the use of X-ray imaging techniques to facilitate the introduction and guidance of devices in the body for diagnostic or treatment purposes;

"ionising radiation" means the transfer of energy in the form of particles or electromagnetic waves of a wavelength of 100 nanometres or less or a frequency of 3×10^{15} hertz or more capable of producing ions directly or indirectly;

"Licensing Authority"—

(a) for the purpose of licensing any practitioner in respect of the administration of radioactive substances means the Secretary of State;

(b) for the purpose of licensing any employer in respect of the administration of radioactive substances means—

(i) in England, the Secretary of State;

(ii) in Scotland, the Scottish Ministers; and

(iii) in Wales, the Welsh Ministers;

"medical exposure" means an exposure coming within any of paragraphs (a) to (e) of regulation 3;

"medical physics expert" means an individual or a group of individuals, having the knowledge, training and experience to act or give advice on matters relating to radiation physics applied to exposure, whose competence in this respect is recognised by the Secretary of State;

"medical radiological" means pertaining to radiodiagnostic and radiotherapeutic procedures, and interventional radiology or other medical uses of ionising radiation for planning, guiding and verification purposes;

"medical radiological procedure" means any procedure giving rise to a medical exposure;

"non-medical imaging exposure" means any deliberate exposure of humans for imaging purposes where the primary intention of the exposure is not to bring a health benefit to the individual being exposed;

"operator" means any person who is entitled, in accordance with the employer's procedures, to carry out practical aspects including those to whom practical aspects have been allocated, medical physics experts and, except where they do so under the direct supervision of a person who is adequately trained, persons participating in practical aspects as part of practical training;

"patient dose" means the dose concerning patients or other individuals undergoing exposures to which these Regulations apply;

"practical aspect" means the physical conduct of a medical exposure and any supporting aspects, including handling and use of medical radiological equipment, the assessment of technical and physical parameters (including radiation doses), calibration and maintenance of equipment, preparation and administration of radio-pharmaceuticals, clinical evaluation and image processing;

"practitioner" means a registered health care professional who is entitled in accordance with the employer's procedures to take responsibility for an individual exposure;

"quality assurance" means all those planned and systematic actions necessary to provide adequate assurance that a structure, system, component or procedure will perform satisfactorily in compliance with generally applicable standards and quality control is a part of quality assurance;

"quality control" means the set of operations (programming, coordinating, implementing) intended to maintain or to improve quality and includes monitoring, evaluation and maintenance at required levels of all characteristics of performance of equipment that can be defined, measured, and controlled;

"radioactive substance" means any substance that contains one or more radionuclides the activity or activity concentration of which cannot be disregarded from a radiation protection point of view;

"radiodiagnostic" means pertaining to in-vivo diagnostic nuclear medicine, medical diagnostic radiology using ionising radiation, and dental radiology;

"radiological installation" means a facility where exposures to which these Regulations apply are performed;

"radiotherapeutic" means pertaining to radiotherapy, including nuclear medicine for therapeutic purposes;

"referrer" means a registered health care professional who is entitled in accordance with the employer's procedures to refer individuals for exposure to a practitioner;

"registered health care professional" means a person who is a member of a profession regulated by a body mentioned in section 25(3) of the National Health Service Reform and Health Care Professions Act 2002(1);

"relevant enforcing authority" means—

(a) in England, the Care Quality Commission (2);

(b) in Scotland, the Scottish Ministers; and

(c) in Wales, the Welsh Ministers;

"unintended exposure" means any exposure to ionising radiation which is significantly different from the exposure intended for a given purpose.

(2) In these Regulations, where an individual is—

(a) an employer;

(b) a referrer;

(c) an operator; or

(d) a practitioner,

and is also an individual coming within at least one other of sub-paragraphs (a) to (d), that individual is subject to each of the duties applying to every person described in a sub-paragraph which also describes that individual.

(1) 2002 c. 17. Section 25 has been amended by paragraph 17 of Schedule 10 and Part 2 of Schedule 15 the Health and Social Care Act 2008 (c. 14), sections 220, 222 and 224 of and paragraphs 56 and 62 of Schedule 15 to the Health and Social Care act 2012 (c. 7), section 5(1) of the Health and Social Care (Safety and Quality) Act 2015 (c. 28), paragraph 1 and 2 of Schedule 4 to the Children and Social Work Act 2017 (c. 16).

(2) Established by section 1 of the Health and Social Care Act 2008 (c. 14).

3. Duties of the Employer

The employer shall ensure that written procedures for medical exposures including the procedures set out in Schedule 1 are in place and:

(a) shall take steps to ensure that they are complied with by the practitioner and operator; or

(b) where the employer is concurrently practitioner or operator, he shall comply with these procedures himself.

The employer shall ensure that written protocols are in place for every type of standard radiological practice for each equipment.

The employer shall establish:

(a) recommendations concerning referral criteria for medical exposures, including radiation doses, and shall ensure that these are available to the referrer

(b) quality assurance programmes for standard operating procedures

(c) diagnostic reference levels for radiodiagnostic examinations falling within regulation 3(a), (b), (c) and (e) having regard to European diagnostic reference levels where available

(d) dose constraints for biomedical and medical research programmes falling within regulation 3(d) where no direct medical benefit for the individual is expected from the exposure.

The employer shall take steps to ensure that every practitioner or operator engaged by the employer to carry out medical exposures or any practical aspect of such exposures:

(a) complies with the provisions of regulation 11(1); and

(b) undertakes continuing education and training after qualification including, in the case of clinical use of new techniques, training related to these techniques and the relevant radiation protection requirements; or

(c) where the employer is concurrently practitioner or operator, he shall himself ensure that he undertakes such continuing education and training as may be appropriate.

Where the employer knows or has reason to believe that an incident has or may have occurred in which a person, while undergoing a medical exposure was, otherwise than as a result of a malfunction or defect in equipment, exposed to ionizing radiation to an extent much greater than intended, he shall make an immediate preliminary investigation of the incident and, unless that investigation shows beyond a reasonable doubt that no such overexposure has occurred, he shall forthwith notify the appropriate authority and make or arrange for a detailed investigation of the circumstances of the exposure and an assessment of the dose received.

The employer shall undertake appropriate reviews whenever diagnostic reference levels are consistently exceeded and ensure that corrective action is taken where appropriate.

4. Duties of the Practitioner, Operator and Referrer

The practitioner and the operator shall comply with the employer's procedures.

The practitioner shall be responsible for the justification of a medical exposure and such other aspects of a medical exposure as is provided for in these Regulations.

Practical aspects of a medical exposure or part of it may be allocated in accordance with the employer's procedures by the employer or the practitioner, as appropriate, to one or more individuals entitled to act in this respect in a recognized field of specialization.

The operator shall be responsible for each and every practical aspect which he carries out as well as for any authorization given pursuant to regulation 6(5) where such authorization is not made in accordance with the guidelines referred to in regulation 6(5).

The referrer shall supply the practitioner with sufficient medical data (such as previous diagnostic information or medical records) relevant to the medical exposure requested by the referrer to enable the practitioner to decide on whether there is a sufficient net benefit as required by regulation 6(1)(a).

The practitioner and the operator shall cooperate, regarding practical aspects, with other specialists and staff involved in a medical exposure, as appropriate.

For the avoidance of doubt, where a person acts as employer, referrer, practitioner and operator concurrently (or in any combination of these roles) he shall comply with all the duties placed on employers, referrers, practitioners or operators under these Regulations accordingly.

5. Justification of Individual Exposures

(1) A person must not carry out an exposure unless—
   (a) in the case of the administration of radioactive substances, the practitioner and employer are licensed to undertake the intended exposure;
   (b) it has been justified by the practitioner as showing a sufficient net benefit giving appropriate weight to the matters set out in paragraph (2);
   (c) it has been authorised by the practitioner or, where paragraph (5) applies, the operator;
   (d) in the case of an exposure taking place in the course of a research programme under regulation 3(c), that programme has been approved by an ethics committee and, in the case of the administration of radioactive substances, approved by an expert committee who can advise on the administration of radioactive substances to humans;
   (e) in the case of an exposure falling within regulation 3(f) (non-medical imaging), it complies with the employer's procedures for such exposures; and
   (f) in the case of an individual of childbearing potential, the person has enquired whether that individual is pregnant or breastfeeding, if relevant.
(2) The matters referred to in paragraph (1)(b) are—
   (a) the specific objectives of the exposure and the characteristics of the individual involved;
   (b) the total potential diagnostic or therapeutic benefits, including the direct health benefits to the individual and the benefits to society, of the exposure;
   (c) the individual detriment that the exposure may cause; and

    (d) the efficacy, benefits and risk of available alternative techniques having the same objective but involving no or less exposure to ionising radiation.

(3) In considering the weight to be given to the matters referred to in paragraph (2), the practitioner justifying an exposure in accordance with paragraph (1)(b) must have regard, in particular to—

    (a) recommendations from appropriate medical scientific societies or relevant bodies where a procedure is to be performed as part of any health screening programme;

    (b) whether in circumstances where there is to be an exposure to a carer or comforter such an exposure would show a sufficient net benefit taking into account—

        (i) the likely direct health benefits to a patient;

        (ii) the possible benefits to the carer or comforter; and

        (iii) the detriment that the exposure might cause;

    (c) in the case of asymptomatic individuals where a medical radiological procedure—

        (i) is to be performed for the early detection of disease;

        (ii) is to be performed as part of a health screening programme; or

        (iii) requires specific documented justification for that individual by the practitioner, in consultation with the referrer, any guidelines issued by appropriate medical scientific societies, relevant bodies or published by the Secretary of State;

    (d) the urgency of the exposure, where appropriate, in cases involving—

        (i) an individual where pregnancy cannot be excluded, in particular if abdominal and pelvic regions are involved, taking into account the exposure of both the person concerned and any unborn child; and

        (ii) an individual who is breastfeeding and who undergoes an exposure involving the administration of radioactive substances, taking into account the exposure of both the individual and the child.

(4) In deciding whether to justify an exposure under paragraph (1)(b) the practitioner must take account of any data supplied by the referrer pursuant to regulation 10(5) and must consider such data in order to avoid unnecessary exposure.

(5) Where it is not practicable for the practitioner to authorise an exposure as required by paragraph (1)(c), the operator must do so in accordance with guidelines issued by the practitioner.

(6) In this regulation—

"ethics committee" means—

    (a) an ethics committee established or recognised in accordance with Part 2 of the Medicines for Human Use (Clinical Trials) Regulations 2004(1);

    (b) the Ethics Committee constituted by regulations made by the Scottish Ministers under section 51(6) of the Adults with Incapacity (Scotland) Act 2000(2); or

(c) any other committee established to advise on the ethics of research investigations in human beings, and recognised for that purpose by or on behalf of the Secretary of State, the Scottish Ministers or the Welsh Ministers; and
"individual detriment" means clinically observable deleterious effects in individuals or their descendants, the appearance of which is either immediate or delayed and, in the latter case, implies a probability rather than a certainty of appearance.

6. Optimization

(1) In relation to all exposures to which these Regulations apply except radiotherapeutic exposures, the practitioner and the operator, to the extent of their respective involvement in an exposure, must ensure that doses arising from the exposure are kept as low as reasonably practicable consistent with the intended purpose.

(2) In relation to all radiotherapeutic exposures the practitioner must ensure that exposures of target volumes are individually planned and their delivery appropriately verified taking into account that doses to non-target volumes and tissues must be as low as reasonably practicable and consistent with the intended radiotherapeutic purpose of the exposure.

(3) Without prejudice to paragraphs (1) and (2), the operator must select equipment and methods to ensure that for each exposure the dose of ionising radiation to the individual undergoing the exposure is as low as reasonably practicable and consistent with the intended diagnostic or therapeutic purpose and in doing so must have regard, in particular to—

(a) quality assurance;

(b) assessment and evaluation of patient dose or administered activity; and

(c) adherence to such diagnostic reference levels for radiodiagnostic examinations falling within regulation 3(a), (b), (e) and (f) as the employer may have established, as set out in the employer's procedures.

(4) For each medical or biomedical research programme falling within regulation 3(c), the employer's procedures must provide that—

(a) the individuals concerned participate voluntarily in the research programme;

(b) the individuals concerned are informed in advance about the risks of the exposure;

(c) the dose constraint set down in the employer's procedures for individuals for whom no direct medical benefit is expected from the exposure is adhered to; and

(d) individual target levels of doses are planned by the practitioner, either alone or with the input of the referrer, for patients who voluntarily undergo an experimental diagnostic or therapeutic practice from which the patients are expected to receive a diagnostic or therapeutic benefit.

(5) In the case of regulation 3(d), the employer's procedures must provide that appropriate guidance is established for the exposure of carers and comforters.

(6) In the case of patients undergoing treatment or diagnosis with radioactive substances, the employer's procedures must provide that, where appropriate, written instructions and information are provided to—

(a) the patient, where the patient has capacity to consent to the treatment or diagnostic procedure;

(b) where the patient is a child who lacks capacity (within the meaning of the Mental Capacity Act 2005(1) in the case of a child aged sixteen or seventeen) so to consent, a person with parental responsibility (within the meaning of the Children Act 1989(2)) for the child; or

(c) where the patient is an adult who lacks capacity (within the meaning of the Mental Capacity Act 2005) so to consent, the person who appears to the practitioner to be the most appropriate person.

(7) The instructions and information referred to in paragraph (6) must—

(a) specify how doses resulting from the patient's exposure can be restricted as far as reasonably possible so as to protect persons in contact with the patient;

(b) set out the risks associated with ionising radiation; and

(c) be provided to the patient or other person specified in paragraph (6) as appropriate prior to the patient leaving the radiological installation where the exposure was carried out.

(8) In complying with the obligations under this regulation, the practitioner and the operator must pay particular attention in relation to—

(a) medical exposures of children;

(b) medical exposures as part of a health screening programme;

(c) medical exposures involving high doses to the individual being exposed;

(d) where appropriate, individuals in whom pregnancy cannot be excluded and who are undergoing a medical exposure, in particular if abdominal and pelvic regions are involved, taking into account the exposure of both the individual and any unborn child; and

(e) where appropriate, individuals who are breastfeeding and who are undergoing a medical exposure involving the administration of radioactive substances, taking into account the exposure of both the individual and the child.

(9) The employer must take steps to ensure that a clinical evaluation of the outcome of each exposure, other than where the person subject to the exposure is a carer or a comforter, is recorded in accordance with the employer's procedures including, where appropriate, factors relevant to patient dose.

7. Clinical Audit

The employer's procedures shall include provision for the carrying out of clinical audit as appropriate.

8. Expert Advice

The employer shall ensure that a medical physics expert shall be involved in every medical exposure to which these Regulations apply in accordance with paragraph (2).

A medical physics expert shall be:

(a) closely involved in every radiotherapeutic practice other than standardized therapeutic nuclear medicine practices

(b) available in standardized therapeutic nuclear medicine practices and in diagnostic nuclear medicine practices

(c) involved as appropriate for consultation on optimization, including patient dosimetry and quality assurance, and to give advice on matters relating to radiation protection concerning medical exposure, as required, in all other radiological practices.

9. Equipment

The employer shall draw up, keep up-to-date and preserve at each radiological installation an inventory of equipment at that installation and, when so requested, shall furnish it to the appropriate authority.

The inventory referred to in paragraph (1) shall contain the following information:

(a) name of manufacturer

(b) model number

(c) serial number or other unique identifier

(d) year of manufacture and

(e) year of installation.

The employer shall ensure that equipment at each radiological installation is limited to the amount necessary for the proper carrying out of medical exposures at that installation.

10. Training

Subject to the following provisions of this regulation no practitioner or operator shall carry out a medical exposure or any practical aspect without having been adequately trained.

A certificate issued by an institute or person competent to award degrees or diplomas or to provide other evidence of training shall, if such certificate so attests, be sufficient proof that the person to whom it has been issued has been adequately trained.

Nothing in paragraph (1) above shall prevent a person from participating in practical aspects of the procedure as part of practical training if this is done under the supervision of a person who himself is adequately trained.

The employer shall keep and have available for inspection by the appropriate authority an up-to-date record of all training undertaken by all practitioners and operators engaged by him to carry out medical exposures or any practical aspect of such exposures or, where the employer is concurrently practitioner or operator, of his own training, showing the date or dates on which training qualifying as adequate training was completed and the nature of the training.

Where the employer enters into a contract with another to engage a practitioner or operator otherwise employed by that other, the latter shall be responsible for keeping the records required by paragraph (4) and shall supply such records to the employer forthwith upon request.

11. Enforcement

The provisions of these Regulations shall be enforced as if they were health and safety regulations made under section 15 of the Health and Safety at Work etc. Act 1974 and, except as provided in paragraph (2), the provisions of that Act, as regards enforcement and offences, shall apply for the purposes of these Regulations.

The enforcing authority for the purposes of these Regulations shall be the appropriate authority.

12. Defence of Due Diligence

In any proceedings against any person for an offence consisting of the contravention of these Regulations it shall be a defence for that person to show that he took all reasonable steps and exercised all due diligence to avoid committing the offence.

II

SCHEDULE 1

Regulation 4(1)

Employer's procedures

The written procedures for medical exposures shall include:

1. procedures to identify correctly the individual to be exposed to ionizing radiation
2. procedures to identify individuals entitled to act as referrer or practitioner or operator
3. procedures to be observed in the case of medico-legal exposures
4. procedures for making enquiries of females of child-bearing age to establish whether the individual is or may be pregnant or breast feeding
5. procedures to ensure that quality assurance programmes are followed
6. procedures for the assessment of patient dose and administered activity
7. procedures for the use of diagnostic reference levels established by the employer for radiodiagnostic examinations falling within regulation 3(a), (b), (c) and (e), specifying that these are expected not to be exceeded for standard procedures when good and normal practice regarding diagnostic and technical performance is applied

8. procedures for determining whether the practitioner or operator is required to effect one or more of the matters set out in regulation 7(4) including criteria on how to effect those matters and in particular procedures for the use of dose constraints established by the employer for biomedical and medical research programmes falling within regulation 3(d) where no direct medical benefit for the individual is expected from the exposure
9. procedures for the giving of information and written instructions as referred to in regulation 7(5)
10. procedures for the carrying out and recording of an evaluation for each medical exposure including, where appropriate, factors relevant to patient dose
11. procedures to ensure that the probability and magnitude of accidental or unintended doses to patients from radiological practices are reduced so far as reasonably practicable.

SCHEDULE 2

Regulation 2(1)

Adequate training

Practitioners and operators shall have successfully completed training, including theoretical knowledge and practical experience, in:

1. such of the subjects detailed in section A as are relevant to their functions as practitioner or operator and
2. such of the subjects detailed in section B as are relevant to their specific area of practice.

A. Radiation Production, Radiation Protection and Statutory Obligations Relating to Ionizing Radiations

1. Fundamental physics of radiation
   1.1. Properties of radiation
         Attenuation of ionizing radiation
         Scattering and absorption
   1.2. Radiation hazards and dosimetry
         Biological effects of radiation
         Risks/benefits of radiation
         Dose optimization
         Absorbed dose, dose equivalent, effective dose and their units
   1.3. Special attention areas
         Pregnancy and potential pregnancy
         Infants and children
         Medical and biomedical research
         Health screening
         High dose techniques

2. Management and radiation protection of the patient
   2.1. Patient selection
      Justification of the individual exposure
      Patient identification and consent
      Use of existing appropriate radiological information
      Alternative techniques
      Clinical evaluation of outcome
      Medico-legal issues
   2.2. Radiation protection
      General radiation protection
      Use of radiation protection devices
      – Patient
      – Personal
      Procedures for untoward incidents involving overexposure to ionizing radiation
3. Statutory requirements and advisory aspects
   3.1. Statutory requirements and non-statutory recommendations
      Regulations
      Local rules and procedures
      Individual responsibilities relating to medical exposures
      Responsibility for radiation safety
      Routine inspection and testing of equipment
      Notification of faults and health department hazard warnings
      Clinical audit

B. Diagnostic Radiology, Radiotherapy and Nuclear Medicine

4. Diagnostic radiology
   4.1. General
      Fundamentals of radiological anatomy
      Fundamentals of radiological techniques
      Production of X-rays
      Equipment selection and use
      Factors affecting radiation dose
      Dosimetry
      Quality assurance and quality control
   4.2. Specialized techniques
      Image intensification/fluoroscopy
      Digital fluoroscopy
      Computed tomography scanning
      Interventional procedures
      Vascular imaging
   4.3. Fundamentals of image acquisition, etc.
      Image quality vs. radiation dose
      Conventional film processing
      Additional image formats, acquisition, storage and display
   4.4. Contrast media
      Non-ionic and ionic

Use and preparation
Contraindications to the use of contrast media
Use of automatic injection devices
5. Radiotherapy
  5.1. General
    Production of ionizing radiations
    Use of radiotherapy
     – Benign disease
     – Malignant disease
     – External beam
     – Brachytherapy
  5.2. Radiobiological aspects for radiotherapy
    Fractionation
    Dose rate
    Radiosensitization
    Target volumes
  5.3. Practical aspects for radiotherapy
    Equipment
    Treatment planning
  5.4. Radiation protection specific to radiotherapy
    Side effects – early and late
    Toxicity
    Assessment of efficacy
6. Nuclear medicine
  6.1. General
    Atomic structure and radioactivity
    Radioactive decay
    The tracer principle
    Fundamentals of diagnostic use
    Fundamentals of therapeutic use
     – Dose rate
     – Fractionation
     – Radiobiology aspects
  6.2. Principles of radiation detection, instrumentation and equipment
    Types of systems
    Image acquisition, storage and display
    Quality assurance and quality control
  6.3. Radiopharmaceuticals
    Calibration
    Working practices in the radiopharmacy
    Preparation of individual doses
    Documentation
  6.4. Radiation protection specific to nuclear medicine
    Conception, pregnancy and breast feeding
    Arrangements for radioactive patients
    Disposal procedures for radioactive waste

SCHEDULE 3

Adequate Training

Practitioners and operators must have successfully completed training, including theoretical knowledge and practical experience, in—

(a) such of the subjects detailed in Table 1 as are relevant to their functions as practitioner or operator; and

(b) such of the subjects detailed in Table 2 as are relevant to their specific area of practice.

Table 1 Radiation Production, Radiation Protection and Statutory Obligations Relating to Ionising Radiations	
Fundamental Physics of Radiation	
Properties of Radiation	Excitation and ionisation
	Attenuation of ionising radiation
	Scattering and absorption
Radiation Hazards and Dosimetry	Biological effects of radiation – stochastic and deterministic
	Risks and benefits of radiation
	Absorbed dose, equivalent dose, effective dose, other dose indicators and their units
Management and Radiation Protection of the individual being exposed	
Special Attention Areas	Pregnancy and potential pregnancy
	Asymptomatic individuals
	Breastfeeding
	Infants and children
	Medical and biomedical research
	Health screening
	Non-medical imaging
	Carers and comforters
	High dose techniques
Justification	Justification of the individual exposure
	Use of existing appropriate radiological information
	Alternative techniques
Radiation Protection	Diagnostic reference levels
	Dose Constraints
	Dose Optimisation
	Dose reduction devices and techniques

Continued

Table 1   Radiation Production, Radiation Protection and Statutory Obligations Relating to Ionising Radiations—cont'd

	Dose recording and dose audit
	General radiation protection
	Quality Assurance and Quality Control including routine inspection and testing of equipment
	Risk communication
	Use of radiation protection devices
Statutory Requirements and Non-Statutory Regulations	
	Regulations
	Non-statutory guidance
	Local procedures and protocols
	Individual responsibilities relating to exposures
	Responsibility for radiation safety
	Clinical audit

Table 2   Diagnostic Radiology, Radiotherapy and Nuclear Medicine

All Modalities	
General	Fundamentals of radiological anatomy
	Factors affecting radiation dose
	Dosimetry
	Fundamentals of clinical evaluation
	Identification of the individual being exposed
Diagnostic radiology	
General	Principles of radiological techniques
	Production of X-rays
	Equipment selection and use
Specialised Techniques	Computed Tomography: advanced applications
	Interventional procedures
	Cone Beam Computed Tomography
	Hybrid imaging
Fundamentals of Image Acquisition etc.	Optimisation of image quality and radiation dose
	Image formats, acquisition, processing, display and storage

Table 2 Diagnostic Radiology, Radiotherapy and Nuclear Medicine—cont'd	
Contrast Media	Use and preparation
	Contraindications
	Use of contrast injection systems
Radiotherapy	
General	Production of ionising radiation
	Treatment of malignant disease
	Treatment of benign disease
	Principles of external beam radiotherapy
	Principles of brachytherapy
	Intra-operative radiotherapy
	Stereotactic radiotherapy and radiosurgery
Specialised techniques	Stereotactic ablative radiotherapy
	Proton therapy
	MR Linac therapy
Radiobiological Aspects for Radiotherapy	Fractionation
	Dose rate
	Radiosensitisation
	Target volumes
	Localisation equipment selection
Practical Aspects for Radiotherapy	Therapy equipment selection
	Verification techniques including on-treatment imaging
	Treatment planning systems
	Side effects—early and late
Radiation Protection Specific to Radiotherapy	Toxicity
	Assessment of efficacy
Nuclear Medicine	
General	Atomic structure and radioactivity
	Radioactive decay
	Principles of molecular imaging and non-imaging exposures
	Principles of molecular radiotherapy
	Dose rate
Molecular Radiotherapy	Fractionation
	Radiobiology aspects

Continued

Table 2   Diagnostic Radiology, Radiotherapy and Nuclear Medicine—cont'd

	Radiosensitisation
	Quantitative imaging – advanced applications
Specialised techniques	Hybrid imaging – advanced applications
	Selective Internal Radiation Therapy
	Types of detection systems
Principles of Radiation Detection, Instrumentation and Equipment	Optimisation of image quality and radiation dose
	Image acquisition, artefacts, processing, display and storage
Radiopharmaceuticals	Calibration
	Working practices in the radiopharmacy
	Preparation of individual doses
Radiation Protection Specific to Nuclear Medicine	Conception, pregnancy and breastfeeding
	Arrangements for radioactive individuals

SCHEDULE 4

Consequential Amendments

Amendment of the Justification of Practices Involving Ionising Radiation Regulations 2004

(1) The Justification of Practices Involving Ionising Radiation Regulations 2004(1) are amended as follows.

(2) For regulation 21 (saving for medical practices) substitute—
"21. Nothing in regulation 4(5) of 5(3) shall prevent anything permitted under regulation 11 of the Ionising Radiation (Medical Exposure) Regulations 2017.".

Amendment of the Human Medicines Regulations 2012

(1) The Human Medicines Regulations 2012(2) are amended as follows.

(2) In regulation 173 (exemption for certain radiopharmaceuticals)—
    (a) in paragraph (d), at the beginning insert "in Northern Ireland";
    (b) after paragraph (d) insert—
        "(e) in England and Wales and Scotland, for administration in accordance with a licence issued under the Ionising Radiation (Medical Exposure) Regulations 2017".

(3) In regulation 240 (radioactive medicinal products)—
- (a) for paragraph (1)(a) substitute—
  "(a) either—
  - (i) in Northern Ireland, a radioactive medicinal product, administration of which results in a medical exposure; or
  - (ii) in England and Wales and Scotland, a radioactive substance, administration of which results in a medical exposure; or";
- (b) in paragraph (2), after "Condition A" insert "in Northern Ireland";
- (c) after paragraph (2) insert—
  "(2A) Condition A in England and Wales and Scotland is that the prescription only medicine is administered by an operator acting in accordance with the procedures and protocols referred to in regulation 6(1) and (4) of the Ionising Radiation (Medical Exposure) Regulations 2017.";
- (d) in paragraph (4), after "condition C" insert "in Northern Ireland";
- (e) after paragraph (4A) insert—
  "(4) Condition C in England and Wales and Scotland is that the IRME practitioner mentioned in paragraph (a) or (b) of paragraph (3) is the holder of a licence issued under the Ionising Radiation (Medical Exposure) Regulations 2017.";
- (f) in paragraph (6) after "Condition C" insert "in Northern Ireland;
- (g) after paragraph (6) insert—
  "(6A) Condition D in England and Wales and Scotland is that the prescription only medicine is not a radioactive substance.".
- (h) for paragraph (7) substitute—
  "(7) In this regulation—
  "IRME practitioner" means—
  - (a) in Northern Ireland, in relation to a medical exposure, a practitioner for the purposes of the Ionising Radiation (Medical Exposure) Regulations 2000;
  - (b) in England and Wales and Scotland, in relation to a medical exposure, a practitioner for the purposes of the Ionising Radiation (Medical Exposure) Regulations 2017; "medical exposure"—
    - (a) in Northern Ireland has the same meaning as in the Ionising Radiation (Medical Exposure) Regulations 2000; and
    - (b) in England and Wales and Scotland has the same meaning as in the Ionising Radiation (Medical Exposure) Regulations 2017; and
    "radioactive medicinal product" means a medicinal product which consists of, contains or generates a radioactive substance so that, when the product is administered, the radiation it emits may be used.".

Amendment of the Ionising Radiations Regulations 2017

(1) The Ionising Radiations Regulations 2017(3) are amended as follows.

(2) In regulation 2(1) (interpretation)—
  (a) omit the definition of "carers and comforters";
  (b) insert after the definition of "calendar year"—
      ""carers and comforters" means individuals knowingly and willingly incurring an exposure to ionising radiation by helping, other than as part of their occupation, in the support and comfort of individuals undergoing or having undergone a medical exposure (other than as a carer and comforter);";
  (c) in the definition of "medical exposure", after paragraph (d) insert—
      "(e) carers and comforters;".
(3) In regulation 3 (application)—
  (a) in paragraph (2), omit "33";
  (b) omit paragraph (4).
(4) Omit regulation 33 (equipment used for medical exposure).
(5) In regulation 35(6) (duties of employees)—
  (a) in sub-paragraph (a), after "overexposure;" insert "or";
  (b) in sub-paragraph (b), omit "or" the second time it appears;
  (c) omit sub-paragraph (c).
(6) In regulation 38(2)(d) (exemption certificates)—
  (a) before "25(2)" insert "and";
  (b) omit "and 33(1)".
(1) S.I. 2004/1769; there are amending instruments but none is relevant.
(2) S.I. 2012/1916 as amended by S.I. 2014/490; there are other amending instruments but none is relevant.
(3) S.I. 2017/1075.

Reference
1. Crown copyright 2017. With the permission of the Controller of Her Majesty's Stationery Office.

Index

A

ABC of resuscitation, 461
Abdomen, ultrasonography of, 19
Abdominal stent grafts, 284–287
Ablative technology
  non-thermal, 201
    irreversible electroporation in,
      204–205
  thermal, 201
    cryoablation in, 203–204
    microwave ablation in, 202–203
    radiofrequency ablation in,
      201–202
Acetylacetonate, 324
Acoustic neuromas, 380
Adenosine, in radionuclide myocardial
  perfusion imaging, 258–259
Adhesive capsulitis, diagnosis and
  distension therapy in, 332
Administration of Radioactive
  Substances Advisory Committee
  (ARSAC), 8
Adrenals
  lesion characterization computed
    tomography, 182
  magnetic resonance imaging of,
    186
Adult advanced life support algorithm,
  462f
Adults with Incapacity (Scotland) Act,
  446
Adults with Incapacity (Scotland) Act
  2000 Codes of Practice, 448
Adverse drug reactions, 466–467
  to contrast media, 466–467
  local anaesthetic toxicity, 468
Air embolus, as catheter complication,
  274
Air enema, 117
Air, in intussusception reduction, 55
ALARP (as low as reasonably practicable
  dose), 2
Alimemazine, 44, 44t
Amplatz coronary artery catheters, 242,
  242f

Anaesthesia
  complications due to, 7
  see also General anaesthesia; Local
    anaesthesia; Sedation
Analgesic drugs, 453
  inhalational, 453
  intravenous, 453–455, 454t
Anaphylaxis, 466–467, 467f
Angiocardiography, 239–241
  contrast medium in, 240, 240t
  equipment for, 240, 240f
  image acquisition for, 241
  indications for, 239
  technique for, 241
Angiography, 167, 275–278
  for brain, 373
  cerebral, 385
    aftercare, 388
    contraindications for, 385
    contrast medium in, 387
    equipment for, 385
    films for, 388
    indications for, 385
    preparation for, 385
    projections in, 387–388
    technique in, 385–387, 386f
  coeliac axis, 167
  computed tomographic, 264
  computed tomography, 183–184
  equipment for, 275
  indications of, 275
  magnetic resonance, 265–266
    of liver, 154
    see also Magnetic resonance
      angiography
  patient preparation for, 275
  peripheral (lower limb) computed
    tomographic, 264–265
  renal, magnetic resonance, 187–188
  superior mesenteric, 167, 298
  technique in, 275–276
Angioplasty, 276–278
  aftercare for, 278
  balloons, 276
  complications in, 278

Note: Page numbers followed by f indicate figures; t, tables.

Angioplasty (*Continued*)
  equipment in, 276–277
  indications for, 276
  patient preparation for, 277
  stents and, venous, 300–301
  technique in, 277–278
Ankle, arthrography for, 344, 344*f*
Anorectal cancer, local staging of,
  magnetic resonance imaging for, 134
Antegrade pyelography, percutaneous,
  191–193
Antibiotic prophylaxis, in barium
  enema, 115
Anticoagulant therapy, interventional
  radiology and, 434
Antiplatelet therapy, interventional
  radiology and, 434
Anus, endoluminal examination of, 123
Anxiety, 11
Anxiolysis, 451
Appendix, ultrasound of, 122
Arachnoiditis, 359
Argon gas, for renal CRYO, 203
Arrhythmias, due to coronary
  arteriography, 244
Arterial system, 263–287
  abdominal stent grafts in, 284–287
  angiography in, 275–278
  angioplasty for, 276–278
  catheter-directed arterial
    thrombolysis in, 280–282
  catheter techniques in
    complications of, 272–274
    see also Catheter techniques
  computed tomographic angiography
    of, 264
  magnetic resonance angiography of,
    265–266
  non-invasive imaging of, 263–266
  peripheral (lower limb) computed
    tomographic angiography of,
    264–265
  stents for, 279–280
  thoracic stent grafts in, 284–287
  vascular access in, 266–272
  vascular embolization in, 282–284
  vascular ultrasound of, 263–264
Arterial thrombus, as catheter
  complication, 273
Arterial toxicity, of intravascular
  contrast media, 25
Arteriovenous fistulae, ultrasound for, 289
Arteriography
  coronary, 241–244
    complications of, 244
    contrast medium in, 242
    equipment for, 242, 242*f*–243*f*
    image acquisition in, 243–244
    indications for, 241–242
    patient preparation for, 243

Arteriography (*Continued*)
  technique for, 243
  inferior mesenteric, 167–171
  pulmonary, 227, 232–233
  renal, 183–184
  for spine, 355
  superior mesenteric, 167–171, 298
Arteriovenous fistula, as catheter
  complication, 274
Artery dissection, as catheter
  complication, 274
Arthrography, 331–334
  aftercare for, 333
  complications of, 333–334
  contraindications for, 332
  contrast medium for, 332–333
  equipment for, 333
  general points of, 330–334
  indications for, 331–332
  patient preparation for, 333
  preliminary images of, 333
  radiographic views of, 333
  site-specific issues for, 334–346
    ankle in, 344, 344*f*
    elbow in, 341–342, 342*f*
    hip in, 335–338, 336*f*–337*f*, 341*f*
    knee in, 334–335, 335*f*
    shoulder in, 338–341, 338*f*, 340*f*
    wrist in, 342–343, 343*f*
Artifacts, in magnetic resonance imaging
  of reproductive system, 216
As low as reasonably practicable dose
  (ALARP), 2, 9
Aseptic technique, 7
Aspiration, 464
Aspirin, 180, 225, 426*t*, 400
Assessment, of capacity, 446–447
  documenting, 449
Atheroembolism, as catheter
  complication, 274
Automated biopsy gun, for breast, 424
Automated blood pressure monitoring, 457
Axillary artery puncture, 273

B
Back pain, 356–357
Bacteraemia, as catheter complication,
  275
Balloon angioplasty, 276–277
Balloon mounted stents, 279
Barium, 99–100, 99*t*
Barium enema, 100, 112–116
Barium follow-through, 99
Barium meal, 99, 104–110, 107*f*
Barium sulphate, 99, 120
Barium swallow, 99
Berenstein catheter, 386*f*
Beta-blockers
  in cardiac computed tomography, 247
  intravascular contrast media and, 29

Bilbao-Dotter tube, 110–111
Bile ducts
    endoscopic retrograde
        cholangiopancreatography of
        contrast medium in, 157
    images in, 158
    ultrasound of
        extrahepatic, 147
        intrahepatic, 147
Biliary calculi, percutaneous extraction
    of retained, 165–167
Biliary system, ultrasound of, 146–148
Biliary tract, 143–174
Biliary tree, computed tomography of,
    149–151
Biopsy
    automated gun, 424
    computed tomography-guided lung,
        223–227
    image-guided breast, 421–427
        equipment of, 424
        indications of, 421
        patient preparation of, 425
        technique for, 427
    omental, 219–220
    percutaneous renal cyst puncture
        and, 191
    percutaneous vertebral, 367–369
Bladder, computed tomography,
    182–184
Bleeding, risk of, 6
Blood–brain barrier imaging, 381
Blood clotting, 6
Blood pressure, automated monitoring
    of, 457–458
Bolus timing, in contrast-enhanced
    cardiac scan, 248
Bone augmentation techniques, 369
Bone scan, radionuclide, 350–353
    additional techniques for, 353
    analysis for, 352
    competing modalities for, 353
    complications of, 353
    contraindications for, 351
    equipment for, 351
    images for, 352
    indications for, 350–353
    patient preparation for, 351
    radiopharmaceuticals in, 351
    technique in, 351–352
Bones and joints, 327–353
    arthrography for, 331–334
        general points in, 330–334
        site-specific issues in, 334–346
    computed tomography for, 328
    imaging modalities for, 327–330
    musculoskeletal magnetic resonance
        imaging for, 329–330
    plain films for, 327
    radionuclide bone scan, 350–353

Bones and joints (*Continued*)
    tendon imaging for, 346–347
    thermoablation of musculoskeletal
        tumours for, 347–350
    ultrasound for, 346–347
Bowel preparation, 6
Brachial artery, for vascular access, 266
Brachial artery puncture, 274
Bradycardia, 466
Brain, 373–388
    acoustic neuromas and, 380
    angiography for, 373
    blood-brain barrier imaging of, 381
    cerebral angiography for, 385
    computed tomography for, 373–374
    dopamine transporter ligand for, 384
    gliomas and, 379
    intracranial haemorrhage and,
        377–378
    magnetic resonance imaging for, 373,
        375–377
    methods of imaging for, 373–375
    plain films for, 374
    positron emission tomography for,
        382–383
    radionuclide imaging for, 373,
        380–385
    regional cerebral blood flow imaging
        for, 380–382
    [201]thallium brain scanning, 383
    ultrasound for, 373–374
Breast, 411–431
    biopsy, image-guided, 421–431
        equipment of, 424
        indications of, 421–428
        patient preparation of, 425–426
        technique for, 427
    calcification, biopsy, 427
    compression of, 415
    imaging methods of, 411–416
    intraoperative sentinel node
        identification of, 420
    magnetic resonance imaging for,
        418–419
    mammography for, 414–416
        equipment of, 414–415
        indications of, 414
        not indicated, 414
        technique for, 415–416
    positron emission tomography
        scanning for, 420
    preoperative localization of, 428–431
    radionuclide imaging of, 420
    ultrasound for, 416–418
Breast carcinoma, sentinel node in,
    322
Bronchospasm, 463–464
Bupivacaine, 453, 454t
Burhenne technique, 165–167
Buscopan, 100–101

C

Calcified biopsy, of breast, 427
Cancer
  cervical, 217
  ovarian, 218
  treatment of, image-guided ablation
    techniques for, 201–207
    cryoablation in, 203–204
    irreversible electroporation in,
      204–205
    microwave ablation in, 202–203
    radiofrequency ablation in,
      201–202
    tips in, 206–207
    types of, 201–206
  see also Tumours
Capacity, 445–446
  acting for person lacking in, 448–449
  assessment of, 446–447
  documenting assessment of, 449
Capsular injuries, in arthrography, 331
Carcinoma, uterine, 218
Cardiac computed tomography, 244–251
  beta-blockers in, 246–247
  contraindications to, 245–246
  indications for, 244–245
  nitrates in, 247
  patient preparation for, 246
  scan protocol for, 247
  technique for, 247
Cardiac imaging see Heart
Cardiac magnetic resonance imaging,
  251–254
  contraindications to, 252
  indications for, 251–254
  patient preparation for, 252
  technique for, 252–254
Cardiovascular emergencies, 465
Cardiovascular toxicity, of intravascular
  contrast media, 25
Catheter-directed arterial thrombolysis,
  280–282
Catheter techniques
  complications of, 272–275
    air embolus, 274
    arterial thrombus, 273
    arteriovenous fistula, 274
    artery dissection, 274
    atheroembolism, 274
    cotton fibre embolus, 274
    distant, 274–275
    haemorrhage/haematoma, 273
    peripheral embolus, 274
    pseudoaneurysm, 273–274
    from technique, 273
  Seldinger, 233
Catheters
  Amplatz coronary artery, 242, 242f
  Berenstein, 386f
  Cournand, 240, 240f

Catheters (Continued)
  impaction of, 275
  JB2, 386f
  Judkins coronary artery, 242, 242f
  knotting, 274
  Mani, 386f
  National Institutes of Health (NIH),
    240, 240f
  pigtail, 240, 240f
  Simmons, 386f
  Tiger II coronary artery, 242–243,
    243f
  transhepatic portal venous, 299–300
  for vascular access, 266–267
  vertebrale, 386f
CCK see Cholecystokinin
Central venography
  inferior vena cavography of,
    296–297
  superior vena cavography of, 296
Cerebral angiography, 385
  aftercare for, 388
  contraindications for, 385
  contrast medium in, 387
  equipment for, 385
  films for, 388
  indications for, 385
  preparation for, 385
  projections in, 387–388
  technique in, 385–387, 386f
Cerebral blood flow imaging, regional,
  380–382
  aftercare for, 382
  analysis for, 382
  complications of, 382
  contraindications for, 381
  equipment for, 381
  images for, 381–382
  indications for, 380
  patient preparation for, 381
  radiopharmaceuticals for, 381
  technique for, 381
Cerebrospinal fluid drain, in thoracic
  stent grafts, 285
Cervical cancer, 217
Cervical myelography, 360–362
  aftercare for, 362
  contrast medium for, 360
  equipment for, 360
  indications for, 360
  lateral cervical C1/2 puncture versus
    lumbar injection in, 360
  by lumbar injection, 365
  patient preparation for, 360
  radiographic views of, 361–362
  technique of, 361
Cervical spine, nerve root blocks for,
  370
Chemical shift imaging, of adrenals,
  186

Children
  barium meal in, 52
  consent of, 5
  hip arthrography for, 335–336
  hip ultrasound for, 346–347
  myelography for, 366
  radionuclide imaging for, 8
  sedation of, 43–45
  ultrasonography for, 20
Chloral hydrate, 44
Cholangiography
  intraoperative, 158
  magnetic resonance, 155
  percutaneous transhepatic, 161
  postoperative (T-tube), 159–160
Cholangiopancreatography
  endoscopic retrograde, 156–163
    in obstructive jaundice, 173
  magnetic resonance, 155
    in non-obstructive jaundice, 173
Cholecystectomy, after ultrasound,
    148
Cholecystokinin (CCK), provocation
    of, 169
Cholesterol embolization, 278
Chronic obstructive pulmonary disease,
    sedation causing, 456
Cleansing bowel preparation, 6
Coaxial needle puncture systems,
    193
Coeliac axis, 167–171
Coeliac axis arteriography, 167
Colonography, computed tomography,
    13, 127–129
  aftercare for, 129
  bowel preparation for, 128
  complications of, 129
  indications of, 127–128
  technique for, 128–129
Colostomy enema, 117
Colour Doppler examination, of venous
    system, 290
Colour Doppler, of arterial system,
    263–264
Common bile duct, ultrasound of,
    146
Common femoral artery, for vascular
    access, 266
Common iliac aneurysm, in abdominal
    stent grafts, 286
Communication, in interventional
    radiology team, 434
Complement activation, 29
Computed tomographic angiography,
    264
  peripheral (lower limb), 264–265
Computed tomographic KUB (CT
    KUB), 182
Computed tomography arthrography,
    332–333

Computed tomography colonography,
    127–129
  aftercare for, 129
  bowel preparation for, 128
  complications of, 129
  indications of, 129–130
  technique for, 130–131
Computed tomography (CT), 11–19
  for acoustic neuromas, 380
  of biliary tree, 149–151
  for bones and joints, 327
  for brain, 374–375
  cardiac, 244–251
    beta-blockers in, 246
    contraindications to, 245–246
    indications for, 244–245
    nitrates in, 247
    patient preparation for, 246
    scan protocol for, 247
    technique for, 247
  colonography, 13
  contrast-enhanced
    multiphasic, 150
    single-phase (portal phase), 150
  in diagnosis of pulmonary emboli,
    231–232
  of gastrointestinal tract, 124–132
    indications of, 124–126
    intraluminal contrast agents,
      125–126
    intravenous contrast, 126–127
    see also Gastrointestinal tract,
      computed tomography of
  for gliomas, 378
  for intracranial haemorrhage,
    377–378
  intravenous contrast medium for,
    11–12
  of liver, 149–151
  in liver tumours, 172
  lung biopsy guided by, 223–227
  of lymph nodes, 320–321
  for obstructive jaundice, 173
  oral contrast medium for, 12–13, 13t
  of pancreas, 151–152
  in pancreatic pseudocysts, 174
  in pancreatitis, 173
  for parathyroid, 402
  patient preparation for, 11
  pelvic scanning in, 13
  of reproductive system, 209
  of salivary glands, 392
    contrast enhanced, 399
  for spine, 356–359
  of thorax, 221–223
  for thyroid, 402
  of urinary tract, 181–182
    adrenal lesion characterization,
      182
    angiography, 183–184

Computed tomography (CT)
(*Continued*)
kidneys, ureters, bladder (KUB),
182
renal lesion characterization,
182–183
standard diagnostic, 181
urogram, 183
of venous system, 291–292
Computed tomography
dacryocystography, for lacrimal
system, 389–391
Computed tomography myelography,
365
Computed tomography pulmonary
angiography (CTPA), 231
multidetector, for pulmonary
embolism, 227
Computed tomography urogram, 183
Computer-aided detection (CAD)
software, mammography, 415
Conduitogram, 190
Connectors, for vascular access, 268
Conray, 22*t*–23*t*
Conscious sedation, 451
Consent, 5–6
of children, 5
express, 5
implied, 5
as legal requirement, 442
patient, 441–450
acting for person lacking in
capacity, 448–449
capacity of, 445
documenting assessment of
capacity by, 449
information for, 444–445
shared decision-making of, 449
supporting patients to make
decisions in, 447–448
standardized preprinted forms, 449
written, 5
Contrast agents
ferromagnetic, 33
intraluminal, 125–126
CT enteroclysis, 126
faecal tagging, 126
full-fat milk, 125
negative oral contrast, 125
osmotic negative contrast agents,
125–126
positive oral contrast, 125
for magnetic resonance imaging, of
gastrointestinal tract, 132
microbubble, 38
paramagnetic, 33*f*, 33
superparamagnetic, 33, 33*f*
in ultrasonography, 38–39
Contrast enema, in neonatal low
intestinal obstruction, 56–57

Contrast-enhanced cardiac scan,
248–251
Contrast-enhanced magnetic resonance
liver imaging, 154
Contrast-enhanced ultrasound, of liver,
145
Contrast-induced nephropathy (CIN),
26
Contrast media, 5–6
in angiocardiography, 239, 240*t*
barium as, 99–100, 99*t*
in Burhenne technique, 165
cervical myelography, 360
in coeliac axis, superior mesenteric,
inferior mesenteric arteriography,
167
complications due to, 7
in endoscopic retrograde
cholangiopancreatography, 156
equipment for, 5
ferromagnetic, 33
gases as, 98
in gastrointestinal tract, 97–98
barium, 99–100, 99*t*
gases, 98
glucagon as, 101–102
hyoscine-N-butylbromide
(Buscopan) as, 100–101
metoclopramide (Maxolon) as, 102
pharmacological agents, 100–102
water-soluble contrast agents,
97–98
in heart imaging, 239
for inferior vena cavography, 296
in internal biliary drainage, 164
intraluminal, 125–126
CT enteroclysis, 126
faecal tagging, 126
full-fat milk, 125
negative oral contrast, 125
osmotic negative contrast agents,
125–126
positive oral contrast, 125
in intraoperative cholangiography,
158
intravascular, 21–39
adverse effects of, 25–32
high osmolar contrast media, 21,
24
historical development of, 21–24,
22*t*–23*t*, 24*f*
ionic compounds and, 21
iso-osmolar contrast media, 24
low osmolar contrast media, 21–24
in magnetic resonance imaging,
32–39
non-ionic dimers and, 24
in pregnancy and lactation, 31
of soft-tissue toxicity, 25
see also Intravascular contrast media

Contrast media (*Continued*)
intravenous, for computed tomography, 11
liver-specific, 154–155
in lumbar myelography, 362
microbubble as, 38
for myelography, 359
oral, for computed tomography, 12, 13t
paramagnetic, 33f, 33
patient preparation for, 5–6
in percutaneous transhepatic cholangiography, 161
for peripheral venography, 294–295
for portal venography, 297
in postoperative (t-tube) cholangiography, 160
risk due to, 4
for superior vena cavography, 296
superparamagnetic, 33, 33f
for transhepatic portal venous catheterization, 300
in ultrasonography, 38–39
volumes of, 5
water-soluble agents, 12, 97–98
Contrast swallow, 50–51
Conventional radiography, 357
Conventional radionuclide brain scanning, 355
Conventional subtraction sialography, for salivary glands, 392–395
Conventional tomography arthrography, 332
Coronary arteriography, 241–244
complications of, 244
contrast medium in, 242
equipment for, 242, 242f–243f
image acquisition in, 243–244
indications for, 241–242
patient preparation for, 243
technique for, 243
Coronary artery disease
2-[18F]fluoro-2-deoxy-D-glucose (18F-FDG) positron emission tomography for, 311
sedation causing, 45–46
Cournand catheter, 240, 240f
Covered stents, 279
Cragg-McNamara catheter, 281
Cryoablation, 203–204
CT *see* Computed tomography
CT-SPECT scanners, 320
CT venography (CTV), 375
Cutting balloon angioplasty (CBA), 277
Cutting needle biopsy needles, for lung biopsy, 224
Cystography, direct radionuclide micturating, 198–199

Cystourethrography, micturating, 198–199
aftercare for, 199
complications of, 199
contraindications for, 198
equipment of, 198
indications for, 198
technique of, 198

D

Dacryocystography, digital subtraction and computed tomography, for lacrimal system, 389–391
Decision-making, shared, 449
Deep sedation, 451
Deep venous thrombosis, MDCT for, 292
Deterministic effects, of radiation risk, 1
Developmental dysplasia of the hip, 346
Diatrizoate, 22t–23t
Diffusion-weighted imaging (DWI), 154
in magnetic resonance imaging, of brain, 377
Digital subtraction dacryocystography, for lacrimal system, 389–391
Digital subtraction sialography, for salivary glands, 393–395
Diodone, 22t–23t
Direct lower limb CT venography, 292
Direct patient care, interventional radiology and, 437
Direct radionuclide micturating cystography, 198–199
Discharge criteria, after sedation, 459
Discitis, 369
Distension therapy, in adhesive capsulitis, 332
Dobutamine, in radionuclide myocardial perfusion imaging, 259
Dobutamine stress imaging, 253
Documentation, nurses role in imaging procedures, 437
Dopamine transporter ligands, 384
Doppler examination, color, of venous system, 290
Doppler ultrasound, for pulmonary embolism, 228
Dose, minimizing of, in radiation, 434–435
Dosimeter badges, 435
Drug coated balloons (DCB), for angioplasty, 276
Drug safety, nurses role in, 439
Drugs, 453
addict, sedation causing, 456
analgesic, 453
local anaesthetic, 453, 454t
sedative, 455–457
Duplex scanning, of venous system, 290

Dynamic method, 347
Dynamic renal radionuclide
  scintigraphy, 196–198
  aftercare for, 198
  analysis of, 197
  complications of, 198
  contraindications for, 196–198
  equipment of, 196
  images of, 197
  indications for, 196
  patient preparation for, 196
  radiopharmaceuticals of, 196
  technique of, 196–198
Dysmotility, 104

E

Echocardiography, for pulmonary
  embolism, 228
Echoplanar imaging, magnetic
  resonance imaging, of brain, 376
Elastography, 417
Elbow, arthrography for, 341–342,
  342f
Elderly patients, at high risk, of
  sedation, 456
Electrocardiograph, 457
Embolism, pulmonary, as venous
  interventions, 227–228
Embolization
  cholesterol, 278
  gonadal vein, 301–302
  vascular, 282–284
Embolus
  peripheral, as catheter complication,
    274
  pulmonary, MDCT for, 292
Emergencies, medical, 461–468
  adverse drug reactions in, 466–467
  aspiration in, 464
  bradycardia as, 466
  bronchospasm as, 463–464
  cardiovascular, 465
  contrast media reaction as, 466–467
  equipment in, 461–463
  hypotension as, 465
  laryngospasm as, 463
  local anaesthetic toxicity as, 468
  pneumothorax in, 464
  respiratory, 463
  respiratory depression in, 463
  tachycardia as, 465–466
Emergency procedures, interventional
  radiology and, 434
Endoleaks, from aortic stent grafts,
  286
Endoluminal examination
  of anus, 122–123
  of oesophagus and stomach, 121
  of rectum, 123

Endoscopic retrograde
  cholangiopancreatography (ERCP),
    156–163
  in obstructive jaundice, 173
Enema
  barium, 112–115
  colostomy, 117–118
Enema variants, 116–119
  air enema, 117
  'instant' enema, 116
Enteroclysis
  CT, 126
  small bowel magnetic resonance, 134
Enterography, small bowel magnetic
  resonance, 134
Environment, maintaining safe, nurses
  role in, 438–439
Equipment
  nurses role, in imaging procedures,
    437–438
  radiographers and, 435–436
ERCP see Endoscopic retrograde
  cholangiopancreatography
Evacuating proctogram, 119–120
Excretion urography, intravenous,
    176–178
  contraindications for, 176
  contrast medium of, 176
  images of, 177–178
  indications for, 176
  patient preparation for, 177
  preliminary images of, 177
  technique of, 177
  variation in, 178
Express consent, 5
External biliary drainage, 164–167
Extrahepatic bile ducts, ultrasound of,
    147–148

F

^{18}F-choline, 312
^{18}F-fluoride, 315
Facet joint arthrography, for spine,
    355
Faecal tagging, 126
Failed back surgery syndrome, 358
Fatal reactions, to intravascular contrast
  media, 28–29
Fédération Internationale de
  Gynécologie et d'Obstétrique
  (FIGO), 217
Female reproductive system
  gynaecological malignancy in, 217
  hysterosalpingography for, 209
  methods of imaging in, 209
Femoral artery, puncture, 167, 269, 273
Fentanyl, 453–454, 454t
Ferromagnetic contrast agents, 33
Ferromagnetic materials, effects of, in
  magnetic resonance imaging, 15

Fetus, radiation effects on, 2–3
FFDM *see* Full-field digital mammography
FIGO *see* Fédération Internationale de Gynécologie et d'Obstétrique
Films, plain, for bones and joints, 327
Filters, inferior vena cava, 302–304
FLAIR sequences (fluid attenuated inversion recovery), in magnetic resonance imaging, of brain, 376
Flumazenil, 455
Fluorine-18 fluorodeoxyglucose (^{18}FDG), 382
2-[^{18}F] fluoro-2-deoxy-d-glucose (^{18}F-FDG), 311
2-[^{18}F]fluoro-2-deoxy-D-glucose (^{18}F-FDG) positron emission tomography, 312–315
Fluoroscopic images, monitoring of, interventional radiology and, 434–435
Fluoroscopy, in intussusception reduction, 54
Frame rate, interventional radiology and, 434–435
Full-fat milk, 125
Full-field digital mammography (FFDM), 414

G
18-gauge sheathed needle, 193
^{67}Ga-gallium citrate, 327
  technique in, 326
Gadolinium-enhanced T1-weighted magnetic resonance imaging, 154
Gadolinium, in MRI, 34–38, 292–293
  adverse reactions of, 35–37, 35*t*
  blood pool agents, 34
  cardiac, 253
  dose of, 34–37
  extracellular fluid (ECF) agents, 34
  liver agents, 34
  in pregnancy and lactation, 37
Galactose monosaccharide microparticles (Echovist), 213
Gallbladder
  function of, assessment of, 168
  ultrasound of, 146
^{68}Gallium-labelled pharmaceuticals, 315
^{67}Gallium radionuclide tumour imaging, 316
Gamma cameras, 9
Gases, as contrast media, 98
Gastric emptying study, radionuclide, 137–140
Gastro-oesophageal reflux study, radionuclide, 136–137
Gastrografin, 97–98

Gastrointestinal bleeding, radionuclide imaging of, 141–142
Gastrointestinal tract, 97–142
  barium enema, 112–115
  barium meal, 104–112, 107*f*
  coeliac axis, 167–171
  colostomy enema, 117–118
  computed tomography of, 124–132
    colonography, 127–129
    indications of, 124–126
    intraluminal contrast agents, 125–126
    intravenous contrast, 126
  contrast enema, in neonatal low intestinal obstruction, 56–57
  contrast media in, 97–98
    barium, 99–100, 99*t*
    gases, 98
    pharmacological agents, 100–102
    water-soluble contrast agents, 97–98
  contrast swallow, 103–104
  enema variants, 116–120
  evacuating proctogram, 119–120
  herniogram, 118–119
  intussusception reduction, 54–55
  loopogram, 118
  magnetic resonance imaging of, 132–136
    anorectal cancer, local staging of, 134
    contraindications of, 132
    contrast agents, 132
    indications of, 132
    motion artefacts in, 132
    perianal fistula, suspected, 133
    pulse sequences in, 133
    small bowel magnetic resonance enteroclysis, 134
    small bowel magnetic resonance enterography, 134
    techniques for, 133–134
  methods of imaging of, 97–103
  radionuclide
    gastric emptying study, 137–140
    gastro-oesophageal reflux study, 136–137
    imaging of gastrointestinal bleeding, 141–142
    Meckel's diverticulum scan, 140–141
  retrograde ileogram, 117
  sinogram, 117
  small bowel enema, 110–112
  small bowel follow-through, 108–110
  superior mesenteric and inferior mesenteric arteriography, 167–171
  ultrasound of, 121–124
    appendix, 122
    endoluminal examination of anus, 123

Gastrointestinal tract (*Continued*)
　endoluminal examination of
　　oesophagus and stomach, 121
　endoluminal examination of
　　rectum, 123–124
　hypertrophic pyloric stenosis, 61
　large bowel, 123
　small bowel, 121–122
　transabdominal examination
　　of oesophagus and stomach,
　　121–123
Gastromiro, 98
Gated blood-pool study, 254
General anaesthesia, 451
　complications due to, 7
General Medical Council (GMC), 441
　information recommended by, 442
　legislation together with, 446
68Germanium, 315
Gliomas, 378
　computed tomography for, 378–379
　magnetic resonance imaging for, 379
Glucagon, 101–102
Glyceryl trinitrate, 247
GMC *see* General Medical Council
Gonad protection, 7
Gonadal vein embolization, as venous
　interventions, 301–302
Gradient-echo T2-weighted sequences, in
　magnetic resonance, of brain, 376
Gradient field, effects of, in magnetic
　resonance imaging, 15–16
Grafts, stent, thoracic and abdominal,
　284–287
Grey-scale US, of arterial system, 263
Guidewires
　for angioplasty, 276
　breakage, 275
　for vascular access, 267–268, 268*f*
Gynaecological malignancy, 217
　cervical cancer, 217
　ovarian cancer, 218–219
　uterine carcinoma, 218

H

Haemangiomas, 172
Haemoptysis, lung biopsy and, 226
Haemorrhage/haematoma, as catheter
　complication, 273
Heart, 239–262
　angiocardiography of, 239–241, 240*f*,
　　240*t*
　computed tomography of, 244–251
　contrast-enhanced scan of, 248–251
　coronary arteriography of, 241–244,
　　242*f*–243*f*
　magnetic resonance imaging of,
　　251–254
　radionuclide ventriculography of,
　　254–257

Hepatic artery, ultrasound of, 145
Hepatic dysfunction, sedation causing, 456
Hepatic veins, ultrasound of, 145
Hepatobiliary agents, 154
Hepatobiliary system
　methods of imaging in, 143–146
　radionuclide imaging in, 168–171
Herniogram, 118–119
Hexabrix, 21, 23–24, 23*t*
High osmolar contrast media (HOCM),
　21, 24, 159
High-pressure balloons, for angioplasty,
　276
High-resolution scan, in computed
　tomography of thorax, 221–223
Hip
　arthrography for, 335–336,
　　336*f*–337*f*, 341*f*
　joint effusion of, 347
　ultrasound, paediatric, 346–347
Histamine release, 29
HMPAO, 325
HOCM *see* High osmolar contrast media
Hybrid systems, 9
Hyoscine-N-butylbromide, 100–103
Hypaque, 22*t*
Hypertrophic pyloric stenosis, 61
Hypotension, 465
Hysterosalpingography, 209–212
　aftercare for, 211
　complications of, 211–212
　contraindications of, 210
　contrast medium of, 210
　equipment of, 210
　images of, 211
　indications of, 209
　patient preparation of, 210
　technique of, 210–211

I

131I-labelled MIBG, 317
123I-orthoiodohippurate (Hippuran),
　196
123I-sodium iodide, 403
Idiosyncratic reactions, to intravascular
　contrast media, 27–29, 28*t*
Ileogram, retrograde, 117
Image guided ablation techniques, for
　cancer treatment, 201–207
　cryoablation in, 203–204
　irreversible electroporation in, 204–206
　microwave ablation in, 202–203
　radiofrequency ablation in, 201–202
　tips in, 206–207
　types of, 201–206
Image-guided breast biopsy, 421–428
　equipment of, 424–425
　indications of, 421
　patient preparation of, 425–426
　technique for, 427–428

Imaging, radionuclide, 8–10
  activity administered, 9
  aftercare for, 10
  for bones and joints, 327
  for brain, 373–374, 380–385
  of breast, 420–421
  complications with, 10
  equipment for, 9
  of gallbladder, 168–171
  of gastrointestinal bleeding, 141–142
  hepatobiliary, 143
  images in, 10
  in infection, 311–326
  of inflammation, 324–326
  of liver, 168–170
  myocardial perfusion, 257–262
  in oncology, 311–326
  for parathyroid, 405–407
  patient positioning in, 10
  radiation safety for, 10
  radioactive injections for, 8–9
  radiopharmaceuticals in, 8–10
  for spine, 355
  of spleen, 170–171
  technique of, 10
  for thyroid, 403–405
  ventriculography, 254–257
Implants, magnetic resonance imaging
      and, 17
Implied consent, 5
[111]In-human immunoglobulin (HIG),
      325
[111]In-labelled leucocytes, 325
[111]In-labelled white cells, technique
      in, 326
[111]In-octreotide, 318
[111]In-oxine, 324
Indirect CT venography, for deep vein
      thrombosis, 292
Inert gas quench, in magnetic
      resonance imaging, 17
Infection, radionuclide imaging in,
      311–326
Inferior mesenteric arteriography,
      121–125, 167
Inferior vena cava filters, as venous
      interventions, 302–304
Inferior vena cavography, 296–297
Infertility, 209
Inflammation, radionuclide imaging of,
      324–326
Inflammatory bowel disease, labelled
      white cell scanning in, 142
Inhalational analgesia, 453
'Instant' enema, 116
Internal biliary drainage, 164–165
Interventional radiology
  nurse role of, 437–439
  radiographer role in, 433–436
  Royal College of Nursing, 437

Intervertebral disc, prolapsed, 358
Intestinal obstruction
  contrast enema in neonatal low,
      56–57
  upper, newborn infants with, 56
Intraarticular chemical therapy, 332
Intraarticular structural abnormalities,
      in arthrography, 331
Intracranial haemorrhage, 377–378
  computed tomography for, 377–378
  magnetic resonance imaging for, 377
Intrahepatic bile ducts, ultrasound of,
      147
Intraluminal contrast agents, 125–126
  CT enteroclysis, 126
  faecal tagging, 126
  full-fat milk, 125
  negative oral contrast, 125
  osmotic negative contrast agents,
      125–126
  positive oral contrast, 125
Intraoperative cholangiography, 158
Intraoperative sentinel node
      identification, 420
Intravascular contrast media, 21–39
  adverse effects of, 25–31
    cardiovascular toxicity, 25
    fatal reactions, 28
    idiosyncratic reactions, 27–28, 28t
    mechanisms of idiosyncratic
      contrast medium reactions, 29
    nephrotoxicity, 26, 27t
    non-fatal reactions, 28–29
    prophylaxis of, 29–31, 31t
    soft tissue toxicity, 25
    thyroid function, 26
    vascular toxicity, 25
  high-osmolar contrast media, 21, 24
  historical development of, 21–24,
      22t–23t, 24f
  ionic compounds and, 21
  iso-osmolar, 24
  low-osmolar contrast media, 21–24
    in magnetic resonance imaging,
      32–38
    see also Magnetic resonance imaging,
      intravascular contrast media in
  non-ionic dimers and, 24
  in pregnancy and lactation, 31
  of soft tissue toxicity, 25
Intravenous analgesia, 453–455
Intravenous contrast, for computed
      tomography of gastrointestinal
      tract, 126
Intravenous excretion urography (IVU),
      176–178
  contraindications for, 176
  contrast medium of, 176
  images of, 177–178
  indications for, 176

Intravenous excretion urography (IVU)
(*Continued*)
  patient preparation for, 177
  preliminary images of, 177
  technique of, 177
  variation in, 178
Intussusception, reduction of, 54–55
Iodine, 21
^{123}Iodine(I)-MIBG, 317
Iodixanol, 22*t*–23*t*, 24
Iohexol, 21–24, 22*t*–23*t*
Iomeprol, 21–24, 22*t*–23*t*
Iomeron, 21–24, 22*t*–23*t*
Ionic contrast media, conventional, 21
Ionising Radiation (Medical Exposure)
  Regulations 2000, 9
Iopamidol, 21–24, 22*t*–23*t*
Iopamiron, 21–24
Iopromide, 21–24, 22*t*–23*t*
Iothalamate, 22*t*–23*t*
Iotrolan, 22*t*–23*t*, 24
Ioversol, 21–24, 22*t*–23*t*
Ioxaglate, 21–24, 22*t*–23*t*
Iron oxide, in magnetic resonance
  imaging contrast agents, 33
  negative agents, 132
  positive agents, 132
  in pregnancy and lactation, 37
Irreversible electroporation, 204–205
Iso-osmolar contrast media, 24
Isopaque, 22*t*
Isovist, 23*t*, 24
Isovue, 21–24, 23*t*

J

Jaundice, investigation of, 172–173
JB2 catheter, 386
Joints, 327–353
  arthrography for, 331–334
    general points in, 330–334
    site-specific issues in, 334–346
  computed tomography for, 328
  imaging modalities for, 327–328
  musculoskeletal magnetic resonance
    imaging for, 329–330
  plain films for, 327
  radionuclide bone scan, 350–353
  tendon imaging for, 346–347
  thermoablation of musculoskeletal
    tumours for, 347–350
  ultrasound for, 346–347
  see also Bones and joints
Joule Thomson effect, in cryoablation,
  203–204
Judkins coronary artery catheters, 242
Justification, of proposed examination, 2

K

Kellett needle, 193
Kidneys, computed tomography, 182

Knee arthrography, 354–355
^{81m}Kr (krypton) gas, 229

L

Lacrimal system, 389, 391
  digital subtraction and computed
    tomography dacryocystography
    for, 389–390
  imaging methods of, 389–390
  magnetic resonance imaging for, 391
Lactation
  intravascular contrast media in, 30
  iodinated contrast in, 31
  magnetic resonance imaging contrast
    agents in, 37
Large bowel, ultrasound of, 123
Laryngospasm, 463
Lasting Power of Attorney (LPA), 448
Lecithin, 315
Left bundle branch block, pulmonary
  arteriography and, 232
Legal advice, 449
Legal regulations, for radiation risk, 2
Leucocyte imaging, radionuclide-
  labelled, 324
Leukoscan, 325
Levovist, 38
'Liberating the NHS, 449
Lidocaine, 453–454
Ligamentous injuries, in arthrography,
  331
Liver, 143–174
  computed tomography of, 149–151,
    172
  magnetic resonance imaging of,
    152–156, 172
  radionuclide imaging of, 168–171
  tumours, investigation of, 171–172
  ultrasound of, 144–146, 172
    contrast-enhanced, 145
Liver-specific contrast agents, 154–155
Local anaesthesia
  complications due to, 7
  drugs for, 453–454
  toxicity of, 468
Local structures, damage to, as catheter
  complication, 273
LOCM *see* Low osmolar iodinated
  contrast material
Long TR sequences, in magnetic
  resonance imaging, of brain, 375
Loopogram, 118
Loose body, in arthrography, 331
Low osmolar iodinated contrast
  material (LOCM), 210
Lower limb
  computed tomographic angiography
    of, 264–265
  peripheral venography of, 293–295
  venous ultrasound, 290–291

Lower limb CT venography, direct, 292
LPA *see* Lasting Power of Attorney
Lumbar myelography, 362–364
   contraindications to, 362
   contrast medium for, 362
   equipment for, 362
   indications of, 362
   patient preparation for, 362
   preliminary images of, 362
   radiographic views of, 364
   technique of, 363–364
Lumbar spine, nerve root blocks for, 370
Lung biopsy, computed tomography-
      guided, 223–227
   aftercare for, 226
   patient preparation for, 225
Lymph glands/nodes
   computed tomography of, 321
   ^{18}F-choline, 315
   2-[^{18}F]fluoro-2-deoxy-D-glucose
      (^{18}F-FDG) positron emission
      tomography, 313–314
   ^{68}gallium-labelled pharmaceuticals,
      315–316
   ^{67}gallium radionuclide tumour
      imaging of, 316
   imaging of, 320–324
   intraoperative sentinel node
      identification of, 420
   magnetic resonance imaging of, 321
   radiographic lymphangiography
      of, 321
   radiography of, 320
   radioiodine
      metaiodobenzylguanidine scan
      of, 316
   radionuclide lymphoscintigraphy of,
      321–324
   somatostatin receptor imaging of,
      319
   ultrasound of, 320–321
Lymphangiography
   magnetic resonance, 323–324
   radiographic, 321
Lymphatic channel
   computed tomography of, 321
   imaging of, 320–324
   magnetic resonance imaging of, 321
   radiographic lymphangiography of,
      321
   radiography of, 320
   radionuclide lymphoscintigraphy of,
      321–324
   ultrasound of, 320–321
Lymphoscintigraphy, radionuclide,
      321–324

M
Magnetic fields, effects of, to magnetic
   resonance imaging, 14–17

Magnetic resonance angiography
   of arterial system, 265–266
   of heart, 254
   of liver, 154
   for pulmonary embolism, 228
   renal, 187–189
Magnetic resonance arthrography, 333
   for bones and joints, 329–330
Magnetic resonance
      cholangiopancreatography
      (MRCP), 155
   in non-obstructive jaundice, 173
Magnetic resonance enteroclysis, small
      bowel, 134
Magnetic resonance imaging (MRI), 14
   for acoustic neuromas, 380
   of adrenals, 186–187
   biological effects of, 14–15
   of bones and joints, 328
   of brain, 373, 375–377
   of breast, 418–419
   cardiac, 251–254
      contraindications to, 252
      indications for, 251–252
      patient preparation for, 252
      technique for, 252–253
   cardiac pacemaker in, effects of, 15
   for cervical cancer, 217–218
   contrast-enhanced, for salivary
      glands, 399
   contrast media in
      gadolinium, 34–37, 292–293
      of gastrointestinal tract, 132–136
      historical development, 32
      mechanism of action, 32–34
      in pregnancy, 37
   controlled access to, 17
   diffusion-weighted imaging in, 154
   electrical devices in, effects of, 15
   ferromagnetic materials in, effects
      of, 15
   gadolinium-enhanced T1-weighted,
      154
   of gastrointestinal tract, 132–136
      anorectal cancer, local staging of,
         134
      contraindications of, 132
      contrast agents, 132
      indications of, 132
      motion artefacts in, 132
      perianal fistula, suspected, 133
      pulse sequences in, 133
      small bowel magnetic resonance
         enteroclysis, 134
      small bowel magnetic resonance
         enterography, 134
      techniques for, 133–135
      see also Gastrointestinal tract;
         magnetic resonance imaging
   for gliomas, 378–379

Magnetic resonance imaging (MRI)
(*Continued*)
gradient field in, effects of, 15–16
implants and, 17
for intracranial haemorrhage,
377–378
intravascular contrast media in,
32–38
gadolinium, 34–37
gastrointestinal, 32
historical development of, 32
mechanism of action, 32–33
in pregnancy, 37
for lacrimal system, 391
of liver, 152–155
liver-specific contrast agents in,
154–155
in liver tumours, 171–172
of lymph nodes, 321
missile effect of, 17
non-biological effects of, 15
for obstructive jaundice, 173
for ovarian cancer, 218–219
of pancreas, 156
of parathyroid, 402
patient preparation for, 14
pregnancy and, 17–18
of prostate, 184–185
for pulmonary embolism, 233–234
pulse sequences in, 152–153
radiofrequency field in, effects of, 16
of reproductive system, 215–219
of respiratory system, 236–237
restricted access to, 17
safety in, 14–19
inert gas quench in, 17
magnetic fields to, effects of,
14–16
noise in, 16–17
recommendations for, 17–18
for salivary glands, 392
for scrotum, 216–217
sedation and monitoring for,
458–459
of sialography, 398
for spine, 356–359
static field in, effects of, 14
for thyroid, 402
of urinary tract, 184–185
for uterine carcinoma, 218
of venous system, 292–293
Magnetic resonance liver imaging,
contrast-enhanced, 154–155
Magnetic resonance
lymphangiography, 323
Magnetic resonance (MR)
cholangiography, 143
Magnetic resonance renal angiography,
187–190
Magnetic resonance urography, 185

Magnetization-prepared rapid-
acquisition gradient echo
(MPRAGE), 379–380
Magnetization-prepared T1-weighted
GRE, 153
Malabsorption, 112
Male, ascending urethrography in,
187–188
Male reproductive system
methods of imaging in, 209
scrotum ultrasonography, 209
Malignancy *see* Tumours
Mammography, 414–416
contrast-enhanced digital, 415
equipment of, 414–415
indications of, 414
not indicated, 414–415
technique for, 415
Mani catheter, 386f
Maximum intensity projection (MIP),
376
Maxolon, 102
Meckel's diverticulum scan,
radionuclide, 140–141
Meconium ileus, 98
Medical emergencies, 461–468
adverse drug reactions in, 466–467
aspiration in, 464
bradycardia as, 466
bronchospasm as, 463–464
cardiovascular emergencies, 465
contrast media reaction as, 466–467
equipment in, 461–462
hypotension as, 465
laryngospasm as, 463
local anaesthetic toxicity as, 468
pneumothorax in, 464
respiratory depression in, 463
respiratory emergencies, 463
tachycardia as, 465–466
Medicines (Administration of
Radioactive Substances)
Regulations 1978 (MARS), 8
Megabecquerel (MBq), 9
Melanoma, injection technique for, 314
Mental Capacity Act 2005, 446
Mesenteric arteriography, superior
mesenteric and inferior, 167–171
Metaiodobenzylguanidine (MIBG) scan,
316
Metoclopramide, 102
Metoprolol, in cardiac computed
tomography, 246
Metrizoate, 22t–23t
Microbubble, as contrast agents, 38–39
Microwave ablation, 202–203
Micturating cystourethrography,
198–199
aftercare for, 198–199
complications of, 199

Micturating cystourethrography
(*Continued*)
  contraindications for, 198
  contrast medium of, 198
  equipment of, 198
  indications for, 198
  patient preparation for, 198
  preliminary image of, 199
  technique of, 198
Midazolam, 455
Midcarpal joint, arthrography for, 343
Monitoring, 457–459
  for magnetic resonance imaging, 458
  sedation and, 451–459
Morphine, 453–454, 454*t*
Morphine, provocation of, 169
Motion artefacts, in magnetic
    resonance imaging, of
    gastrointestinal tract, 132
MR (magnetic resonance) enteroclysis,
    134
MRCP *see* Magnetic resonance
    cholangiopancreatography
MRI *see* Magnetic resonance imaging
Multidetector CT cholangiography, 142
Multidetector CT (MDCT), 291–292
Multiparametric imaging, 184
Multiphasic contrast-enhanced
    computed tomography, 150–151
Multiplanar imaging, 292–293
Musculoskeletal magnetic resonance
    imaging, 329–330, 329*t*
Musculoskeletal tumours,
    thermoablation of, 347–350
  biopsy of, 349
  complications of, 350
  contraindications for, 349
  equipment for, 349
  indications for, 348
  introduction of, 347–350
  post-radiofrequency ablation care
    for, 350
  procedure for, 349
  rationale for, 348
  thermoablation of, 349
  thermocoagulation of, 348–349
Myelography
  cervical, 360–362
    aftercare for, 362
    contrast medium for, 360
    equipment for, 360
    indications of, 360
    lateral cervical C1/2 puncture *versus*
      lumbar injection in, 360–361
    by lumbar injection, 365
    patient preparation for, 360
    radiographic views of, 361
    technique of, 361–362
  computed tomography, 365
  lumbar, 362–365

Myelography (*Continued*)
    contraindications to, 362
    contrast medium for, 362
    equipment for, 362
    indications of, 362
    patient preparation for, 362
    preliminary images of, 362
    radiographic views of, 364
    technique of, 363–365
  paediatric, 366–367
  for spine, 355, 360–370
Myocardial perfusion
  magnetic resonance imaging, 251
  radionuclide imaging, 257–261

N
Naloxone, 454–455
Nasolacrimal drainage apparatus,
    methods of imaging for, 389–390
National Institutes of Health and
    Excellence (NICE), 374
National Institutes of Health (NIH)
    catheter, 240, 240*f*
Needle, for vascular access, 267
Negative oral contrast, 125–126
Neonatal low intestinal obstruction,
    contrast enema in, 56–67
Nephrogenic systemic fibrosis (NSF),
    35–36
Nephrolithotomy, percutaneous,
    193–196
  aftercare for, 195
  complications of, 194
  contraindications for, 194
  contrast medium of, 194
  equipment of, 194
  indications for, 194–196
  patient preparation for, 194
  technique of, 194–195
Nephrostomy, percutaneous antegrade,
    191–193
Nephrotoxicity, of intravascular
    contrast media, 26–27, 27*t*
Nerve root blocks
  cervical spine, 370
  lumbar spine, 370
  for spine, 370
Neurology, 2-[18F]fluoro-2-deoxy-
    D-glucose (18F-FDG) positron
    emission tomography for, 311
Newborn infants, with upper intestinal
    obstruction, 53
Niopam, 21–24, 22*t*–23*t*
Nitrates, in cardiac computed
    tomography, 244
Noise, in magnetic resonance imaging,
    16
Non-echoplanar imaging, in magnetic
    resonance imaging, of brain, 376

Non-thermal ablative technology, 201
  irreversible electroporation in,
    204–205
Non-image guided technique, of
  vascular access, 270–272
  computed tomographic angiography,
    264
    peripheral (lower limb), 264–265
  magnetic resonance angiography,
    265–266
  vascular ultrasound, 263–264
Non-invasive imaging, of arterial
  system, 263–266
Non-ionic contrast media, 21–24
Non-obstructive jaundice, investigation
  of, 173
Nurse, role of, in interventional
  radiology, 436–439
  assisting with imaging procedures, 438
  carrying out specific interventions, 439
  preparing patients, 437–438
  safe environment, maintaining, 438
  safely caring for patients, 438
  supporting patients, 438

O

Obstruction, intestinal
  low, contrast enema in neonatal,
    56–57
  upper, newborn infants with, 53
Obstructive jaundice, investigation of,
  173
Octreotide, 319
Oesophageal transit, 137
Oesophagus
  endoluminal examination of, 121
  pathology of, contrast swallow for, 103
  perforation of, 103
  transabdominal examination of, 121
  ultrasonography of, 19
Omental biopsy, 219
Omnipaque, 21–24, 22t–23t
Opioid drugs, 453–455, 454t
Optiray, 21–24, 22t–23t
Osmotic negative contrast agents, 125
Ovarian cancer, 218

P

Paediatric myelography, 366
Paediatrics see Children
Pain block, in arthrography, 332
Pancreas, 143–174
  computed tomography of, 151–152
  endoscopic retrograde
    cholangiopancreatography of
    contrast medium in, 157
    images in, 158
  magnetic resonance imaging of, 156
  methods of imaging, 143
  ultrasound of, 148–149

Pancreatic pseudocysts, investigation
  of, 173
Pancreatitis, investigation of, 173
Para-articular cyst, in arthrography,
  331–334
Paramagnetic contrast agents, 33, 33f
Parathyroids, 389–407
  computed tomography for, 402
  magnetic resonance imaging for, 402
  methods of imaging for, 399–3402
  radionuclide imaging of, 403–405
  ultrasound for, 400
Parotid gland, preliminary images
  of, for conventional and digital
  subtraction sialography, 393
Patient consent, 441–449
  acting for person lacking in capacity,
    448–449
  capacity of, 446
  documenting assessment of capacity
    by, 449
  information for, 444–445
  shared decision making of, 449
  supporting patients to make decisions
    in, 447–448
  voluntariness of, 441–442
  see also Consent
Patient immobilisation, during
  radionuclide imaging, 10
Patients
  in imaging procedures, 437–438
  preparation of
    for computed tomography-guided
      lung biopsy, 223
    for radionuclide lung ventilation/
      perfusion imaging, 228
Pelvic scanning, in computed
  tomography, 13
Pelvis, ultrasonography of, 19–20
Percutaneous antegrade pyelography
  and nephrostomy, 191–193
  aftercare for, 193
  complications of, 193
  contraindications for, 192
  contrast medium of, 192
  equipment of, 192
  indications for, 192
  patient preparation for, 192
  technique of, 192–193
Percutaneous extraction, of retained
  biliary calculi, 165–167
Percutaneous nephrolithotomy, 193–196
  aftercare for, 195
  complications of, 194
  contraindications for, 194
  contrast medium of, 194
  equipment of, 194
  indications for, 194
  patient preparation for, 194
  technique of, 194

Percutaneous omental biopsy, 219
Percutaneous renal cyst puncture and
    biopsy, 191
Percutaneous transhepatic
    cholangiography, 161
Percutaneous vertebral biopsy, 367–369
Perianal fistula, for magnetic resonance
    imaging, 133
Peripheral embolus, as catheter
    complication, 274
Peripheral (lower limb) computed
    tomographic angiography, 264–265
Peripheral MR venography (MRV), 292
Peripheral venography
  of lower limb, 293–295
    aftercare for, 294
    complications in, 294–295
    contraindications for, 293
    contrast medium for, 294
    equipment for, 294
    images in, 294
    indications for, 293
    method of, 293
    patient preparation in, 294
    technique for, 294
  of upper limb, 295
    aftercare for, 295
    complications in, 295
    contrast medium for, 295
    equipment for, 295
    indications for, 295
    method of, 295
    patient preparation in, 295
    technique for, 295
PET computerized tomography, of
    reproductive system, 217
PET-CT, 9
PET (positron emission tomography) see
    Positron emission tomography
Pethidine, 453–454, 454t
Phaeochromocytoma, 102
Pharmaceuticals, in radionuclide
    imaging
  myocardial perfusion, 257–258
  ventriculography, 254
Phosphatidylcholine, 315
Physicists, radiographers and, 435
Pigtail catheter, 240, 240f
Plain computed tomography, heart, 247
Plain film chest radiograph, for
    pulmonary embolism, 227
Plain film radiography, for urinary
    tract, 176
Plain films, 176
  for bones and joints, 327
  for salivary glands, 392
'Plain old balloon angioplasty' (POBA),
    276
Pneumatic reduction, of
    intussusception, 54–55

Pneumothorax, 464
  lung biopsy for, 225–1226
Point resolved spectroscopy (PRESS),
    379
Portal phase contrast-enhanced
    computed tomography, 150
Portal vein, ultrasound of, 144
Portal venography, 297–299
  aftercare for, 299
  complications in, 299
  contrast medium for, 297
  equipment for, 298
  images in, 299
  indications for, 297
  methods of, 297
  patient preparation in, 298
  technique for, 298–299
Portal venous catheterization,
    transhepatic, 299–300
Positive oral contrast, 125
Positron emission tomography (PET), 9,
    311–314
  acceptance of, 311
  for brain, 382–383
  for breast, 420
  [18F]-choline, 312
  [18F]-fluoride, 315
  2-[[18F]fluoro-2-deoxy-D-glucose
    ([18F]-FDG) positron emission
    tomography, 312–314
  [68]gallium-labelled pharmaceuticals,
    315
  [67]gallium radionuclide tumour
    imaging, 316
Positron emission tomography scanner
    (PET-CT), 9
Postcholecystectomy, 156
Postembolization syndrome, 283
Postoperative (t-tube) cholangiography,
    159–160
Power Doppler, of arterial system, 264
Pregnancy
  intravascular contrast media in, 30t
  iodinated contrast in, 31
  magnetic resonance imaging and, 18
  magnetic resonance imaging contrast
    agents in, 37
  radiation risk during, 3
Preliminary images, 6
Premedication, 6
Proctogram, evacuating, 119
Prostate, magnetic resonance imaging
    of, 184
Prostate-specific membrane antigen
    (PSMA), imaging of, [68]gallium-
    labelled pharmaceuticals, 315
Prosthesis assessment, in arthrography,
    332
Pseudoaneurysm, as catheter
    complication, 273

Pseudocysts, pancreatic, 174
Pulmonary arteriography, 232–233
  for pulmonary embolism, 227
Pulmonary embolism
  diagnosis of, computed tomography
    in, 231–232
  imaging methods for, 227–235
  magnetic resonance of, 232–233
  as venous interventions, 300–301
Pulmonary haemorrhage, local, lung
    biopsy for, 226
Pulse oximetry, 457
Pulse sequences, in magnetic resonance
    imaging, 152–153
  of gastrointestinal tract, 133
  of reproductive system, 209
Pulsed-wave Doppler, of arterial system,
    263
Pyelography, percutaneous antegrade,
    191–192
Pyeloureterography, retrograde,
    189–194
Pyloric stenosis, hypertrophic, 61

R
Radial artery, for vascular access, 266
Radiation
  ALARP dose of, 2
  deterministic effects of, 1–2
  hereditary effects of, 1
  justification of, 2
  legal regulations for, 2
  during pregnancy, 4
  risk due to, 1–4
  stochastic effects of, 2
Radiation protection supervisor (RPS),
    435
Radiation safety, for radionuclide
    imaging, 10
Radiocarpal joint, arthrography for,
    342–343
Radiofrequency ablation, 201–202
Radiofrequency field, effects of, in
    magnetic resonance imaging, 16
Radiographers
  outside angiographic suite, 436
  physicists and, 435
  PPE and, 435
  preprocedural role of, 433–434
  role of, in interventional radiology,
    433–436
  in theatre, 428–429
Radiographic lymphangiography, of
    lymph nodes, 321
Radiography
  conventional, 357
  of lymph nodes, 320
  plain film chest, for pulmonary
    embolism, 227–228
  plain film, for urinary tract, 176

Radioiodine metaiodobenzylguanidine,
    316–318
Radioisotope-guided occult lesion
    localization using Iodine-125, seeds
    ("ROLLIS"), 420
Radiology, 1–9
  aftercare for, 7
  complications of, 7–8
  contraindications to, 1–4
  images in, 7
  indications of, 1
  interventional
    nurse role of, 436–439
    radiographer role in, 433–436
    Royal College of Nursing, 437
  preliminary images in, 6
  risk due to contrast medium, 4–5
  risk due to radiation, 1–4
  technique of, 7
Radionuclide bone scan, 350–353
  additional techniques for, 353
  analysis for, 352
  competing modalities for, 353
  complications of, 353
  contraindications for, 351
  equipment for, 351
  images for, 352–353
  indications for, 350–352
  patient preparation for, 351
  radiopharmaceuticals in, 351
  technique in, 351
Radionuclide gastric emptying study,
    137–139
Radionuclide gastro-oesophageal reflux
    study, 136–138
Radionuclide imaging, 8–10
  activity administered, 9
  aftercare for, 10
  for bones and joints, 327
  for brain, 373–374, 380–384
  of breast, 414
  for children, 9
  complications with, 10
  equipment for, 9
  of gallbladder, 168–170
  of gastrointestinal bleeding, 141–142
  gastrointestinal tract see
    Gastrointestinal tract,
    radionuclide
  hepatobiliary, 168–170
  images in, 10
  in infection, 311–326
  of inflammation, 324–325
  of liver, 168–169
  myocardial perfusion, 257–261
    aftercare for, 261
    analysis in, 260
    complications of, 261
    contraindications to, 257
    equipment for, 258

Radionuclide imaging (*Continued*)
images in, 260
indications for, 257–261
patient preparation for, 258
radiopharmaceuticals for, 257–258
technique for, 258–260
in oncology, 311–326
for parathyroid, 405–407
patient positioning in, 10
radiation safety for, 10
radioactive injections for, 8
radiopharmaceuticals in, 8–10
for spine, 355
of spleen, 170–171
technique of, 10
for thyroid, 402–408
ventriculography, 254–256
aftercare for, 256
analysis for, 256
complications of, 256
contraindications to, 254
equipment for, 255
images in, 255
indications for, 254–256
patient preparation for, 255
radiopharmaceuticals for, 254
technique for, 255–256
Radionuclide-labelled leucocyte
imaging, 324
Radionuclide lung ventilation/
perfusion imaging, 228–230
radiopharmaceuticals for, 228
Radionuclide lymphoscintigraphy, of
lymph nodes, 321–324
Radionuclide Meckel's diverticulum
scan, 140–141
Radionuclide micturating cystography,
direct, 198–199
Radionuclide scintigraphy
dynamic renal, 196–198
Radiopharmaceuticals, 170
in radionuclide imaging
of gallbladder, 173
hepatobiliary, 168
of liver, 171
of spleen, 170
RE cell agents *see* Reticuloendothelial
(RE) cell agents
Recombinant tissue plasminogen
activator (rt-PA), 280
Recovery, from sedation, 455
Rectum, endoluminal examination of,
123
Regional cerebral blood flow imaging,
380–382
aftercare for, 382
analysis for, 382
complications of, 382
contraindications for, 381
equipment for, 381

Regional cerebral blood flow imaging
(*Continued*)
images for, 381
indications for, 380
patient preparation for, 381
radiopharmaceuticals for, 381
technique for, 381
Relative percentage washout (RPW),
181
Remifentanil, 455
Renal angiography, magnetic
resonance, 187–188
Renal artery stenosis, 196–198
Renal cyst puncture and biopsy,
percutaneous, 191
Renal failure, sedation causing, 456
Renal lesion characterization computed
tomography, 181
Renal vein thrombosis, 180
Reproductive system, 209–219
computerized tomography of, 215
female
gynaecological malignancy, 217
hysterosalpingography for, 209
methods of imaging in, 209
ultrasound of, 214–215
magnetic resonance imaging of,
215–217
male
methods of imaging in, 209
scrotum ultrasonography, 209
omental biopsy of, 219
uterine artery embolization in, 216
Respiratory depression, 463
Respiratory emergencies, 463
Respiratory system, 221–234
computed tomography-guided lung
biopsy of, 223–226
imaging of, methods for, 221
magnetic resonance imaging of,
236–237
pulmonary arteriography of,
232–233
pulmonary embolism and
diagnosis of, computed
tomography in, 231–232
magnetic resonance of, 233–234
methods of imaging of, 227–234
radionuclide lung ventilation/
perfusion imaging of, 228–230
thorax and, computed tomography
of, 221–223
Resuscitation, ABC of, 463
Retained biliary calculi, percutaneous
extraction of, 165–166
Reticuloendothelial (RE) cell agents,
155
Retrograde ileogram, 117–118
Retrograde pyeloureterography,
189–193

Right-sided percutaneous femoral arterial approach, in uterine artery embolization, 216
Right ventricular end-diastolic pressure, elevated, pulmonary arteriography and, 232
Rotational movement, 15
Royal College of Nursing, 437

S

Salivary glands, 392–399
  computed tomography for, 398
  magnetic resonance imaging for, 398
  methods of imaging for, 392–395
  plain films for, 392
  sialoscintigraphy for, 392
  ultrasound for, 392
Sampling needle, for lung biopsy, 224–225
Scan protocol, for cardiac computed tomography, 247
Sciatica, 356–357
Scintigraphy
  dynamic renal radionuclide, 196–198
  static renal radionuclide, 196–197
Scrotum
  magnetic resonance, 209
  methods of imaging in, 209
  ultrasound of, 215
Scrub practitioner, nurses role, in imaging procedures, 438
Sedation, 451–456, 452f
  of children, 455–456, 454t
  complications of, 455–456
  discharge criteria after, 459
  drugs for, 455–456
  for magnetic resonance imaging, 458
  monitoring and, 457–459
  recovery from, 459
Seldinger technique, pulmonary arteriography and, 233
Self-expanding stents, 279
Sentinel node
  imaging of, in radionuclide lymphoscintigraphy, 323
  localization of, 322
Sentinel node identification, intraoperative, 420
Shared decision making, 449
Short tau inversion recovery (STIR), 153
Short TR sequences, in magnetic resonance imaging, of brain, 375
Shoulder, arthrography for, 338–341, 340f–341f
  technique for, 338–341
    anterior, fluoroscopic guided, 338–339, 338f
    posterior, fluoroscopic guided, 339–340, 340f
    ultrasound guided, posterior, 340–341, 341f

Sialoscintigraphy, for salivary glands, 392
Silk tube, 110
Simmons catheter, 386f
Single-phase (portal phase) contrast-enhanced computed tomography, 150
Single photon emission computed tomography (SPECT), 9, 195, 256, 260–261
Sinogram, 117–120
Skin sepsis, at needle puncture site, 4
Slipped femoral capital epiphysis, 347
Small bowel enema, 97, 110–112
Small bowel follow-through, 108–109
Small bowel magnetic resonance enteroclysis, 134
Small bowel magnetic resonance enterography, 134
Small bowel transit time (SBTT), 102
Small bowel, ultrasound of, 121–122
Sodium acetrizoate, 21
Sodium iodide, 21, 22t–23t
Solutrast, 21–24
Somatostatin, 318
Somatostatin receptor imaging, 319–320
SonoVue, 38
SPECT-CT, 9
SPECT scanners, 318
Spine, 355–370
  arteriography for, 355
  back pain and sciatica in, 356–357
  bone augmentation techniques for, 369
  cervical myelography for, 360–362
  computed tomography for, 357–359
  computed tomography myelography for, 359
  conventional radiography for, 357
  discography for, 355
  facet joint arthrography for, 355
  facet joint/medial branch blocks for, 367
  imaging of, 356–359
  magnetic resonance imaging for, 356–359
  myelography for, 355, 359–367
  nerve root blocks for, 370
  paediatric myelography for, 366–367
  percutaneous vertebral biopsy for, 367–369
  plain films for, 355
  radionuclide imaging for, 355
  ultrasound for, 356
Spleen
  radionuclide imaging of, 168–169
  ultrasound of, 146
Standard gadolinium extracellular agents, 154

Static (Graf) method, 347
Static renal radionuclide scintigraphy, 196–198
Stent grafts, thoracic and abdominal, 284–287
Stents, 278–280
  aftercare for, 279
  balloon mounted, 279
  complication in, 280
  covered, 279
  equipment for, 279
  indications for, 278
  patient preparation for, 279
  self-expanding, 279
  technique in, 279
Stimulated echo acquisition mode (STEAM), 379
STIR see Short tau inversion recovery
Stochastic effects, of radiation, 2
Stomach
  endoluminal examination of, 121
  transabdominal examination of, 121
Stress regimen, in radionuclide myocardial perfusion imaging, 258
Submandibular gland, preliminary images of, for conventional and digital subtraction sialography, 394
Superior mesenteric angiography, 298
Superior mesenteric arteriography, 122, 167
Superior vena cavography, 296
Superparamagnetic contrast agents, 33, 33f
Susceptibility-weighted imaging, in magnetic resonance imaging, of brain, 376

T
T-tube cholangiography, 159–160
T1-W GRE fat-suppressed volume acquisition, 153
T1-weighted magnetic resonance imaging, gadolinium-enhanced, 154
T1-weighted spoiled gradient echo (GRE), 152
T2-weighted spin echo (SE), 153
Tachycardia, 465–466
Taps, for vascular access, 268
^{99m}Tc, 228
^{99m}Tc-colloid, for lymphatic drainage/lymphoedema, 322–323
^{99m}Tc-dimercaptosuccinic acid (DMSA), 195–196
^{99m}Tc-DTPA, 229–230
^{99m}Tc-ethyl cysteinate dimer (ECD), for regional cerebral blood flow imaging, 381
^{99m}Tc-hexamethylpropylenea-mineoxime, for regional cerebral blood flow imaging, 381

^{99m}Tc-hexamethylpropylenea-mineoxime (HMPAO)-labelled leucocytes, 325
^{99m}Tc-HMPAO-labelled white cells, technique in, 326
^{99m}Tc-human immunoglobulin (HIG), 325
^{99m}Tc-MAG-3 (mercaptoacetyltriglycine), 196
^{99m}Tc-methoxyisobutylisonitrile, 405
  in radionuclide myocardial perfusion imaging, 257–258
^{99m}Tc-MIBI rest/stress test, 259
^{99m}Tc-pertechnetate, 403–404
^{99m}Tc-sulesomab, 325
^{99m}Tc-Technegas, 229
^{99m}Tc-tetrofosmin, 405
  in radionuclide myocardial perfusion imaging, 257
^{99m}Technetium (Tc)-nanocolloidal albumin, 322
Tendon imaging, for bones and joints, 346–347
Tendon injuries, in arthrography, 331
Testes, methods of imaging in, 209
Tetrofosmin rest/stress test, 259
^{201}Thallium brain scanning, 383
Theatre, 434–436
Thermal ablative technology, 201
  cryoablation in, 203–204
  microwave ablation in, 202–203
  radiofrequency ablation in, 201–202
Thermoablation, of musculoskeletal tumours, 347–350
  biopsy of, 349
  complications of, 350
  contraindications for, 349
  equipment for, 349
  indications for, 348
  introduction of, 347–350
  post-radiofrequency ablation care for, 350
  procedure for, 349
  rationale for, 348
  thermoablation of, 349–350
  thermocoagulation of, 348
Thermocoagulation, 348
Thoracic stent grafts, 284–286
Thorax, computed tomography of, 221–223
Thrombolysis
  catheter-directed arterial, 280–282
  as venous interventions, 304–305
Thrombosis, venous, ultrasound for, 289
Thrombus
  arterial, as catheter complication, 273
  aspiration of, in angioplasty, 276

Thyroid, 389–409
  computed tomography for, 402
  magnetic resonance imaging for, 402
  methods of imaging for, 399–401
  radionuclide imaging of, 403–405
  ultrasound for, 401–402
Thyroid function, intravascular contrast
    media on, 26–27
Thyrotoxicosis, 30t
Tiger II coronary artery catheter,
    242–243, 243f
Tissue characterization, in cardiac
    magnetic resonance imaging,
    252–253
^{201}Tl-thallous chloride, 405
  in radionuclide myocardial perfusion
    imaging, 257
Tomosynthesis, 415
Toxicity, local anaesthetic, 468
Tracheo-oesophageal fistula in infants, 51
Trans-splenic approach, in portal
    venography, 298–299
Transabdominal examination, of
    oesophagus and stomach, 121
Transhepatic cholangiography,
    percutaneous, 161
Transhepatic portal venous
    catheterization, 299–300
Translational movement, 15
Transoesophageal echocardiography, 20
Triclofos, 456
Tropolonate, 324
Tumours
  ^{18}F-choline imaging for, 315
  2-[^{18}F]fluoro-2-deoxy-D-glucose
    (^{18}F-FDG) positron emission
    tomography for, 312–313
  ^{68}gallium-labelled pharmaceuticals
    imaging for, 315–316
  ^{67}gallium radionuclide tumour
    imaging for, 316
  liver, investigation of, 171–172
  radioiodine
    metaiodobenzylguanidine scan
    for, 316
  somatostatin receptor imaging for, 319
  thermoablation of musculoskeletal,
    347–350
    biopsy of, 349
    complications of, 350
    contraindications for, 349
    equipment for, 349
    indications for, 348
    introduction of, 347–350
    post radiofrequency ablation care
      for, 350
    procedure for, 349
    rationale for, 348
    thermoablation of, 349–350
    thermocoagulation of, 347–348

U
Ultrasonography, 19–20
  of abdomen, 19
  for children, 20
  contrast agents in, 38
  endoscopic, 20
  patient preparation for, 19–20
  of pelvis, 19–20
Ultrasound (US)
  of biliary system, 146–148
  for bones and joints, 328, 346–347
    developmental dysplasia, 346
    dynamic method, 347
    hip-joint effusion, 347
    indications for, 346
    slipped femoral capital epiphysis,
      347
    static (Graf) method, 347
    technique for, 347–348
  of brain, 374
  for breast, 416–417
  of common bile duct, 146
  for female reproductive system, 216
  of gallbladder, 146–148
  of gastrointestinal tract, 121
    appendix, 122
    endoluminal examination of anus,
      123
    endoluminal examination of
      oesophagus and stomach, 121
    endoluminal examination of
      rectum, 123
    hypertrophic pyloric stenosis, 61
    large bowel, 123
    small bowel, 121–122
    transabdominal examination
      of oesophagus and stomach,
      121–122
  of hepatic artery, 145–146
  of hepatic veins, 145
  intussusception and, 61–63
  of liver, 144–146
    contrast-enhanced, 145
  in liver tumours, 170–172
  lower limb venous, 290–291
    equipment for, 291
    indications for, 291
    technique of, 290–291
  of lymph nodes, 320
  in non-obstructive jaundice, 173
  in obstructive jaundice, 173
  for ovarian cancer, 218
  of pancreas, 148–149
  in pancreatic pseudocysts, 174
  in pancreatitis, 174
  for parathyroid, 399
  of portal vein, 145
  for salivary glands, 392
  for scrotum, 209, 214
  for spine, 356

Ultrasound (US) (*Continued*)
  of spleen, 146
  for thyroid, 400
  upper limb venous, 291
    equipment for, 291
    indications for, 291
    technique of, 291
  of urinary tract, 178–180
    contraindications for, 179
    equipment of, 179
    indications for, 178–180
    patient preparation for, 179
    technique of, 179
  vascular, 263–264
  for vascular access, 266
  of venous system, 289–291
    colour Doppler, 290
    duplex scanning, 290
Ultravist, 21–24, 22*t*–23*t*
Upper intestinal obstruction, newborn
    infants with, 53
Upper limb
  peripheral venography of, 295
  venous ultrasound, 291
Ureters, computed tomography, 183
Urethrography, ascending, in male,
    187–188
Urinary tract, 175–199
  ascending urethrography in the male,
    187–188
  computed tomography of, 181–184
  conduitogram for, 190
  direct radionuclide micturating
    cystography for, 198–199
  dynamic renal radionuclide
    scintigraphy for, 196–198
  imaging methods in, 176–178
  intravenous excretion urography for,
    176–178
  magnetic resonance imaging of,
    184–185
  micturating cystourethrography for,
    198–199
  percutaneous antegrade
    pyelography and nephrostomy
    for, 191–192
  percutaneous nephrolithotomy for,
    191–196
  percutaneous renal cyst puncture and
    biopsy for, 191
  plain film radiography for, 176
  renal arteriography for, 183–184
  retrograde pyeloureterography for,
    189–193
  ultrasound of, 179–180
Urograffin, 22*t*–23*t*
Urography
  intravenous excretion, 176–178
  magnetic resonance, 185–186
US *see* Ultrasound

Uterine artery embolization, in
    reproductive system, 215–217
  clinical indications of, 215–216
Uterine carcinoma, 218

V
Varicose veins, ultrasound for, 289
Vascular access, 266–272
  aftercare for, 272
  equipment in, 267–268
    catheters, 268
    connectors, 268
    guidewires, 267, 268*f*
    needle, 267
    taps, 269
    ultrasound, 267
    vascular sheaths, 267–268
  patient preparation in, 266–267
  relative contraindications of, 269
  in stent grafts, 285
  technique in, 269–270, 271*f*
Vascular embolization, 282–283
Vascular sheaths, for vascular access,
    267–268
Vascular toxicity, of intravascular
    contrast media, 25
Vascular ultrasound, 263–264
Veins
  gonadal, embolization, 301–302
  varicose, ultrasound for, 289
Venography
  central, 296
    inferior vena cavography, 296–297
    superior vena cavography, 296
  peripheral, 293–299
    of lower limb, 293–295
    of upper limb, 295
  portal, 297–298
Venous angioplasty and stents, as
    venous interventions, 300–301
Venous interventions, 300–301
  gonadal vein embolization, 301–302
  inferior vena cava filters, 302–304
  pulmonary embolism, 306–307
  thrombolysis, 304–305
  venous angioplasty and stents,
    300–301
Venous system, 289–308
  central venography of, 296
  computed tomography of, 291–292
  magnetic resonance of, 292–293
  methods of imaging, 289
  peripheral venography of, 293–299
  portal venography of, 297–298
  transhepatic portal venous
    catheterization of, 299–300
  ultrasound of, 289–290
  venous interventions, 300–301
Venous thrombosis, ultrasound for,
    289

Venous toxicity, of intravascular contrast media, 25
Ventilation/perfusion (V/Q) radionuclide scanning, for pulmonary embolism, 227
Ventriculography, radionuclide, 254–256
Vertebrale catheter, 386*f*
Visipaque, 22*t*–23*t*, 24
Vitamin K, for abnormal prothrombin time, 161
Volume scan, in computed tomography of thorax, 222

Voluntariness, 441–442
Vomiting, after oral sedation, 45

W
Warfarin, 425*t*
Water-soluble contrast agents, 97–98
Wrist, arthrography for, 342–343, 343*f*
Written consent, 5, 219

X
^{133}Xe (xenon) gas, 229